Asthma Reviews

Volume 2

Asthma Reviews

Volume 2

Edited by

JOHN MORLEY
Sandoz AG, CH-4002 Basel
Switzerland

ACADEMIC PRESS
Harcourt Brace Jovanovich, Publishers
London San Diego New York Berkeley
Boston Sydney Tokyo Toronto

ACADEMIC PRESS LIMITED
24/28 Oval Road,
London NW1 7DX

United States Edition published by
ACADEMIC PRESS INC.
San Diego, CA 92101

This book is printed on acid-free paper ∞

British Library Cataloguing in Publication Data

Is available

ISBN 0–12–040922–4

Typeset by Photo·Graphics, Honiton, Devon
Printed in Great Britain at the University Press, Cambridge

Contributors

I. Akutsu, Department of Allergy and Clinical Immunology, Dokkyo University School of Medicine, Tochigi 321–02, Japan

R. C. Benyon, Department of Microbiology and Infectious Diseases, Faculty of Medicine, The University of Calgary Health Sciences Centre, 3330 Hospital Drive N.W., Calgary, Alberta T2N 4N1, Canada

M. C. Berenbaum, Department of Experimental Pathology, St Mary's Hospital Medical School, London W2, UK

M. K. Church, Clinical Pharmacology and Medicine I, University of Southampton, Centre Block, Southampton General Hospital, Southampton, Hampshire S09 4XY, UK

T. Fukuda, , Department of Allergy and Clinical Immunology, Dokkyo University School of Medicine, Tochigi 321–02, Japan

P. J. Gardiner, Bayer UK, Stoke Court, Stoke Poges, Slough, Bucks SL2 4LY, UK

S. T. Holgate, Clinical Pharmacology and Medicine I, University of Southampton, Centre Block, Southampton General Hospital, Southampton, Hampshire S09 4XY, UK

M. A. Lowman, Department of Microbiology and Infectious Diseases, Faculty of Medicine, The University of Calgary Health Sciences Centre, 3330 Hospital Drive N.W., Calgary, Alberta T2N 4N1, Canada

S. Makino, Department of Allergy and Clinical Immunology, Dokkyo University School of Medicine, Tochigi 321–02, Japan

T. Numao, Department of Allergy and Clinical Immunology, Dokkyo University School of Medicine, Tochigi 321–02, Japan

D. Pavia, Clinical Research Department, Medical Division, Boehringer Ingelheim Limited, Ellesfield Avenue, Bracknell, Berks RG12 4YS, UK

A. N. Payne, Department of Pharmacology, Wellcome Research Laboratories, Langley Court, Beckenham, Kent BR3 3BS, UK

P. H. Rees, Department of Microbiology and Infectious Diseases, Faculty of Medicine, The University of Calgary Health Sciences Centre, 3330 Hospital Drive N.W., Calgary, Alberta T2N 4N1, Canada

Preface

Asthma Reviews arose as a consequence of organizing a course each year on the pharmacology of asthma. In selecting topics for the course, emphasis was given to developments in those areas of asthma research that were in an active phase; in this way, it was possible to review key areas for the non-specialist. Additionally, less popular areas of research were reviewed periodically in order to provide a background for debate and to encourage investigators to reconsider their research priorities in asthma.

In the present volume this policy has been maintained, with contributions from Gardiner, Benyon *et al.* and Fukuda *et al.*, dealing with areas that are central to the research effort of many laboratories. By way of contrast the contributions of Payne, Berenbaum and Pavia have covered topics, whose technical difficulties are sufficient to deter many investigators. I hope that the present volume will contribute to asthma research and therapy by adding to the body of current knowledge, and that the diversity of topics will ensure that most clinicians and research investigators, whose special interest is asthma, will find something new and interesting.

Basel, Switzerland *J. Morley*

Contents

1

Inhaled aerosols: clinical and experimental applications in relation to asthma

Adrian N. Payne

Department of Pharmacology, Wellcome Research Laboratories, Langley Court, Beckenham, Kent BR3 3BS, UK

I INTRODUCTION

Administration of anti-asthmatic drugs as inhaled aerosols offers many theoretical advantages over systemic therapy. By inhalation high therapeutic levels can be achieved at small doses and systemic drug concentrations are thus reduced. Consequently there is a lower incidence of systemic side-effects than with other routes of administration. As the drug is delivered directly to the site of action within the airways, the inhaled route also offers the benefit of a rapid onset of action. In addition, some anti-asthmatic drugs (e.g. sodium cromoglycate) are only effective by inhalation.

Historically, the origins of inhalation therapy can be traced back to the Ancient Egyptians (see review by Sakula, 1988). One of the ways that they treated a respiratory disease, which we would probably recognize today as asthma, was the inhalation of the emanations from herbal extracts placed on heated bricks. More recently, in the nineteenth century, the smoking of cigarettes containing pharmacologically active botanical extracts (e.g. the anti-cholinergic stramonium) incorporated with the tobacco was a popular form of treatment. The introduction of metered-dose inhalers (MDIs) in the 1960s, revolutionized the ergonomics of inhalation therapy. As a result, inhaled aerosol drug presentations have

ASTHMA REVIEWS VOLUME 2
ISBN 0-12-040922-4

become a mainstay in the contemporary treatment of asthma (Newhouse and Dolovich, 1986).

The inhaled route can also be used to facilitate experimental studies, such as determining the effects on airway calibre and reactivity of various putative pharmacological mediators of asthma. Because of obvious ethical and practical considerations many of these studies are carried out in species other than man. After surveying briefly the clinical use of inhaled aerosols in asthma therapy, this review will consider the general principles of their generation and characterization, and describe some examples of their administration in experimental studies in laboratory animals.

II AEROSOL THERAPY IN ASTHMA

A Current status

Inhaled aerosols are currently used both acutely and chronically in therapy of asthma, especially in the UK (Clarke, 1986). A range of sympathomimetic and anti-cholinergic bronchodilators are currently available in aerosol presentations, as well as "anti-allergic" agents and corticosteroids. In many cases these drugs are used in combination to achieve the desired therapeutic profile (Shenfield, 1982; Skorodin, 1986), for example, sympathomimetics and corticosteroids.

B Sympathomimetics

Where the predominant cause of reduced airway calibre is bronchial smooth muscle contraction (e.g. the early asthmatic response), by their potent bronchodilator action, those inhaled β-adrenoceptor stimulants currently available as inhaled aerosols can provide rapid symptomatic relief for up to 4 hours, with relatively minimal systemic effects (Skidmore, 1984). For example, after inhalation of the β_2 selective agonist salbutamol, peak bronchodilation can be achieved within 10–15 minutes, as opposed to up to 2 hours following oral administration (Ruffin *et al.*, 1977). This class of anti-asthmatic drugs can also be useful prophylactically, e.g. in preventing exercise-induced asthma (Bakran *et al.*, 1980).

Inhaled β-adrenoceptor stimulants are less effective where airway inflammation is a major factor (e.g. the late asthmatic response) and increasing emphasis is being placed on the potentially life-threatening role of this component in asthma (Payne, 1988). Indeed, although never proven, overdependence on the palliative effects of inhaled sympathomimetics may have contributed to the rise in asthma mortality soon after their introduction into clinical use in the 1960s (Anon, 1976). Similarly, concern has been expressed that new long-acting β-adrenoceptor stimulants may be used inappropriately by asthmatics and thereby mask the underlying pathology of the disease (Abbott, 1988).

C Anti-cholinergics

In the western world, anti-cholinergic drugs such as atropine and its derivatives have been used to treat asthma since the seventeenth century (Gandevia, 1975). By inhalation atropine is an effective, if variable, bronchodilator drug of moderate potency with a slow onset of action (Pakes, 1984). Although less common when given by inhalation, atropine can produce unpleasant side effects, such as drying of the mouth and increased sputum viscosity. A quarternary derivative of atropine, ipratropium bromide, is more bronchoselective and has fewer systemic side-effects (Ruffin *et al.*, 1977). However, like atropine, the protective effect of ipratropium against experimentally-induced bronchoconstriction (e.g. antigen challenge) is somewhat variable and generally less effective in this situation than inhaled β-adrenoceptor stimulants (Pakes, 1984).

D Anti-allergics

An example of this class of drug is sodium cromoglycate (SCG). SCG is poorly absorbed orally, but by inhalation it is an effective prophylactic drug in certain subsets of asthmatics (Buckle, 1984). It has no direct bronchodilator action. SCG was initially presumed to act by preventing mediator release from mast cells (Cox, 1967). However, it is now thought unlikely that such an action could totally explain its clinical efficacy, and other mechanisms such as inhibition of pulmonary sensory C-fibre discharge may be involved (Church, 1986; Richards *et al.*, 1986).

A new drug in this category is nedocromil sodium (NS), which, like SCG, is a chromone derivative. NS is equipotent with SCG in classical anti-allergic screens (Riley *et al.*, 1987). In experimental studies, inhaled NS has been found to prevent asthmatic bronchoconstriction following various provocation stimuli (Cairns and Orr, 1987). It has recently been licensed in the UK for prescription as a MDI presentation for asthma prophylaxis.

E Corticosteroids

By inhalation, topically acting corticosteroids such as betamethasone, beclomethasone, and budesonide have proven utility in the maintenance therapy of asthma, particularly when other treatment regimes (e.g. inhaled sympathomimetics) have failed (Crompton, 1983). Whilst inhaled steroids have no direct bronchodilator effect, they block late-onset asthmatic responses (Dahl and Johansson, 1982) and prevent and reverse the development of airway hyperreactivity (Sotomayor *et al.*, 1984; Fabbri *et al.*, 1985).

Side-effects (oral candidiasis, hoarseness) of inhaled steroids are minor in comparison with the major problems associated with continued systemic steroid therapy, such as suppression of the hypothalamic pituitary axis (Brogden, 1983; Cochrane 1983). In this respect, the high therapeutic index of inhaled steroids is perhaps one of the best practical examples, to date, of the realization of the advantages of inhalation therapy.

III GENERAL PROPERTIES OF AEROSOLS

A Definition of an aerosol

An aerosol can be defined as a system of finely-divided liquid droplets or solid particles in gaseous suspension. For this suspension to be relatively stable, the aerosol particles must be sufficiently small to remain airborne for some period of time and yet large enough not to diffuse like molecules of gas. Hence most aerosol particles fall within the range 0.01–100 μm (Fuchs, 1964; Morrow, 1981). However, the most desirable particle size range for therapeutic inhaled aerosols is 1–5 μm. The actual size and density of the particles that form the aerosol will influence their physical behaviour within the respiratory tract. This will in turn play a major role in determining the site and amount of material, and (in the case of medical aerosols) drug, deposited within the bronchial tree.

B Particle size distribution

1 Aerodynamic diameter

Aerosols are termed monodisperse if the aerosol particles are of uniform size and shape, and either poly- or heterodisperse if the particles are not. Pharmaceutical aerosols are typically polydisperse and may contain nonspherical particles of variable density. A major determinant of the pulmonary deposition of inhaled aerosols is the aerodynamic properties of the constituent particles. The theoretical concept of "aerodynamic diameter" is often used to predict the likely particle deposition pattern. Aerodynamic diameter is defined as the physical diameter of a unit density (1 g cm^{-3}) sphere that would have exactly the same aerodynamic properties as the particle being considered. This concept is useful in that aerosol particles having varying sizes, shapes and densities can be compared in terms of their relative aerodynamic diameter, and thus inertial behaviour. As the volume of a sphere increases with the cube of its diameter, so the largest particles within a polydisperse medical aerosol will contain most of the drug mass. Consequently the amount of material deposited in the lungs is usually proportional to particle mass rather than particle number.

2 *MMAD and GSD*

The two parameters of the particulate characteristics of an inhaled aerosol considered most useful for predicting deposition patterns in the lung are the mass median aerodynamic diameter (MMAD), and in those aerosols displaying a unimodal log normal particle size distribution, the associated geometric standard deviation (GSD). The MMAD is the mid-point of aerosol mass, i.e. the aerodynamic diameter of the particle above which 50% of the aerosol mass resides. The GSD is an indication of the dispersion of aerodynamic diameters of particles within the aerosol, and is derived from the ratio of the particle size, with a cumulative value of 84.1% of the total particle number, to that of the median size (cumulative value of 50%). GSD has no units and must, by definition, always be greater than unity. Perfectly monodisperse aerosols rarely exist and for practical purposes aerosols with a GSD of less than 1.2 are usually considered to fall within this category.

If the particle size profile of an aerosol describes a log normal distribution, it follows that the particle mass, particle surface area and any other properties that are power functions of particle size are similarly distributed. These distributions are interrelated by the Hatch–Choate equations (Mercer *et al.*, 1972). The various size parameters that can be computed using these equations are shown in Fig. 1.

3 *Aerosol measurement systems*

Various techniques are available for measuring the size distribution of aerosol particles. These range from cascade impactors (Fuchs, 1978), to

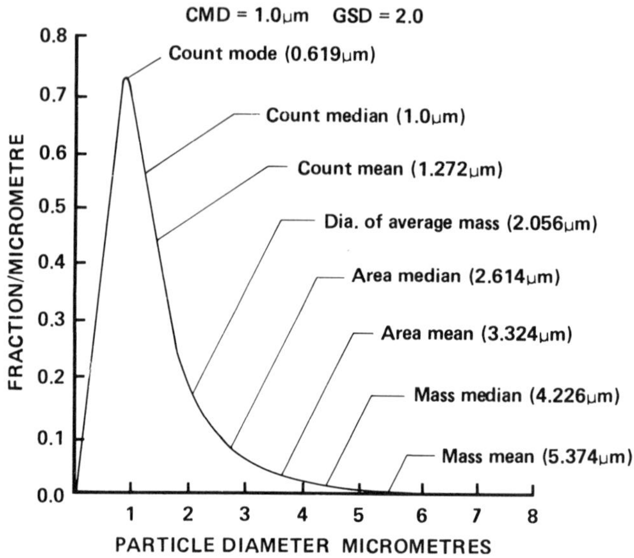

Fig. 1 The size distribution (particle diameter) of an aerosol of which the particle size profile is log normally distributed. When particle diameter is plotted on a linear scale (as shown), the distribution curve is skewed. If diameter was plotted on a logarithmic scale, the distribution curve would appear symmetric and be bell-shaped. Using the Hatch–Choate equations, which are applicable for any log-normal distribution (see text), various particle size parameters can be calculated as indicated along the curve. CMD = count median diameter, GSD = geometric standard deviation. (From Brain and Valberg, 1979).

more sophisticated devices such as single particle aerodynamic relaxation time (SPART) analysers (Hiller *et al.*, 1981), aerodynamic particle sizers (Bouchikhi *et al.*, 1988) and those based on Fraunhofer diffraction (Malvern particle sizers). When conducting particle size measurements, it is important to monitor the relative humidity. This is because in a high humidity environment (e.g. within the respiratory tract) the particles may grow in size, by absorbing water after leaving the aerosol generating device (Ferron, 1977).

IV AEROSOL GENERATION

A Basic principles

Aerosols can be produced by two basic principles. These are first, condensation of vapour molecules and second, comminution of either solids or liquids into small particles. Condensation is generally unsuitable for the generation of therapeutic aerosols, because the low vapour pressure of most drugs used for this purpose means that they undergo thermal degradation before sufficient vapour for condensation is available. Comminution (to reduce to minute particles) is used to produce aerosols of both liquid and solid matter. With liquids, energy is required to overcome surface tension forces. This energy is usually provided by either compressed air (jet nebulizers) or high frequency ultrasound vibrations (ultrasonic nebulizers). With solids, comminution is generally performed by micronization following which an aerosol is produced by dispersion, either by chlorofluorocarbon propellants (pressurized metered-dose inhalers) or inhaled air (dry powder inhalers).

B Aerosol generating devices

1 Jet nebulizers

Jet nebulizers are commonly used to generate therapeutic aerosols. Usually these types of nebulizers use the Rayleigh stream principle, whereby a jet of compressed air at a pressure of 35–270 kPa is used to entrain and shatter a stream of liquid containing the drug in solution. An example of one of these devices is shown in Fig. 2(a). By means of the Bernoulli effect, the fluid to be nebulized is drawn up a feed tube into the jet stream by the negative static pressure (with respect to ambient atmospheric pressure) created by the jet of air expanding as it leaves the nebulizer orifice. The fragmented liquid then impinges on one or a series of proximal baffles that further disrupt the jet stream, yielding a greater amount of inhalable (<5 μm) particles and returning larger particles to the liquid reservoir for re-nebulization.

Aerosol output from jet nebulizers is usually proportional to the flow rate of compressed air through the device (Clay *et al.*, 1983). Under optimal flow conditions, and depending on the actual type of device and the surface tension and density of the liquid being nebulized, the aerosol particles produced by jet nebulizers generally have a MMAD in the range 1.2–6.9 μm with a GSD 1.7–2.2 (Mercer, 1981). While these types of nebulizers produce appropriate particle size distributions for inhalational therapy, because of losses in the apparatus, dead space in the reservoir and the fact that nebulization is continuous whereas inspiration is intermittent, only about 12% of the nebulized drug is deposited in the lung (Lewis *et al.*, 1982a).

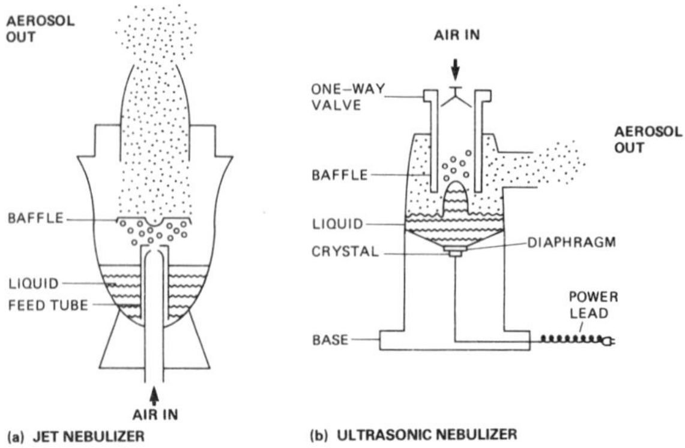

Fig. 2 (a) Cross-sectional diagram of a typical jet nebulizer. Liquid is drawn up the feed tube by the stream of compressed air entering at the bottom of the device. The entrained liquid fragments into droplets, the larger of which impinge on the baffle, smaller droplets are carried away in the exiting airstream and subsequently inhaled.

(b) Schematic diagram showing the working principles of an ultrasonic nebulizer. The high frequency vibrations (typically 1–2 MHz) of a piezo-electric crystal are transmitted, via a diaphragm, to the liquid in the aerosol reservoir. The resulting standing wave in the liquid creates a fountain of liquid droplets, the smaller of which are carried away in the inhaled airstream. Larger droplets impinge on the baffle assembly and are returned to the reservoir for re-nebulization.

2 *Ultrasonic nebulizers*

Ultrasonic nebulizers use a standing wave of high frequency ultrasound, produced by a piezo-electric crystal vibrating typically in the range of 1–2 MHz in an electric field. A cross section of a nebulizer of this type is shown in Fig. 2(b). Transduction of the high frequency energy to the liquid to be nebulized causes the free surface of this liquid to oscillate, due to adiabatic compressions and rarefactions. This results in the production of small surface waves (Faraday Crispations) that form a liquid geyser, at the apex of which fine droplets are released. Airflow through the device is then used to carry the smaller droplets away as an aerosol for inhalation. The mean particle size is inversely proportional to the operating frequency of the piezo-electric crystal, and will also depend on the surface tension and density of the liquid to be nebulized. MMADs of the liquid droplets produced at the outlet of ultrasonic nebulizers typically are in the range 3.7–10.5 μm with GSDs 1.4–2.0 (Mercer, 1981).

3 *Metered-dose inhalers*

Pressurized metered-dose inhalers (MDIs) became available in the UK in the 1960s and overcame, to a large extent, the problems of portability of other nebulizers available at that time. MDIs are essentially self-contained hermetically sealed nebulizers holding usually 100–200 doses of the active constituent, usually in the form of a micronized suspension in chlorofluorocarbon propellants with added surfactants. A cross section of one of these devices, illustrating its operating principles, is shown in Fig. 3(a). When the aerosol is actuated by depressing the valve stem, the contents of the metering chamber, which may be up to 5 mg of active material, are discharged into the mouthpiece. The exiting micronized drug particles are enclosed within droplets of propellant. Whilst some of

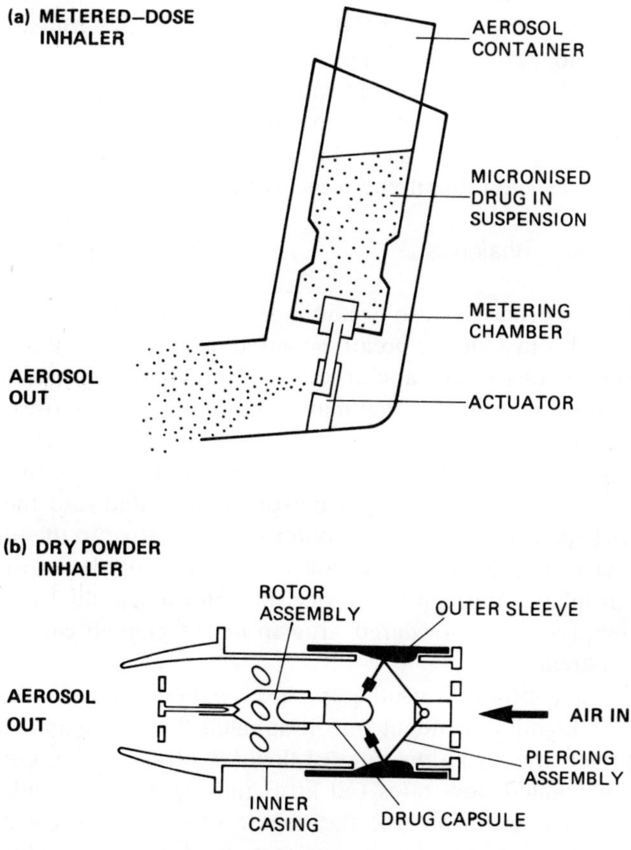

Fig. 3 (a) Cross sectional diagram of a pressurized metered dose inhaler (MDI). Depression of the aerosol container delivers a metered dose (typically 0.1–1 mg) of micronized drug together with propellant.

(b) An example of a dry powder inhaler. Inhaling through the device rotates the rotor assembly in which a drug capsule is mounted and pierced before inspiration. The powdered drug is emptied out into the inhaled airstream by centrifugal force.

this propellant vaporizes rapidly on leaving the actuator orifice (a process termed flashing), leaving free particles of active drug, it may take many seconds for the remaining propellant to evaporate (Clarke and Newman, 1981). Hence, the resulting aerosol may contain a wide range of particle sizes (MMAD typically 1.5–4.3 μm, GSD 1.5–3.9; Lourenco and Cotromanes, 1982; Kim *et al.*, 1985).

There are two basic drawbacks with current MDI devices. First, the extremely high velocity (exceeding 30 m s^{-1}) of the droplets leaving the actuator orifice, with a resulting propensity for oropharyngeal deposition. Consequently, even under optimal conditions, only 9–10% of the output of a MDI is available to the pulmonary airways (Newman *et al.*, 1981). Second, as the output of a MDI is delivered in the course of a vital capacity manoeuvre rather than tidal breathing, it is important to synchronize the aerosol discharge with inspiration. As a result there have been several attempts to overcome these problems by incorporating auxiliary delivery systems, such as reservoir bottles, spacer tubes, breath actuator devices and rebreathing bags (Tobin *et al.*, 1982, Newman, 1984).

4 Dry powder inhalers

Anti-asthmatic drugs can also be administered by inhalation as dry powder aerosols. In this instance, a breath-actuated insufflator is used to generate an aerosol by dispersing a unit dose of previously comminuted drug together with any excipients that may be required (e.g. lactose) to achieve the necessary dispersal characteristics. An example of such a device is the "Spinhaler", the design of which is shown in Fig. 3(b). In this device a gelatin capsule containing SCG powder is mounted into the hub of a propellor-shaped rotor. Sliding an outer sleeve relative to the inner casing of the device pierces two small holes in the end of the capsule. When the patient inhales through the device the rotor assembly rotates rapidly, thereby emptying the powdered drug from the pierced capsule into the inhaled airstream.

Because dry powder insufflators are "patient driven" the delivery efficiency is highly dependent on the inhaled flow rate, and the capsule may empty erratically at low rates of flow (30 litres min^{-1}). On the other hand, high inhaled flow rates (60 litres min^{-1}) may, depending on the actual type of device, increase the degree of oropharyngeal deposition. Hence, as little as 5% of active drug may reach the lungs. However, dry powder insufflators do overcome, to a large extent, the problem of synchronizing inspiration with actuation.

Recent innovations in the design of dry-powder inhalers include the "Diskhaler", where the powered drug is packaged in cartridge form, and the "Turbohaler" in which a small unit dose is scraped from a compressed plug of drug and then dispersed by a turbulent stream of inhaled air.

V LUNG DEPOSITION

A The respiratory tract

In the present context, deposition refers to the collection and initial pattern of regional distribution of inhaled aerosol particles within the lung. The majority of therapeutic aerosols are administered during mouth, rather than nose, breathing. For the purposes of discussing their deposition, the respiratory tract (excluding the nasal passages) can be sub-divided into three distinct anatomical zones:

(i) Oropharyngeal; mouth to larynx
(ii) Tracheobronchial; trachea to terminal bronchioles
(iii) Respiratory; respiratory bronchioles, alveoli.

Most theoretical models used to assess the probable regional deposition pattern of inhaled aerosols are based on symmetric (regular dichotomy) lung models, such as that described by Weibel (1963), represented schematically in Fig. 4; according to this model each airway is assumed to divide equally into two equivalent branches. The term "generation" is used to describe each successive branching. Although airway diameter decreases towards the lung periphery, because of increasing airway number the overall cross-sectional area of the airways becomes progressively larger, resulting in a greater surface area for aerosol deposition. In a normal human lung the total pulmonary surface area is about 70 m^2.

B Deposition mechanisms

The two principal mechanisms applicable to the pulmonary deposition of therapeutic inhaled aerosols are inertial impaction and gravitational sedimentation. These and other mechanisms of lesser importance, are described briefly below. For a comprehensive account of the deposition of aerosol particles in the respiratory tract, the reader is referred to reviews by Brain and Valberg (1979), Newman *et al.* (1982), Agnew (1984) and Newman (1985).

Factors that affect the lung deposition of inhaled aerosols include particle size, inhalation mode, airway geometry and degree of airway

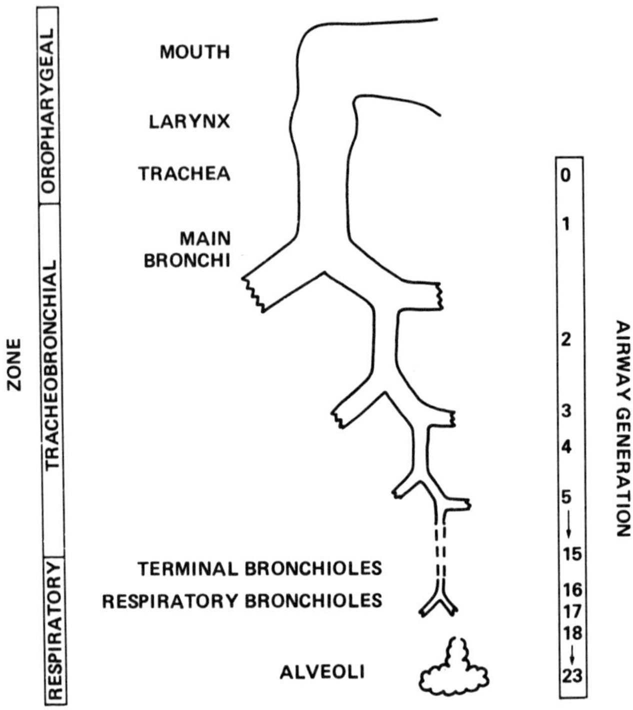

Fig. 4 Schematic representation of the symmetric (regular dichotomy) model of airway branching as proposed by Weibel (1963). (Adapted from Newman *et al.*, 1982).

obstruction. Because of the variable influence of these factors, exposure to an aerosol does not adequately define the dose delivered, nor does it specify the anatomic distribution of that dose.

1 *Inertial impaction*

Inertial impaction is the major mechanism of deposition of those inhaled particles with an equivalent aerodynamic diameter greater than 3 μm (Raabe *et al.*, 1986). It occurs primarily in the oropharyngeal and tracheobronchial zones. Depending on inhalation flow and particle density, this mechanism of deposition may also be significant for any particle larger than 1 μm in diameter (Hatch and Gross, 1964).

Inertial impaction occurs where the aerosol particles are unable, because of their inertia, to follow changes in the direction of the inhaled airstream.

As a consequence the particles collide with the airway wall, for example at the back of the throat, and at the carina. As already noted, oropharyngeal deposition is a particular problem with MDI devices because of the high velocity of the aerosol cloud leaving the actuator orifice.

2 *Gravitational sedimentation*

Gravitational sedimentation pertains to those aerosol particles that are either sufficiently small, or have sufficiently low velocity, to escape inertial impaction and penetrate to the more distal tracheobronchial zone and the respiratory zone. In these zones the movements in air flow are small relative to those in the upper airways and particles can settle onto the airway walls through the influence of the Earth's gravity. The rate of gravitational settling of small particles is proportional to the square of their aerodynamic diameter, which for a 5 μm diameter aerosol particle is approximately 0.7 mm s^{-1} (Newman, 1985). Slow, steady breathing and/or breath-holding increase the opportunity for gravitational sedimentation due to the consequent increased intra-pulmonary residence time of the aerosol particles.

3 *Other mechanisms*

Other mechanisms that are of secondary importance in respect of the lung deposition of therapeutic inhaled aerosols include Brownian diffusion (significant only for particles with aerodynamic diameters less than 0.5 μm), interception (important for fibrous aerosols) and electrostatic attraction.

C Clearance and retention

To re-cap, lung *deposition* refers to the initial regional distribution of inhaled aerosol particles on the surface of the airways. The amount of aerosol material which is subsequently retained is influenced by *clearance*. This term is used to describe collectively the processes of translocation, transformation and removal of deposited particles from deposition sites within the respiratory tract. Hence, *retention* (the amount of aerosol material present in the lungs at any one time) is the result of deposition minus clearance. Important physiological mechanisms of clearance include sneeze, cough and mucociliary transport, the ultimate mechanism being systemic clearance via the circulation (Silbaugh, 1987).

VI EXPERIMENTAL APPLICATIONS IN LABORATORY ANIMALS

A General considerations

As with any experimental procedure certain basic factors have to be taken into account in designing studies with inhaled aerosols. Bearing in mind the possibility of environmental contamination with aerosols of test substances of undefined toxicology, safety is of primary importance. Thus, adequate precautions should be taken, such as using appropriate exposure chambers, filters and masks to ensure that the investigator does not become the subject of the experiment in question.

Pharmacological, as opposed to toxicological, studies primarily employ either jet or ultrasonic nebulizers. As these devices generate aerosols from liquids, it is important that the drug or test substance is soluble in aqueous solution. This can sometimes be facilitated by judicious addition of small amounts of organic solvents (e.g. propylene glycol) and surfactants (e.g. Tween 80). Whilst aerosols of drug suspensions (e.g. beclomethasone diproprionate) can also be generated, the drug particles must be sufficiently small to be encapsulated in liquid droplets of aerosol carrier. Stability is also an important factor as the test substance may be sensitive to aeration (in jet nebulizers) or heating (in ultrasonic nebulizers).

In man, inhaled aerosols are administered either passively in the course of normal tidal breathing, or actively during a vital capacity manoeuvre. Given that active administration involves some degree of co-operation and synchronization on the part of the subject, most studies using conscious animals are conducted using passive inhalation. Due to the consequent high by-pass ratio, drug wastage can be a problem. In addition, because of differences in breathing patterns, airway geometry, and lung size in relation to body weight, as well as individual variability, it cannot be assumed that different species or even different animals of the same species, receive identical doses when breathing the same aerosol (Brain and Valberg, 1979). Also, most animals are primarily nose breathers. This will influence the pulmonary penetration of aerosol particles due to the resulting nasopharyngeal deposition and very little aerosol mass in relation to the total aerosol output may in fact reach the lungs (see below). For this reason, in conscious animals, particularly larger species (e.g. dogs), inhaled aerosols are sometimes administered via either a previously created tracheostomy or endotracheal tube (Lewis *et al.*, 1982b). In anaesthetized animals, this method of administration is routine. The aerosolized material can then be administered unhindered into the lungs ("direct inhalation"), in the course of either spontaneous breathing or during mechanical ventilation.

B Deposition studies

Small rodents such as rats and guinea-pigs are often the subject of lung function studies involving the use of inhaled aerosols, such as investigating the effects of aerosolized bronchodilators, and challenging previously sensitized animals with aerosolized antigen (see below). In advance of these studies it is useful to have some background information concerning the likely deposition patterns of the aerosol being administered, particularly when non-tracheotomized conscious animals are used. For this purpose, as in man, radioaerosols (Newman, 1984) are often employed. The methodology for using radioactive tracers in this respect is well established (see Thomas and Lie, 1963; Thomas, 1969; Berteau and Bierman, 1977; Sweeny *et al.*, 1983; Raabe *et al.*, 1977). In our own studies (Gazeley *et al.*, 1986), we exposed either conscious or anaesthetized rats in a "head-only" configuration to a polydisperse radioaerosol of distilled water containing a tracer amount (0.3 mCi ml^{-1}) of ^{99}m technicium pertechnetate. The aerosols were generated using a jet nebulizer, which produced particles ranging 0.7–15 μm with a count mode of 0.9 μm, MMAD of 9.0 μm and GSD of 2.2.

As shown in Table 1, there was relatively little deposition and subsequent retention of radioaerosol mass in the lower respiratory tract (LRT) compared with either the head region or gastrointestinal tract (GIT). Although the overall count rate was less in anaesthetized animals, as might be expected owing to reduced ventilation, deposition in the LRT was similar to that in conscious animals. However, there was a marked reduction in radioemission from the GIT, the most obvious explanation

Table 1 γ-radioemission (c s^{-1}) from individual organs dissected from the carcasses of rats that had been previously exposed in a "head-only" configuration for 10 minutes to an aqueous radioaerosol of ^{99}m technetium pertechnetate (0.3 mCi ml^{-1}) either when conscious or anaesthetized. All values represent the mean, ± s.e. mean, count rate from organs taken from 5 animals (Data from Gazeley *et al.*, 1986).

Region/Organ	*Conscious*	*Total (%)*	*Anaesthetized*	*Total (%)*
Head	1116 (± 206)	36.8	724 (± 53)	73.6
Thorax	380 (± 73)	12.5	135 (± 26)	13.8
Trachea	32 (± 15)	1.1	15 (± 9)	1.6
Lungs	134 (± 44)	4.5	60 (± 9)	6.2
Oesophagus	135 (± 18)	4.5	5 (± 2)	0.6
Stomach	1169 (± 621)	38.6	29 (± 19)	3.0
Duodenum	29 (± 20)	1.0	5 (± 1)	0.5
Heart	28 (± 11)	1.0	6 (± 2)	0.7

for this being a depression of the swallowing reflex. These results highlight the fact that in conscious rodents the major proportion of aerosol mass is swallowed rather than delivered to the lungs. This is an important consideration when interpreting experimental results, especially when dealing with orally active compounds.

Where it is not possible to use an isotopic method, providing the particle size distribution is known, a reasonably good estimate of regional deposition and retention fraction can be derived from first principles, based on published data (see references above). In either case, the dose (D) can be estimated by application of the following formula:

$$D = \frac{C \times t \times \alpha \times V_{\mathrm{m}}}{w} \mathrm{kg}^{-1}$$

C = the concentration of drug in the inspired air; t = time of administration; α = retention fraction; V_{m} = minute volume (usually on the basis of Guyton, 1947); w = body weight of the animal.

C Bronchodilator studies

An example of the use of aerosols in animal studies, which at the same time has an obvious clinical parallel, is the pharmacological investigation of the bronchodilator effects of an inhaled β-adrenoceptor agonist such as salbutamol. The protective (anti-bronchoconstrictor) effect of this drug can be readily demonstrated, for instance in conscious guinea-pigs, by using a jet nebulizer and a simple exposure chamber. The results from such an experiment are shown in Fig. 5. In this experiment, the pharmacological effect was determined by visual assessment of the attenuation (following drug pre-treatment) of respiratory symptoms resulting from bronchial provocation with an aerosol of 5-HT. Increased measurement sophistication can be introduced if required, by mounting the animal in either a single or double chamber plethysmograph box during the experiment, so deriving objective mechanical indices of lung function such as airways resistance and specific airways conductance (Pennock *et al.*, 1979).

In an artificially respired anaesthetized preparation, the bronchodilator effect of a β-agonist aerosol can be demonstrated using the technique shown in Fig. 6. In this technique an ultrasonic nebulizer incorporated in the ventilator circuit is used to generate and administer the aerosol by "direct inhalation" via a tracheal cannula. Detailed instructions for

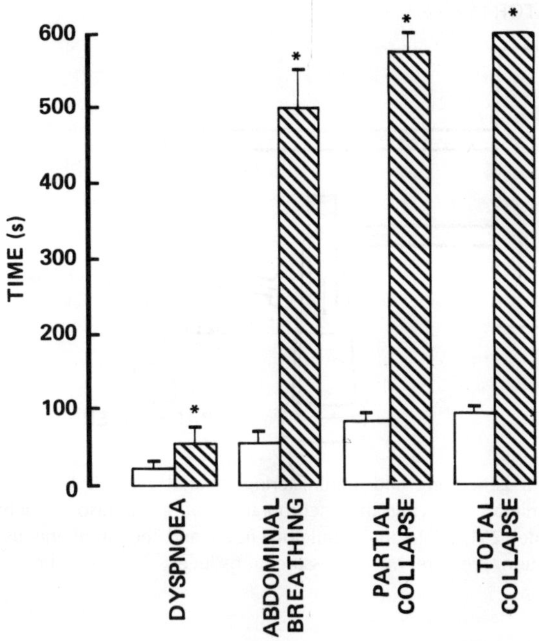

Fig. 5 Protective effect (elongation of onset time) of prior exposure to an aerosol of salbutamol against visually scored respiratory symptoms resulting from subsequent exposure of conscious guinea-pigs to 5-HT aerosol. Animals inhaled either saline aerosol (open columns) or salbutamol (100 μg ml^{-1}) aerosol (hatched columns) for 2 minutes immediately prior to exposure to an aerosol of 5-HT (300 μg ml^{-1}, 10 minutes). Turret jet-nebulizers (air flow 4 l min^{-1}, pressure 14 p.s.i.), were used to generate the aerosols and each animal was exposed individually in a whole body configuration in a 2.5 l perspex chamber. Each column represents the mean result from a group of 5 animals, vertical bars indicate s.e.m., * = $p<0.05$ vs saline exposure.

adapting an ultrasonic nebulizer for this purpose can be found elsewhere (Lees and Payne, 1986). The use of this type of nebulizer avoids the problem of the positive pressure artefact, which would otherwise be introduced into the ventilation circuit system by the use of a jet nebulizer. This consideration is especially important when pulmonary inflation pressure is itself being monitored as an index of intra-thoracic airway calibre. The inhibition of 5-HT-induced bronchospasm in an anaesthetized guinea-pig by "direct inhalation" of isoprenaline is shown in Fig. 7. This figure also illustrates the increased bronchoselectivity and longer duration of action of isoprenaline when inhaled compared with that seen following its systemic administration.

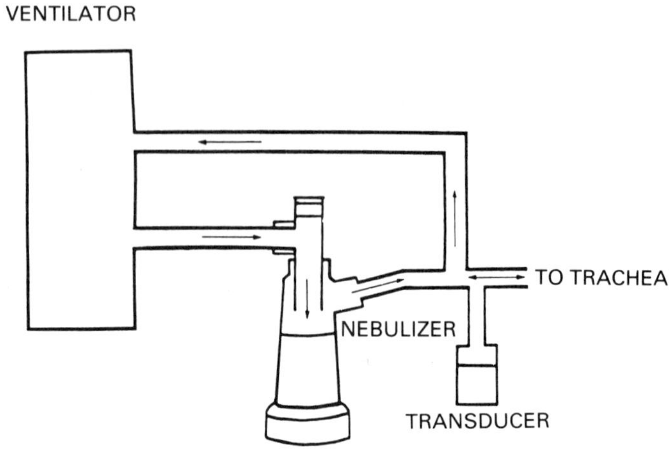

Fig. 6 Method for generating and administering inhaled aerosols by "direct inhalation" in anaesthetized animals showing the incorporation of an ultrasonic nebulizer (DeVilbiss Pulmosonic Model 2512) into the ventilator circuit and the simultaneous measurement of pulmonary inflation pressure by a pressure transducer. Arrows indicate the direction of airflow.

Using essentially the same methods as described above, jet and ultrasonic nebulizers can be used to administer pharmacological aerosols to a variety of species and for sensitizing and/or challenging animals with antigens (Weissberg *et al.*, 1978; Spannhake *et al.*, 1980; Lewis *et al.*, 1982b; Fitzgerald *et al.*, 1985; Lagente *et al.*, 1987; Lees and Payne, 1987; see below). Other published methods of administering aerosols to laboratory animals include the use of synchronized intratracheal aerosol generating systems (Schreck *et al.*, 1986) and forced insufflation of micronized drug powders (Schiantarelli *et al.*, 1982).

D Bronchial anaphylaxis in guinea-pigs

Despite well recognized immunopharmacological differences to the human disease, bronchial anaphylaxis in sensitized guinea-pigs remains a popular laboratory model of allergic asthma (Kallos and Kallos, 1984). However, in many instances the route of antigen challenge used is systemic. A more obvious analogy to man is where the challenge route is by inhalation. In the same way as described above for giving salbutamol by "direct inhalation", an in-line ultrasonic nebulizer can be used to generate and

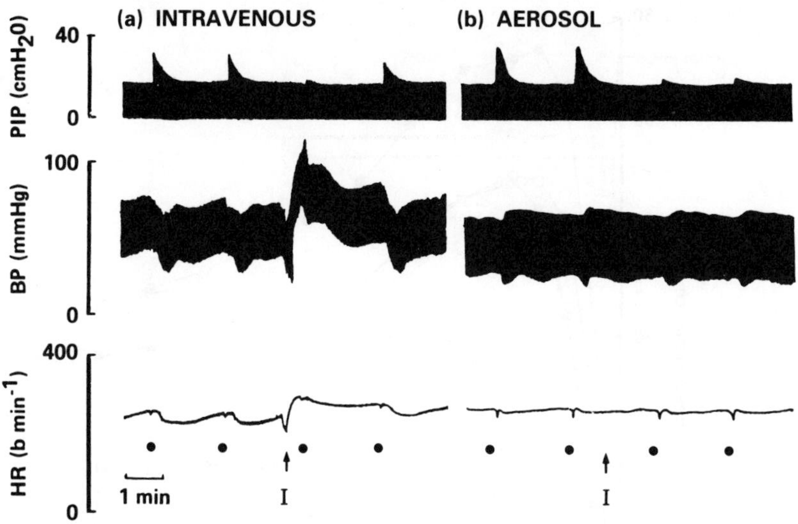

Fig. 7 Comparative cardiovascular effects of intravenous and inhaled isoprenaline (I) at doses giving equivalent initial inhibition of the bronchoconstrictor effect of i.v. 5-HT (0.1 μg kg^{-1}) in pump-ventilated anaesthetized guinea-pigs: (a) isoprenaline (0.03 μg kg^{-1}) i.v. (b) isoprenaline 3 μg ml^{-1} solution by direct inhalation for 10 seconds, (approx. administered dose 0.01 μg kg^{-1}) 1 minute before 5-HT. Note absence of cardiovascular effects and longer duration of bronchodilator action of inhaled isoprenaline. PIP = pulmonary inflation pressure, BP = blood pressure, HR = heart rate.

administer aerosolized ovalbumin in order to provoke anaphylactic bronchoconstriction *in vivo* and *in vitro* in guinea-pigs previously actively sensitized to this antigen (Payne and Nucci, 1987). Using this method, aerosol challenge provokes concentration related anaphylactic bronchoconstriction as shown in Fig. 8. Accompanying cardiovascular effects are much reduced compared with i.v. challenge, and furthermore, there is no concomitant fall in either circulating leukocyte or platelet count, illustrating the local nature of the immunological response. This experimental model is amenable to pharmacological modulation (Daffonchio *et al.*, 1987a) and has been used with success in determining the bronchial effects of a novel series of 5-lipoxygenase inhibitors (Payne *et al.*, 1988). In this instance, the animals were pre-treated with mepyramine and indomethacin to exclude respectively the bronchoconstrictor contribution of histamine and cyclo-oxygenase products of arachidonic acid metabolism and reveal a predominantly leukotriene-dependent bronchoconstriction.

As the effects of aerosol challenge are pulmonary rather than systemic, this route of antigen administration is particularly useful when the effects

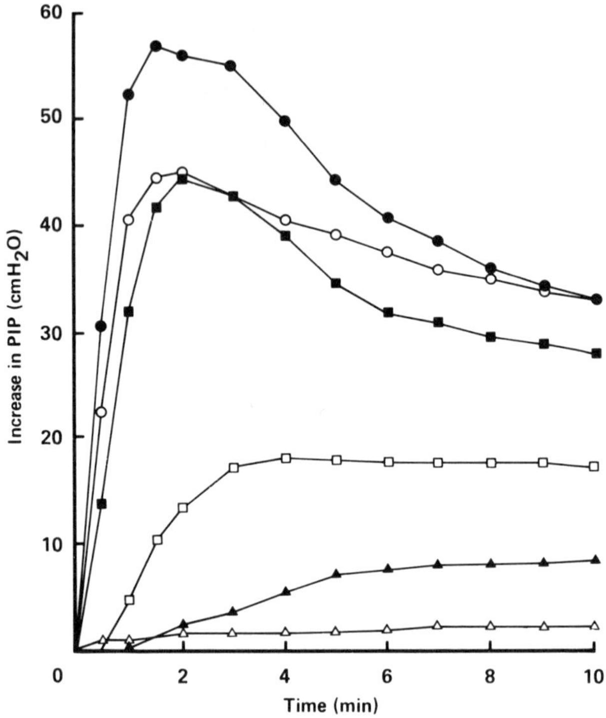

Fig. 8 Magnitude and time course of the rise in pulmonary inflation pressure (PIP) provoked by 5 s challenge of actively-sensitized anaesthetized guinea-pigs with aerosols generated from stock solutions of increasing concentrations of ovalbumin antigen (△), 0.03 mg ml^{-1}; (▲), 0.1 mg ml^{-1}; (□), 0.3 mg ml^{-1}; (■), 1.0 mg ml^{-1}; (○), 3.0 mg ml^{-1}; (●), 10 mg ml^{-1}. The aerosols were generated and administered by "direct-inhalation" using an in-line ultrasonic nebulizer. Each point represents the mean result from individual groups of five animals. S.e. means have been omitted for clarity but for any single point did not exceed 5.0 cm H_2O. (From Daffonchio *et al.*, 1987a).

of a potential anti-asthmatic drug given itself as an aerosol are being evaluated. In this case, two separate nebulizers (one containing the antigen, the other containing the drug) can be mounted in parallel and switched in and out of the ventilation circuit as required.

E Airway hyperreactivity

A non-specific enhancement of bronchial smooth muscle responsiveness (airway hyperreactivity) to inhaled pharmacological and environmental

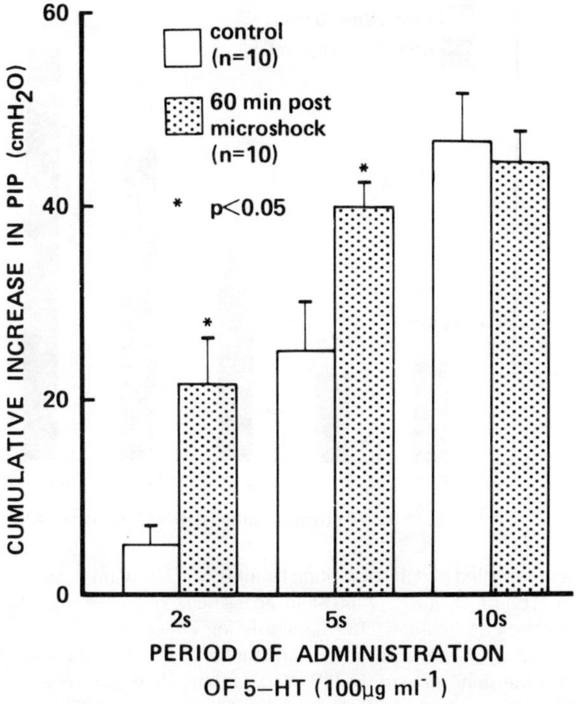

Fig. 9 Effect of aerosol challenge with a submaximal (microshock) dose of ovalbumin aerosol (0.3 mg ml^{-1}, 5 s) on airway reactivity to inhaled 5-HT in anaesthetized guinea-pigs. Reactivity to inhaled 5-HT was assessed 1 hour after antigen challenge. All aerosols were generated and administered by "direct inhalation" using an in-line ultrasonic nebulizer. Each column represents the mean result from n animals as indicated. Vertical bars indicate s.e. mean. (Data from Daffonchio *et al.*, 1987b).

stimuli is a cardinal feature of asthma (Boushey *et al.*, 1980). It has been suggested that this phenomenon occurs as a result of underlying bronchial inflammation (Robinson and Holgate, 1985; O'Bryne, 1986). As such, both clinical and animal studies have linked the development of airway-hyperreactivity primarily to the late (inflammatory), rather than the early (bronchoconstrictor), phase of the asthmatic response to provocation stimuli (Cockcroft *et al.*, 1977; Cartier *et al.*, 1982; Marsh *et al.*, 1985; Murphy *et al.*, 1986). Apart from anaphylactic bronchoconstriction, aerosol challenge of sensitized guinea-pigs also causes pulmonary recruitment of leukocytes (Dunn *et al.*, 1988; Hutson *et al.*, 1988). In addition, there appears to be a relationship between leukocyte infiltration and the development of airway hyperreactivity to i.v. spasmogens (Daffonchio *et*

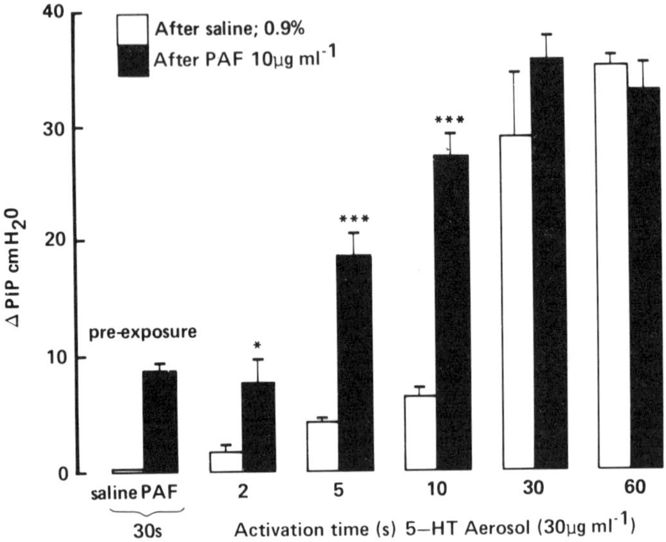

Fig. 10 Effect of inhaled platelet activating factor (PAF) (10 μg ml^{-1}, 30 s) on airway reactivity to inhaled 5-HT (30 μg ml^{-1}, 2–60 s) in anaesthetized guinea-pigs. Reactivity to inhaled 5-HT was assessed 15 minutes after administering either saline (open columns; n = 5) or PAF (filled columns; n = 5) aerosol by "direct inhalation". As indicated, PAF (but not saline) itself caused a transient increase in PIP. Vertical bars show s.e. mean. * = $p<0.05$, *** = $p<0.001$ versus saline control. (Data from Fitzgerald *et al.*, 1987b).

al., 1988). Using the "direct-inhalation" method (see above), following aerosol challenge it is also possible to demonstrate in anaesthetized animals the development of airway hyperreactivity to inhaled bronchoconstrictors such as 5-HT, as shown in Fig. 9. Whilst the relevance of such acute changes in reactivity to the chronic hyperreactivity exhibited by asthmatics remains to be established, it is of interest that in a recent clinical study it was found that bronchial reactivity increased soon after the early asthmatic response in dual-responding subjects (Thorpe *et al.*, 1987). Thus, an acute change in airway reactivity might be, in certain conditions, a possible cause of the late asthmatic response rather than a resulting factor.

Changes in airway reactivity to inhaled spasmogens similar to those occurring after antigen challenge can be demonstrated experimentally both in animals and in man following inhalation of aerosolized platelet activating factor (PAF) (Cuss *et al.*, 1986; Fitzgerald *et al.*, 1987a,b; Fig. 10). This effect is thought to be due to high local concentrations of inhaled PAF causing epithelial damage, which may be analogous to the focal epithelial denudation seen in asthmatic airways (Laitinen *et al.*, 1985). Studies such as these represent pertinent examples of the experimental application of inhaled aerosols in investigating the role of putative mediators such as PAF in asthma.

VII CONCLUDING REMARKS

The science of aerosol generation, and its application to clinical therapeutics has, not surprisingly, advanced greatly since the times of the Ancient Egyptians. Providing one is aware of the practical limitations (especially in terms of quantifying dosage) as well as the potential advantages, inhalation offers a highly exploitable route for the delivery of anti-asthmatic drugs direct to their site of action, in the lungs, with minimal systemic side-effects. At the same time, because this route of administration offers direct access to the region of the lung where a primary lesion of asthma may occur, i.e. damage to the airway epithelium, the use of inhaled aerosols as experimental tools has obvious potential in both clinical and animal studies into the pathophysiology of the disease itself.

REFERENCES

Abbott, A. (1988). *Tr. Pharm. Sci.* **9,** 149–150.
Agnew, J.E. (1984). In *Aerosols and the Lung: Clinical and Experimental Aspects* (Eds S.W. Clarke and D. Pavia), pp. 49–70. Butterworths, London.
Anon, (1976). *Drug Ther. Bull.* **14,** 21–22.
Bakran, I., Jnr, Vrhovac, B. and Plavsic, F. (1980). *Int. J. Clin. Pharm. Ther. Tox.* **18,** 442–446.
Berteau, P.E. and Bierman, A.H. (1977). *Tox. Appl. Pharmacol.* **39,** 177–183.
Bouchikhi, A., Becquemin, M.H., Bignon, J., Roy, M. and Teillac, A. (1988). *Eur. Respir. J.* **1,** 547–552.
Boushey, H.A., Holtzman, M.J., Sheller, J.R. and Nadel, J.A. (1980). *Am. Rev. Resp. Dis.* **121,** 389–413.
Brain, J.D. and Valberg, P.A. (1979). *Am. Rev. Resp. Dis.* **120,** 1325–1373.
Brogden, R.N. (1983). In *Steroids in Asthma, a Reappraisal in the Light of Inhalation Therapy* (Ed. T.J.H. Clark), pp. 121–134. Adis Press, Auckland.
Buckle, D.R. (1984). In *Development of Anti-Asthma Drugs* (Eds D.R. Buckle and H. Smith), pp. 261–296. Butterworths, London.
Cairns, H. and Orr, T.S.G. (1987). *Int. Arch. Allergy appl. Immunol.* **82,** 513–517.
Cartier, A., Thomson, N.C., Frith, P.A., Roberts, R. and Hargreave, F.E. (1982). *J. Allergy Clin. Immunol.* **70,** 170–171.
Clarke, T.J.H. (1986). *Chest* **90,** 67S–70S.
Clarke, T.J.H. and Newman, S.P. (1981). *Chest* **80,** (suppl.) 907–908.

Church, M.K. (1986). *Agents and Actions* **18,** 288–293.
Clay, M.M., Pavia, D., Newman, S.P. and Clarke, S.W. (1983). *Thorax* **38,** 755–759.
Cochrane, G.M. (1983). In *Steroids in Asthma, a Reappraisal in the Light of Inhalation Therapy* (Ed. T.J.H. Clark), pp. 103–120. Adis Press, Auckland.
Cockcroft, D.W., Ruffin, R.E., Dolovich, J. and Hargreave, F.E. (1977). *Clin. Allergy* **7,** 503–513.
Cox, J.S.G. (1967). *Nature, Lond.* **81,** 1328–1329.
Crompton, G.K. (1983). In *Steroids in Asthma, a Reappraisal in the Light of Inhalation Therapy* (Ed. T.J.H. Clark), pp. 166–192. Adis Press, Auckland.
Cuss, F.M., Dixon, C.M.S. and Barnes, P.J. (1986). *Lancet* **i,** 189–192.
Daffonchio, L., Lees, I.W., Payne, A.N. and Whittle, B.J.R. (1987a). *Br. J. Pharmacol.* **91,** 701–708.
Daffonchio, L., Lees, I.W., Payne, A.N. and Whittle, B.J.R. (1987b). *Br. J. Pharmacol.* **90,** 141p.
Daffonchio, L., Lees, I.W., Payne, A.N. and Whittle, B.J.R. (1988). *Br. J. Pharmacol.* **94,** 663–668.
Dahl, R. and Johansson, S.A. (1982). *Eur. J. Resp. Dis.* **63,** (suppl. 122) 167–175.
Dunn, C.J., Elliott, G.A., Oostveen, J.A. and Richards, I.M. (1988). *Am. Rev. Resp. Dis.* **137,** 541–547.
Fabbri, L.M., Chiesura-Corona, P., Dal Vecchio, L., Di Giacomo, G.R., Zocca, E., De Marzo, N., Mastrelli, P. and Mapp, C.E. (1985). *Am. Rev. Resp. Dis.* **132,** 1010–1014.
Ferron, G.A. (1977). *J. Aerosol Sci.* **8,** 251–267.
Fitzgerald, M.F., Parente, L. and Payne, A.N. (1985). *Prostaglandins* **30,** 707.
Fitzgerald, M.F., Lees, I.W., Parente, L. and Payne, A.N. (1987a). *Br. J. Pharmacol.* **90,** 112p.
Fitzgerald, M.F., Lees, I.W., Parente, L. and Payne, A.N. (1987b). *Bull. Eur. Phys. Resp.* **23,** (suppl. 12) 315S.
Fuchs, N.A. (1964). *The Mechanics of Aerosols.* Pergamon Press, Oxford.
Fuchs, N.A. (1978). In *Fundamentals of Aerosol Science* (Ed D.T. Shaw), pp. 1–83. John Wiley, New York.
Gandevia, B. (1975). *Postgrad. Med. J.* **51,** (suppl. 7) 13–20.
Gazeley, M.J.S., Lees, I.W., Payne, A.N., Webbon, P.M. and Woolley, G.E. (1986). *Br. J. Pharmacol.* **87,** 122p.
Guyton, A.C. (1947). *Am. J. Physiol.* **150,** 70–77.
Hatch, T.F. and Gross, P. (1964). *Pulmonary Deposition and Retention of Inhaled Aerosols.* Academic Press, New York.
Hiller, F.C., Mazumder, M.K., Wilson, J.D., Renninger, R.G. and Bone, R.C. (1981). *Chest* **80,** (suppl.) 901–903.
Hutson, P.A., Church, M.K., Clay, T.P., Miller, P. and Holgate, S.T. (1988). *Am. Rev. Resp. Dis.* **137,** 548–557.
Kallos, P. and Kallos, L. (1984). *Int. Arch. Allergy appl. Immunol.* **73,** 77–85.
Kim, C.S., Trujillo, D. and Sackner, M.A. (1985). *Am. Rev. Resp. Dis.* **132,** 137–142.
Laitinen, L.A., Heino, A., Laitinen, A., Kava, T. and Haahtela, T. (1985). *Am. Rev. Resp. Dis.* **131,** 599–606.
Lagente, V., Moncada, S., de Nucci, G. and Payne, A.N. (1987). *Br. J. Pharmacol.* **90,** 35p.
Lees, I.W. and Payne, A.N. (1986). *Br. J. Pharmacol.* **87,** 225p.
Lees, I.W. and Payne, A.N. (1987). *Br. J. Pharmacol.* **92,** 642p.
Lewis, R.A., Cushley, M.J., Fleming, J.S. and Tattersfield, A.E. (1982a). *Am. Rev. Resp. Dis.* **125,** 94.

Lewis, A.J., Dervinis, A. and Rosenthale, M.E. (1982b). *Eur. J. Pharmacol.* **80,** 171–184.
Lourenco, R.V. and Cotromanes, E. (1982). *Arch. Intern. Med.* **142,** 2163–2172.
Marsh, W.R., Irvin, C.G., Murphy, K.R., Lyn Behrens, B. and Larsen, G.L. (1985). *Am. Rev. Resp. Dis.* **131,** 875–979.
Mercer, T.T. (1981). *Chest* **80,** (suppl.) 813–818.
Mercer, T.T., Morrow, P.E. and Staber, W. (1972). *Assessment of Airborne Particles.* Charles C. Thomas, Springfield, Ill.
Morrow, P.E. (1981). *Chest* **80,** 809–813.
Murphy, A.R., Wilson, M.C., Irvin, C.G., Glezen, L.S., Marsh, W.R., Haslett, C., Henson, P.M. and Larsen, G.L. (1986). *Am. Rev. Resp. Dis.* **134,** 62–68.
Newhouse, M. and Dolovich, M. (1986). *Respiration* **50** (suppl. 2), 123–130.
Newman, S.P. (1984). In *Aerosols and the Lung: Clinical and Experimental Aspects* (Eds S.W. Clarke and D. Pavia), pp. 71–91. Butterworths, London.
Newman, S.P. (1985). *Chest* **88,** 152S–160S.
Newman, S.P., Pavia, D., Moren, F., Shenan, N.F. and Clarke, S.W. (1981). *Thorax* **36,** 52–55.
Newman, S.P., Agnew, J.E., Pavia, D. and Clarke, S.W. (1982). *Clin. Phys. Physiol. Meas.* **3,** 1–20.
O'Byrne, P.M. (1986). *Chest* **90,** 575–577.
Pakes, G.E. (1984). In *Development of Anti-asthma Drugs* (Eds D.R. Buckle and H. Smith), pp. 159–183. Butterworths, London.
Payne, A.N. (1988). In *Asthma: Basic Mechanisms and Therapeutic Perspectives* (Eds J.R. Vane, G.A. Higgs, S.A. Marsico and G. Nistico), pp. 151–182. Pythagora Press, Rome and Milan.
Payne, A.N. and de Nucci, G. (1987). *J. Pharm. Meth.* **17,** 83–90.
Payne, A.N., Garland, L.G., Lees, I.W. and Salmon, J.A. (1988). *Br. J. Pharmacol.* **94,** 540–546.
Pennock, B.E., Cox, C.P., Rogers, R.M., Cain, W.A. and Wells, J.H. (1979). *J. Appl. Physiol.; Respirat. Environ. Exercise Physiol.* **46,** 399–406.
Raabe, O.G., Howard, R.S. and Cross, C.E. (1986). In *Bronchial Asthma* (Ed. M.E. Gershwin), pp. 495–514. Grune and Stratton, London and New York.
Raabe, O.G., Yeh, H-C., Newton, G.J., Phalen, R.F. and Velasquez, D.J. (1977). In *Inhaled Particles IV* (Ed. W.H. Walton), pp. 3–22. Pergamon Press, New York.
Richards, I.M., Dixon, M., Jackson, D.M. and Vendy, K. (1986). *Agents and Actions* **18,** 294–300.
Riley, P.A., Mather, M.E., Keogh, R.W. and Eady, R.P. (1987). *Int. Arch. Allergy. Appl. Immunol.* **82,** 108–110.
Robinson, C. and Holgate, S.T. (1985). *J. Allergy Clin. Immunol.* **76,** 140–144.
Ruffin, R.E., Fitzgerald, J.P. and Rebuck, A.S. (1977). *J. Allergy Clin. Immunol.* **59,** 136–141.
Sakula, A. (1988). *J. Roy. Coll. Phy. Lon.* **22,** 36–44.
Schreck, R.M., Sekuterski, J.J. and Gross, K.B. (1986). In *Aerosols: Formation and Reactivity, 2nd Int. Aerosol Conf. Berlin*, pp. 301–304. Pergamon Journals, London.
Schiantarelli, P., Bongrani, S., Papotti, M. and Cadel, S. (1982). *J. Pharm. Meth.* **8,** 9–17.
Shenfield, G.M. (1982). *Drugs* **24,** 414–439.
Silbaugh, S.A. (1987). In *Current Topics in Pulmonary Pharmacology and Toxicology Vol. II* (Ed. M.A. Hollinger), pp. 96–106. Elsevier, Amsterdam.
Skidmore, I.F. (1984). In *Development of Anti-asthma Drugs* (Eds D.R. Buckle and H. Smith), pp. 185–204. Butterworths, London.
Skorodin, M.S. (1986). *Am. J. Med.* **81,** (suppl. 5A) 8–15.

Sotomayor, H., Badier, M., Vervloet, D. and Orehek, J. (1984). *Am. Rev. Resp. Dis.* **130,** 56–58.

Spannhake, E.W., Hyman, A.L. and Kadowitz, P.J. (1980). *J. Pharm. Exp. Ther.* **212,** 584–590.

Sweeny, T.D., Brain, J.D. and LeMott, S. (1983). *J. Appl. Physiol.; Respirat. Environ. Exercise Physiol.* **54,** 37–44.

Thomas, R.L. (1969). *Health Physics* **16,** 417–428.

Thomas, R.L. and Lie, R. (1963). *Procedures and Equipment used in Inhalation Studies on Small Animals.* AEC Research and Development Report, LF11, Lovelace Foundation, Albuquerque, New Mexico, USA.

Thorpe, J.E., Steinberg, D., Bernstein, L.L. and Murlas, C.G. (1987). *Chest* **91,** 21–25.

Tobin, M., Jenouri, G., Danta, I., Kim, C.S., Watson, H. and Sackner, M.A. (1982). *Am. Rev. Resp. Dis.* **126,** 670–675.

Weibel, E.R. (1963). *Morphometry of the Human Lung.* Springer-Verlag, Berlin.

Weissberg, R.M., Bradshaw, J.B. and Garay, G.L. (1978). *J. Pharm. Exp. Ther.* **205,** 246–254.

2

Synergy in the pathogenesis and treatment of asthma

M.C. Berenbaum

Department of Experimental Pathology, St. Mary's Hospital Medical School, London W2, UK

I INTRODUCTION

Interactions between biologically active agents are classified as synergistic (when the agents work together to produce their effects), antagonistic (when they work against each other) or zero-interactive (when they do neither of these). Such interactions are clearly important in asthma for a number of reasons.

Firstly, many of the pathogenetic mechanisms in the disease appear to be governed by synergistic or antagonistic interactions between biological mediators (Barnes *et al.*, 1988). Mechanisms in which interactions are believed to be important include bronchoconstriction (Barnes *et al.*, 1984; Fuller *et al.*, 1986; Heaton *et al.*, 1984; Leff and Munoz, 1981; Leff, 1988; Mazzoni *et al.*, 1985; Watson *et al.*, 1988), release of mast cell mediators (Marquardt *et al.*, 1978; Nishizuka, 1984; Peters *et al.*, 1982), platelet activation (De Chauffoy de Courcelles *et al.*, 1987; Grant and Scrutton, 1980; Kaibuchi *et al.*, 1983; Haslam *et al.*, 1985; Ware *et al.*, 1987), immunological responses (Berenbaum *et al.*, 1976; Bich-Thuiy and Fauci, 1986; Ennist *et al.*, 1987; Fernandez-Botran *et al.*, 1988) and acute inflammatory reactions (Archer *et al.*, 1984, 1987; Bachelet *et al.*, 1988; Basran *et al.*, 1982; De Maeyer and De Maeyer-Guignard, 1988; Hellewell

ASTHMA REVIEWS VOLUME 2
ISBN 0-12-040922-4

and Williams, 1988; Williams, 1979; Williams and Morley, 1973; Williams and Peck, 1977).

Secondly, many asthmatic patients require combinations of drugs, for example, combinations of β_2-agonists and theophylline or combinations of these with corticosteroids, as the pharmacological interactions between these may confer therapeutic advantage. Britton *et al.* (1988) found that 40–50% of patients on asthma medication were taking three or four such drugs, and Lindsay (1988) noted that 98 of 100 patients he had treated recently required drug combinations rather than single agents.

Thirdly, many patients take other drugs, not directly related to the asthmatic state, but for coincident diseases (cardiac failure, respiratory infection, etc), or for indications such as insomnia. For example, some of the patients of Weinberger and Bronsky (1974) had, not only the combinations of ephedrine and theophylline that were on trial, but also isoproterenol for treatment of acute symptoms, as well as antacids, acetaminophen, hydroxyzine and penicillin or erythromycin. Although combinations of these kinds are not given with the intention of producing a pharmacological interaction, such interactions may nevertheless occur and are generally adverse. For example, administration of phenobarbital accelerates the catabolism of steroids and, in steroid-dependent asthmatic patients, has led to increased bronchospasm, deterioration in spirometric test results and increased peripheral blood eosinophilia, effects that were reversed when phenobarbital was withdrawn (Brooks *et al.*, 1972). Interactions of this sort are especially important in patients on theophylline, which has a narrow therapeutic range and serious toxicity. Blood theophylline may be raised to levels that induce grand mal seizures by concurrent administration of antibiotics, especially erythromycin (Pfeifer *et al.*, 1978; Raoof *et al.*, 1987; Rieder and Spino, 1988; Takagi *et al.*, 1988; Weinberger *et al.*, 1976; Wijnands *et al.*, 1984; Zarowitz *et al.*, 1981) and of cimetidine (Jackson *et al.*, 1981; Weinberger *et al.*, 1981), while administration of phenytoin accelerates clearance of the drug and results in low blood levels (Marquis *et al.*, 1982). Multiple drug taking is particularly common among the elderly, on average, 20% of them are taking three or more prescribed drugs, and in individuals referred to a geriatric service the proportion rises to 50% (Gilchrist *et al.*, 1987; Cartwright and Smith, 1988).

Thus, synergy and antagonism, and methods for their analysis and measurement are of great importance in the pathogenesis and management of asthma, and the question arises as to the precise meaning of these terms.

At the outset of this review, a distinction must be made between conventional synergy and antagonism, which are the interactions between two or more biologically active agents in producing single specified effects, such as bronchodilatation or tachycardia, and so-called "therapeutic synergy" (Steen, 1978), which concerns the relations between these interactions in respect of two or more different types of effects (such as bronchodilatation *and* tachycardia) in one and the same individual. As has been pointed out by Shenfield (1982), in connection with the enhanced bronchodilatation that may be produced by combinations of two or more drugs, "whether this enhancement is truly synergistic or merely additive does not matter to the patient." What matters is a desirable therapeutic outcome, which must be defined in terms of all the important effects, beneficial and adverse, produced by the administered drugs.

This topic will be considered in detail below. For the present, it will suffice to point out that, in order to understand the complex interrelations between two or more different types of effect, it is necessary to understand the individual interactions themselves. Thus, the study of therapeutic synergy and therapeutic outcome must be based firmly on the study of interactions in respect of individual effects.

II MECHANISTIC AND EMPIRICAL MODELS OF INTERACTIONS

First let us examine the idea that synergy and antagonism may be defined in terms of mechanisms of action, i.e. they occur when a combination produces an effect greater or less than that which would be expected from an accurate understanding of the mechanisms of action of the agents. If the effect of the combination is what is expected from these mechanisms, it is deemed to show zero interaction. For instance, we might know that drugs A and B both act on the same receptor site, we might have good information about their respective concentration–effect relations at that site, we might know that these relations follow the law of mass action, and so on. Then, using all this information, we might attempt to predict quantitatively the effect of a particular combination of the agents. If our understanding of the mechanisms is adequate, then our prediction might well be correct and, according to this approach, the interaction would be classified as being zero interaction. On the other hand, if the combination turned out to have a significantly greater or lesser effect than expected, it would be classified as being synergistic or antagonistic. However, there is a flaw in this approach, for instance, if the combination is more effective than expected from a supposedly good understanding of the mechanisms of action of the agents, it follows that this understanding is imperfect. The mechanisms would be investigated further and previously unknown features of those mechanisms might be discovered that would be sufficient to explain the observed effect. But then, according to this approach, the interaction would be categorized as zero interaction. In other words, this approach implies that synergy and antagonism are artefacts arising out of incomplete knowledge and with sufficient investigation all such interactions may be made to vanish.

Evidently, interactions cannot be usefully categorized in this way and, consequently, they are usually classified by considering quantitative phenomena only, i.e. by examining the relationship between the effect of the combination and the effects of its constituents or, more comprehensively, by looking at the relationship between the composition and effect of the combination and the dose–effect curves of the individual agents. This approach takes no account of underlying mechanisms of action and so is empirical.

In the literature on asthma, the almost universally accepted definition of synergy is based on the summative criterion, which is that when the agents in a combination do not interact pharmacologically to produce its effect, then this should simply be the sum of the effects of the constituents

$$E(A,B) = E(A) + E(B) \quad (1)$$

Thus, synergy is said to be present when $E(A,B) > E(A) + E(B)$ and antagonism when $E(A, B) < E(A) + E(B)$ (Anderson *et al.*, 1981; Archer *et al.*, 1984; Basran *et al.*, 1982; Bertelli *et al.*, 1973; Campbell, 1979; Campbell *et al.*, 1977; Dale and Penfield, 1984; Hanna and Roth, 1979; Kreisman *et al.*, 1981; Leff and Munoz, 1981; Lightbody *et al.*, 1978; Marlin *et al.*, 1979a, 1979b; Trotman *et al.*, 1978). The summative criterion is also implied in the use of analysis of variance to classify interactions (Anderson *et al.*, 1981; Beck *et al.*, 1985; Bryant, 1985; Campbell *et al.*, 1977; Grandordy *et al.*, 1988; Kreisman *et al.*, 1981; Lefcoe *et al.*, 1982; Myers *et al.*, 1986; Pierce *et al.*, 1957; Rebuck *et al.*, 1983; Reisman *et al.*, 1988; Sims *et al.*, 1978) and, with this statistical method, interaction is *defined* as departure from simple summation of effects.

Although the summative criterion is virtually the only one used by investigators of asthma, this is not because there is a general consensus among pharmacologists that this is the correct criterion for assessing interactions, or because it is particularly appropriate to this field. In fact, there is no general agreement and at least eight different criteria are currently in use (Berenbaum, 1989). The principal reason for the fairly consistent usage of the summative criterion in the asthma literature is that workers in this field appear to have shown relatively little curiosity about the problems involved in assessing drug interactions, to have been largely unaware of the extensive disagreement on the matter that pervades the wider literature and have adopted an approach that superficially appears simple and straightforward, but which is in fact usually invalid.

A simple example will demonstrate the difficulties that arise out of the summative definition of zero interaction. Suppose we have two drug solutions, labelled A and B respectively. The identity of the drugs is unknown, but their dose–response curves for effects on FEV_1 (Forced Expiratory Volume in 1 s) are as shown in Fig. 1.

Suppose it is found that 1 mg/kg of either A or B alone increases FEV_1 by 5%, whereas a combination of 1 mg/kg A and 1 mg/kg B increases FEV_1 by 35%. According to the summative criterion, A and B are undoubtedly synergistic. At this stage we learn that A and B are in fact one and the same drug, and the dose–response curve confirms that, although 1 mg of this drug increases FEV_1 by only 5%, 2 mg/kg causes an increase of 35%. Two conclusions are possible: either the drug is synergistic with itself (i.e. a sham "combination" of 1 + 1 mg/kg of the drug gives a greater response than expected), or the criterion of zero interaction used is incorrect. The former is not tenable because the effect of a sham "combination" of one and the same agent can only be precisely that expected from its dose–response curve, and so only the latter conclusion remains.

A similar dilemma would arise on comparing the effects of single doses of 0.5 mg/kg, each produce no measurable effect, a sham "combination"

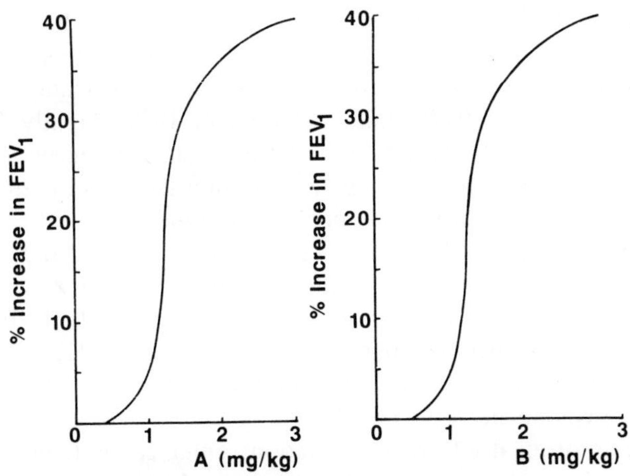

Fig. 1 In this figure A and B are the same drug, so interaction is absent. The effect of any sham "combination" of A and B can simply be read off either dose–response curve and, with the curves shown here, the summative criterion does not hold in general (*see* text).

of both of these together, which, according to the summative criterion should also have no effect, in fact increases FEV_1 by 5%.

Consider also a combination of 1.5 mg/kg A and 1.5 mg/kg B. Each of these doses alone produces a 30% increase in FEV_1, but the combination produces a 40% increase, so its effect is clearly less than the sum of the effects of its constituents. Again, as it turns out we are dealing with a single drug only, and therefore cannot conclude that the effect of the sham "combination" is less than expected from the dose–response curve of the drug, we must conclude that the criterion used was wrong.

In this field, the only other common approach to defining interactions is to use the terms synergy and antagonism without defining them, the authors apparently believing that the conclusion is obvious from the data, and being under the mistaken impression that there is a general consensus as to the meaning of the terms (Ardlie *et al.*, 1987; Baraban *et al.*, 1985; De Chauffoy de Courcelles *et al.*, 1987; Evans *et al.*, 1980; Fujimura *et al.*, 1986; Kaliner *et al.*, 1971; Taylor *et al.*, 1965; Vargaftig *et al.*, 1982; Ware *et al.*, 1987; Watson *et al.*, 1988).

III TERMINOLOGY

Confusion arises, not only out of failure to define the terms used to classify interactions, but also out of the use of the same term in different ways. A term often misused in this way is additivism. In the asthma literature, an additive response generally means one in which the effect of a combination is obtained by adding the effects of its constituents, i.e. the summative criterion holds (Bruderman *et al.*, 1983; Campbell, 1979; Dyson and Campbell, 1977; Hanna and Eyre, 1979; Lightbody *et al.*, 1978; Shenfield, 1982). However, in the pharmacological literature generally, additivism more often means zero interaction, and other usages involve assessing lateral shifts or changes in the slopes of the dose–response curve (Advenier *et al.*, 1988; Bongrani *et al.*, 1981; Leopold and Handslip, 1979; Pöch, 1981; Pöch and Holtzmann, 1980; Pöch and Zimmermann, 1988). The word is also used in connection with so-called "functional additivism", a mechanism in which two agonists act on different receptors (Undem and Adams, 1988). Because of these multiple definitions, the term will be avoided here.

Other terms often used are potentiation, enhancement, amplification and augmentation, which are generally undefined by the users, but mean simply increase of a response. Some authors use these terms to mean merely that the response of a combination exceeds that of each of its constituents (a hardly surprising effect that would occur in any case even with a "combination" of one and the same agent). Others use the terms to mean that the effect of a combination exceeds the sum of the effects of its constituents. In both cases the terms are sometimes used interchangeably with synergy. These sources of confusion will be avoided in this review, in which interactions will be classified into three types only—zero interaction, in which a response is precisely what is expected, synergy, in which it exceeds expectation and antagonism, in which it is less. The crux of the matter, which will now be considered, is clearly—what is to be expected?

IV EMPIRICAL EXPECTATIONS AND THE ISOBOLE METHOD

A The isobole method

Let us examine the situation in Fig. 1 in another way. A graph is drawn (Fig. 2(a)), the axes of which are respectively the dose-axes of A and B (which are known to be one and the same drug). Points on the graph represent particular combinations of A and B, e.g. a point with co-ordinates (1,2) represents a combination of 1 mg/kg A with 2 mg/kg B.

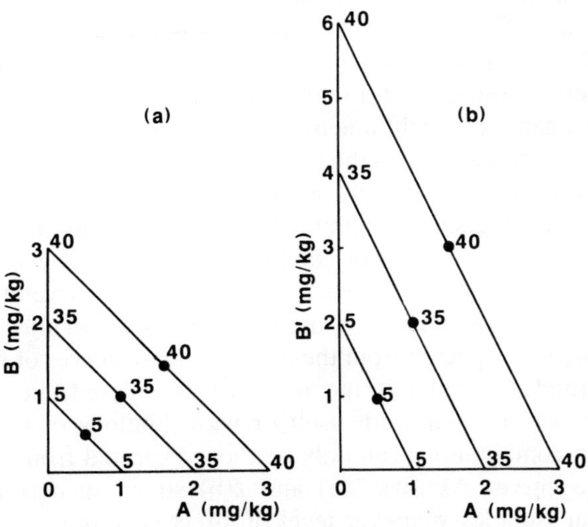

Fig. 2 (a) Construction of isoeffect curves (isoboles) for combinations of A and B. (b) Construction of isoeffect curves for combinations of A and B′.

On this graph insert along the dose-axes the effects obtained with the agents alone (read off the dose–response curves in Fig. 1) and, at the points with the appropriate coordinates, insert the effects obtained with the sham "combinations". Isoeffect curves (isoboles) are drawn, joining all points of equal effects, and it appears that the isobole for 35% increase in FEV_1, which passes from the point representing 2 mg/kg A on the A dose-axis, through the point representing the combination of 1 mg/kg of each of A and B, to the point representing 2 mg/kg B on the B dose-axis, is a straight line. Moreover, all the other points on this line, e.g. with coordinates (0.1, 1.9), (1.25, 0.75), represent combinations in which the total dose of agent is 2 mg/kg, and so all have this same effect. Similarly, the isobole for 40% increase of FEV_1, which passes from the point representing 3 mg/kg A through that representing combination (1.5, 1.5) to the point representing 3 mg/kg B, is a straight line, and similarly the isobole for a 5% increase is a straight line. Thus, irrespective of the level of effect chosen, the isobole is a straight line.

In this diagram, A and B have identical dose–response curves (in fact, they are one and the same agent), so we next consider the effect of changing the dose–response curve of B by diluting this drug two-fold with some inert material. The diluted drug will be called B′. It should be noted that the dose–response curves of A and B′ are similar, i.e. they could be superimposed simply by a uniform contraction of the dose-axis for B by half, or a uniform two-fold expansion of the dose-axis for A.

The effect of the manoeuvre is shown in Fig. 2(b). The combination of 1 mg/kg A with 2 mg/kg B′ must have the same effect as a combination of 1 mg/kg A with 1 mg/kg B (because 2 mg of B′ is merely 1 mg B plus some inert material) and 4 mg/kg B′ must have the same effect as 2 mg/kg B so, again, a straight line isobole is produced for a 35% increase in FEV_1. For the same reason, the isoboles for 40% increase and for 5% increase in FEV_1 are also straight lines.

As A and B are the same drug and B′ is also this drug merely diluted with inert material, the effects of combinations of A and B or of A and B′ can only be those expected from the dose–response curve of this drug.

If zero interaction is defined as the situation in which the effect of a combination is that expected from the dose–response curves of the agents, then an appropriate model is the one just considered, i.e. the sham "combination" of an agent with itself or with dilutions of itself, as the effects of such combinations can only be those expected from the agent's dose–response curve. As Figs 2(a) and 2(b) show, such combinations generate linear isoboles whatever level of effect is chosen.

In the model constructed above the sham agents had dose–response curves that were either identical or similar (superimposable by a linear scaling of the dose-axes). However, it can be proved by an extension of this model that linear isoboles are generated by zero-interactive combinations irrespective of whether the dose–response curves are similar or not; in fact, the shapes of these curves are quite irrelevant (Berenbaum, 1985, 1989).

Thus, a combination of different agents is defined as zero-interactive if its effect is that expected from the dose–response curves of the agents (considered purely quantitatively and without reference to mechanisms of action), such expectation being unambiguously described by the generation of a linear isobole for the observed effect. The features of synergy and antagonism are readily deduced (Fig. 3). A synergistic combination is more effective than expected, so less of the agents are required to produce a given effect. Accordingly, the isobole for that effect is concave-up with respect to the origin. Conversely, in antagonism the combination is less effective than expected, so more of the agents are needed to produce the given effect and the isobole is concave-down with respect to the origin.

The isobole method was first described by Fraser (1870–1, 1872) and developed by Loewe and his colleagues (Loewe, 1928, 1953, 1957; Loewe and Muischnek, 1926). However, the method did not come into general use until about 80 years after its introduction (Nichols, 1948; Chen and Ensor, 1953; Elion *et al.*, 1954). It has not appeared in the literature on the pathogenesis or treatment of asthma, and the only isobole published on a related subject is that of Hayashi *et al.* (1988) on the effects of

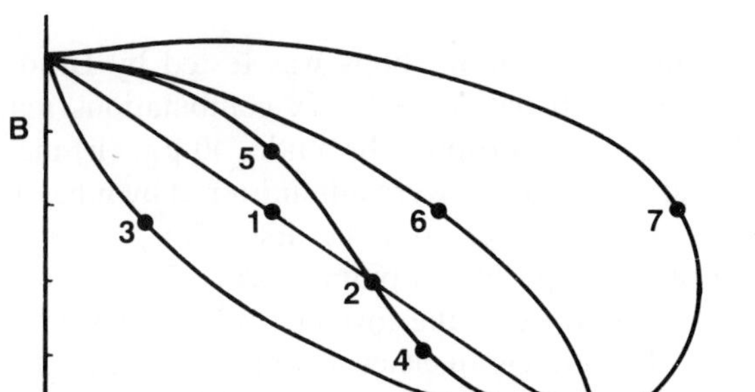

Fig. 3 Isoboles for zero interaction, synergy and antagonism. Combinations 1 and 2 on the linear isobole are zero-interactive. Combinations 3 and 4 below the zero interaction line are synergistic. Combinations 5, 6 and 7 above this line show antagonism. Note that an isobole need not follow a consistent course, e.g. combinations 2, 4 and 5 all have the same effect but one shows synergy, one zero interaction and one antagonism.

combinations of α_1- and β-adrenoceptor agonists against induced cardiac arrythmias. The isobole method is simple and powerful and its introduction into the study of interactions in asthma is long overdue.

B Comments on the isobole method

1 *Useful experimental designs*

A variety of experimental designs has been used in studies of interactions between agents involved in the pathogenesis or treatment of asthma, and the application of the isobole method to the data obtained with these may be illustrated by the following examples:

(1) Blumenthal (1980) treated asthmatic children with 5-week courses of aminophylline, salbutamol and a combination of both. Each child had all three regimens. The constituents of the combination given to each patient contained half the dose of the drugs given singly. (There was considerable interpatient variation in dosage, which weakens the experiment, but this will be ignored for the purpose of this example.) The effects of the full doses of single agents and the combination of half-doses are shown in Fig. 4. The isoboles for the effects of the combinations are concave-up for all four responses. Thus, the interactions are conclusively classified as synergistic, although each isobole is based on only three determinations and the effects of the constituents of the combination were not assessed.

(2) A greater number of combinations was tested by Bruderman *et al.* (1983), who treated each patient with six combinations made up from two of the following: (i) ipratropium bromide, 40 μg, (ii) metaproterenol 1.25 mg and (iii) placebo. Drugs were administered by inhaler, the second of the pair being given an hour after the first. Thus, patients were given a total of either 40 or 80 μg ipratropium, 1.25 or 2.5 mg metaproterenol or the combination of 40 μg of the former with 1.25 mg of the latter (or in reverse order). The effects of placebo only were not determined.

Figure 5 shows results as areas under the FEV_1 time–response curves over a 6-hour period (expressed in arbitrary units). When ipratropium was given before metaproterenol (Fig. 5(a)), the single doses of 80 μg ipratropium or 1.25 mg metaproterenol had less effect on FEV_1 than the combination of half-doses of each, so the isobole for the effect of the combination is concave-up, indicating synergy. (The effects of 40 μg metaproterenol or 1.25 mg ipratropium alone are irrelevant to this

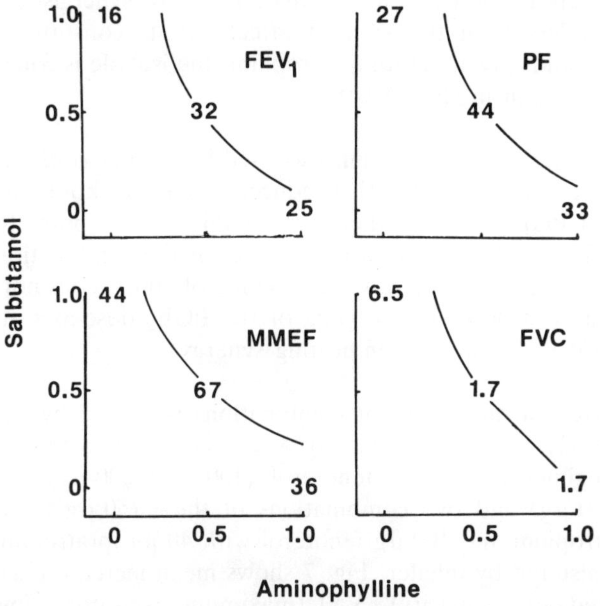

Fig. 4 Effects of combinations of aminophylline and salbutamol in asthmatic children (Blumenthal, 1980, Table 3). Doses varied between patients, but in each case the constituents of the combination contained half the dose of each drug given singly, and so dosage is expressed as a fraction of the full individual dose. For all four measures, the effect of the combination (0.5, 0.5) exceeded that of the full dose (1.0) of salbutamol and exceeded or equalled that of the full dose (1.0) of aminophylline, so all isoboles are concave-up, indicating synergy.

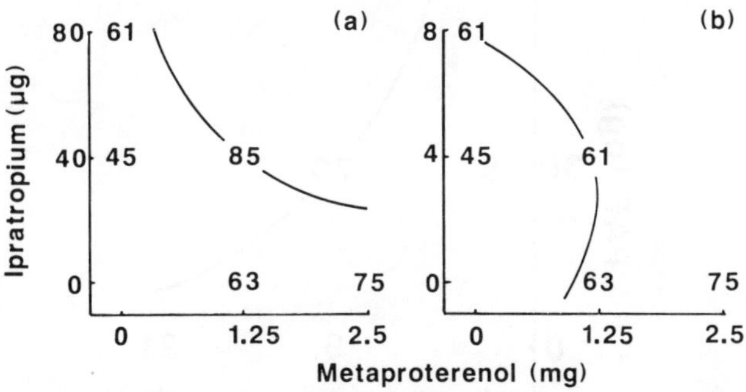

Fig. 5 Effects of combinations of metaproterenol and ipratropium bromide on FEV_1 expressed as areas under 6-hour FEV_1 time–response curves (arbitrary units) (Bruderman *et al.*, 1983, Figs. 1–3). (a) Ipratropium bromide given 1 hour before metaproterenol. (b) Metaproterenol given 1 hour before ipratropium bromide. The combination of 1.25 mg metaproterenol with 40 μg ipratropium bromide is, in fact, less effective than 1.25 mg metaproterenol alone.

analysis, except to show that a combination may be synergistic even when its effect is less than the sum of effects of its constituents). When metaproterenol is given before ipratropium, the isobole is concave-down, indicating antagonism (Fig. 5(b)).

(3) A similar experimental design was used by Archer *et al.* (1984), who measured the volumes of wheals produced in human skin by intradermal injections of PGE_2, PAF-acether or a combination of both. Results are shown in Fig. 6. The isobole for the effect of the combination of 30 ng PAF with 0.5 μg PGE_2, i.e. a wheal volume of 70 μl, does not reach the PAF dose-axis at doses up to 60 ng or the PGE_2 dose-axis at doses up to 1 μg, so it is concave-up, indicating synergy.

(4) A different arrangement of combinations was used by Elwood and Abboud (1982), who treated each of a series of stable asthmatic patients with six regimens: placebo, fenoterol (100 and 200 μg), ipratropium bromide (40 μg) and two combinations of these (50 μg fenoterol with 20 μg ipratropium and 100 μg fenoterol with 40 μg ipratropium). Drugs were administered by inhaler. Fig. 7 shows mean increase (%) in FEV_1, FVC (forced vital capacity), $\dot{V}50$ (maximum expiratory flow at 50% FVC), and SGaw (specific airway conductance) over a 9-hour period. The authors thought the low-dose combination might be synergistic, but believed that they could not assess this possibility as they did not determine the effects of the low doses on their own. However, Fig. 7

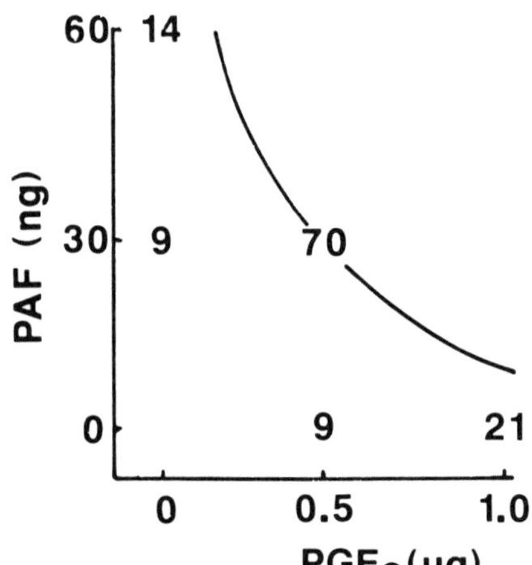

Fig. 6 Induction of wheals in human skin by PGE_2 and PAF (Archer *et al.*, 1984, Table 2).

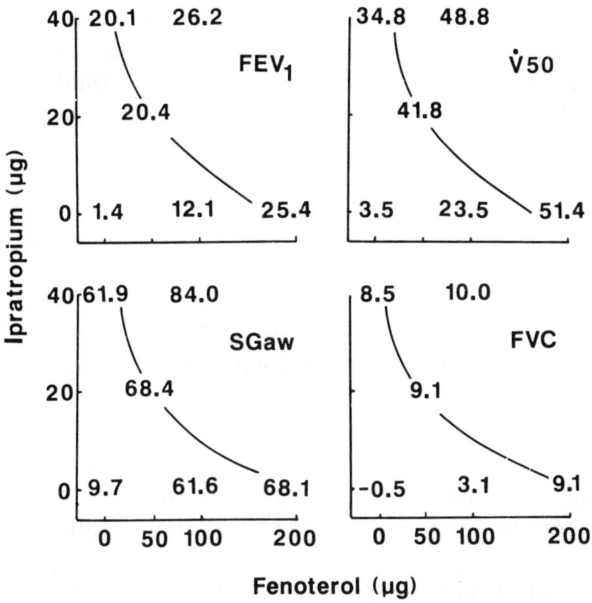

Fig. 7 Effects of combinations of fenoterol and ipratropium bromide in stable asthmatics (Elwood and Abboud, 1982, Table III). For all four measures, the effect of the combination of 50 μg fenoterol with 20 μg ipratropium bromide exceeded that of 40 μg iptratropium bromide and exceeded or equalled that of 200 μg fenoterol, so all isoboles are concave-up, indicating synergy.

shows that the isoboles for the effects of the low-dose combination showed synergy for all these effects, and that the effects of the low doses on their own would have been irrelevant to this assessment.

As these examples show, relatively little information may be needed in order to decide whether synergy or antagonism is shown. It is not necessary to have complete dose–response curves of the agents as has been asserted (Mitchell, 1976; Chou and Talalay, 1981, 1984). All that may be required are upper or lower limits for the isoeffective doses of the individual agents. If these are high enough or low enough to show that the isobole is concave-up or concave-down (as is the case in all the examples discussed above), then a decision that the combination shows synergy or antagonism may be made.

However, the experimental designs used in these examples are not always successful in this respect. For example, if in Fig. 5 the effect of the combination had been less than that of 2.5 mg metaproterenol but more than that of 1.25 mg, the isobole would have ended on the metaproterenol dose-axis somewhere between these two doses, but whether it was concave-up, straight or concave-down could not have been determined. The success of these designs, therefore, depends on the experimental results and they may fail if the interaction is insufficiently marked.

In order to be assured of being able to decide the nature of an interaction and to quantify it (see below), it is necessary to determine precisely where an isobole meets the respective dose-axes, that is, to know what doses of the agents on their own produce the effect of the combination. This usually requires determination of the dose–response curves over the relevant range of effects (but not necessarily complete curves). Examples of the procedure are as follows:

(1) Olsson (1972) measured the LD50 for mice of theophylline, (−)-noradrenaline and combinations of these. Results are shown in Fig. 8, and it is evident that the isobole for the LD50 shows marked antagonism.

(2) Undem and Adams (1988) measured contractions in guinea-pig tracheal segments induced by histamine, leukotriene E_4 (LTE_4) and

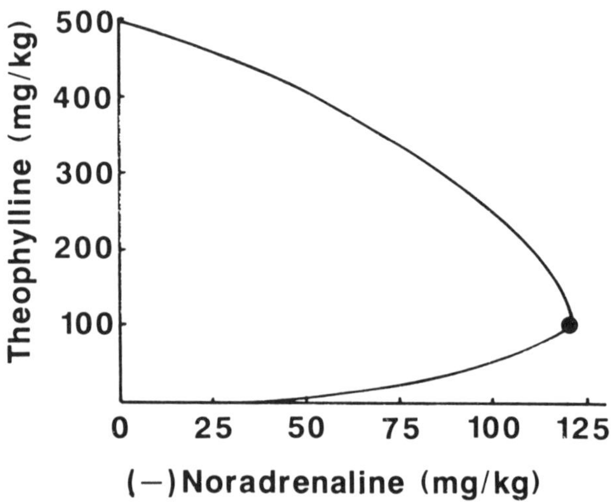

Fig. 8 LD50 isobole for combinations of (−)-noradrenaline and theophylline in mice (Olsson, 1972, Table 1). The LD50 of (−)-noradrenaline is 28 mg/kg and that of theophylline 500 mg/kg. The same effect is produced by a combination of 121 mg/kg (−)-noradrenaline and 100 mg/kg theophylline, so the isobole is concave-down with respect to the origin, indicating antagonism.

combinations of these. The dose–response curves for the separate agents are shown in Fig. 9(a), and also the effects of three combinations of histamine (10^{-7}, 3×10^{-7} and 10^{-6} M) with 10^{-8} M LTE_4. The combinations produced respectively 42%, 50% and 60% of maximal contraction, and the isoboles for these effects are shown in Fig. 9(b). The ends of the isoboles on the respective concentration-axes are located by reading off the dose–response curves in Fig. 9(a) the concentrations

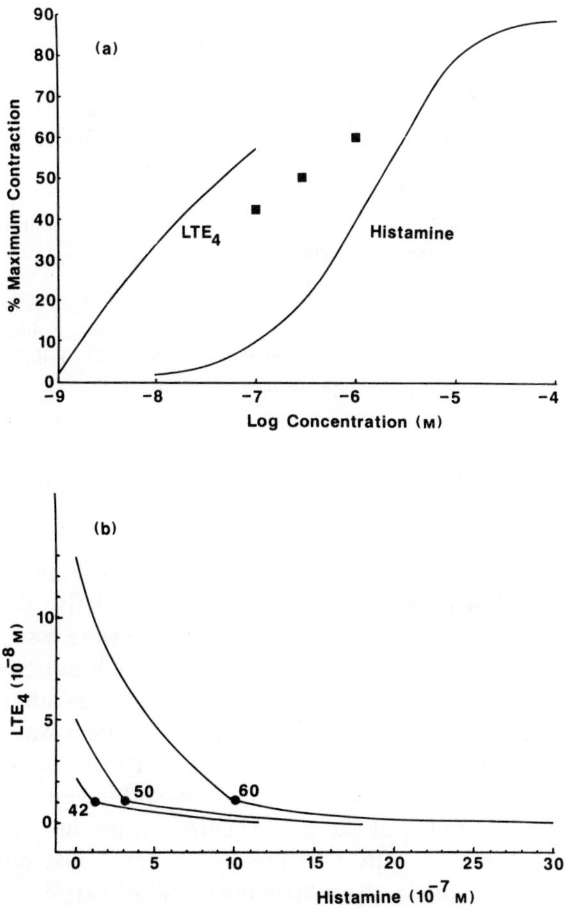

Fig. 9 (a) Dose–response curves for contraction of guinea-pig tracheal segments induced by histamine and LTE_4 (Undem and Adams, 1988, Fig. 1A). (The effect of LTE_4 was not measured at concentrations above 10^{-7} M.) ■ = effects of combinations of histamine 10^{-7}, 3×10^{-7} and 10^{-6} M with 10^{-8} M LTE_4. (b) Isoboles for the effects of the three combinations shown in (a).

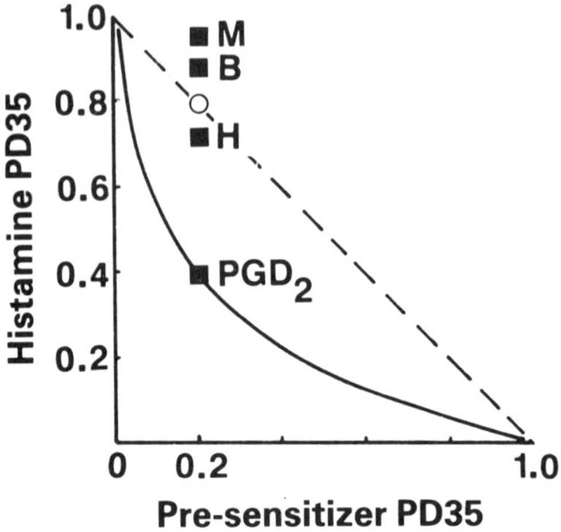

Fig. 10 Effects of combinations of histamine with histamine (H), methacholine (M), bradykinin (B) and PGD_2 on specific airway conductance (Fuller *et al.*, 1986, Fig. 2a). The expected PD35 of histamine after pre-sensitization is indicated by the point (○) on the linear zero interaction line, and, in fact, the observed value when histamine itself is the pre-sensitizer is probably within the limits of experimental error for this point. Methacholine and bradykinin have little effect, if any, on the expected PD35 of histamine, but PGD_2 reduces it substantially, indicating synergy, as shown by the concave-up isobole for the PD35 effect.

of these agents that on their own had the same effects. All three isoboles are concave-up, indicating synergy.

(3) The final example to be examined here is that of Fuller *et al.* (1986), who used the following experimental design. Cumulative dose-responses to histamine, PGD_2, bradykinin and methacholine were assessed in stable atopic asthmatic subjects to find the dose that reduced SGaw by 35% (the PD35). Subsequently, 0.2 PD35 of each agent was administered and then increasing doses of histamine, until a PD35 effect was produced by the combination. The results are shown in Fig. 10. If there had been no interaction, another 0.8 PD35 of histamine would have been required to supplement the 0.2 PD35 of the pre-sensitizer to produce a combination with a PD35 effect. The effect of pre-administered histamine is almost exactly as predicted (for a sham "combination" of two doses of one and the same agent must be zero-interactive). The effects of bradykinin and methacholine are slightly less than expected, but departure from expectation is probably not statistically significant in these cases. However, with PGD_2, substantially less histamine was required than expected, and so the two agents act synergistically in causing bronchoconstriction.

2 2 × 2 and 2 × n arrays

In contrast to the experimental designs described above there are others that, although widely used, are inherently incapable in most circumstances of providing the information sought. One of the most frequently used of such designs is a 2 × 2 array of combinations, i.e. the agents are given alone and together in fixed doses so that the four points representing the tested regimens (including controls) lie at the corners of a rectangle (Anderson *et al.*, 1981; Baadsgard *et al.*, 1985; Campbell *et al.*, 1977, De Chauffoy de Courcelles *et al.*, 1987; Douglas *et al.*, 1979; Evans *et al.*, 1980; Hahn *et al.*, 1970; Heaton *et al.*, 1984; Howarth *et al.*, 1982; Hughes *et al.*, 1982; Kreisman *et al.*, 1981; Mitchell *et al.*, 1979; Myers *et al.*, 1986; Pierce *et al.*, 1957).

For example, Campbell *et al.* (1977) gave patients single doses of either aminophylline (250 mg i.v.) or isoprenaline (about 0.17 mg by inhaler) or both, and measured changes in maximum expiratory flow rate at 50% forced vital capacity ($\dot{V}max_{50}$). The results, shown in Fig. 11, were claimed to show synergy because analysis of variance showed that the effect of the combination significantly exceeded the sum of the effects of the individual drugs. However, use of analysis of variance is based on the assumption that the dose–response curves of the agents are linear. No information about this was obtained in this experiment and, in fact, dose–response curves of the agents relevant to this review are rarely linear (see below). As Fig. 11 shows, it is not possible to say, with the limited information that this experimental design yields, whether the isobole for the effect of the combination is concave-down, straight or concave-up and, thus, it is not possible to determine the nature of the interaction.

An experimental design in which one of the agents is tested at more than one level but the other at only one (2 × *n* array) may also be insufficient to determine the nature of an interaction. For example, Lichtenstein and Margolis (1968) measured the inhibition of antigen-induced histamine release from human leucocytes by exposure to a range of concentrations of theophylline with or without 10^{-6} M ephedrine, and claimed that the interaction was synergistic, apparently because combinations produced definite inhibition, even when the agents on their own at the same concentrations as used in the combination did not. However, the results in Fig. 12 show that it is impossible to ascertain the shapes of the isoboles, because only one concentration of ephedrine was tested.

These two examples invalidate the suggestion that 2 × 2 or 2 × *n* experimental designs may provide evidence of synergy, i.e. the individual

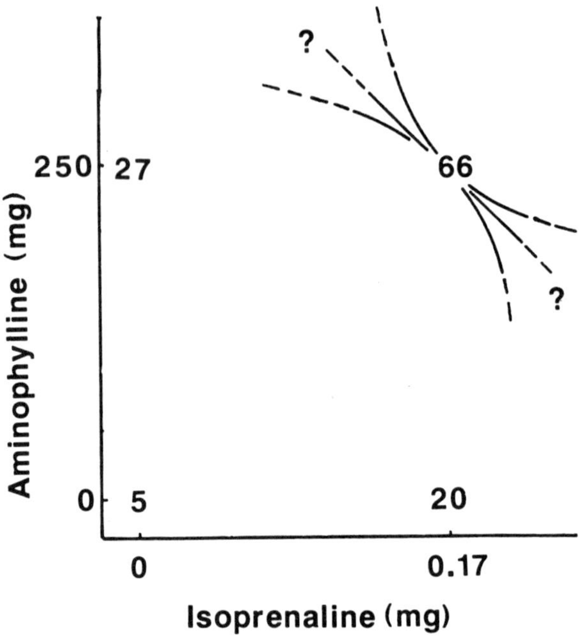

Fig. 11 Effect of a combination of isoprenaline (0.16–0.17 mg by inhaler) and aminophylline (250 mg i.v.) on $\dot{V}max_{50}$ (peak increases (%) are shown). A 2 × 2 factorial experimental design is used (Campbell *et al.*, 1977, Fig. 1).

drugs on their own are ineffective in the dose given, but the combination of these doses produces a significant effect. However, designs of these types may be able to reveal antagonism when this is marked, i.e. when the effect of a combination is less than that of one of its constituents, for then some lower dose of this constituent will be iso-effective with the combination and so the isobole for this effect must be concave-down with respect to the origin.

3 *Heterergic combinations*

The simplest types of interaction between two agents are those in which only one agent has the effect being measured and the other does not, acting only to increase or decrease the effect of the active agent. Combinations of this type may be termed heterergic (Loewe, 1953), in contrast with homergic interactions in which both agents can produce the effect being measured. The simplicity in determining the nature of any interaction with heterergic combinations derives from the fact that, if

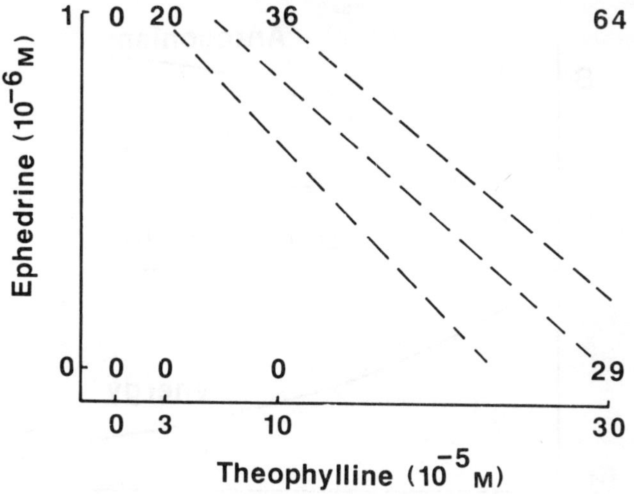

Fig. 12 Effects of combinations of theophylline (3, 10 and 30 × 10^{-5} M) and ephedrine (10^{-6} M) on antigen-induced histamine release from human leucocytes, using a 2 × 4 experimental design (Lichtenstein and Margolis, 1968, Table II). Results shown are inhibition of release (%). Tentative and incomplete isoboles are drawn for 20%, 29% and 36% inhibition but, because ephedrine was tested at one level only, it is impossible to determine the direction of the isoboles above this level, and to say whether they are concave-up, straight or concave-down. Thus, the nature of the interaction between the two agents cannot be determined using this experimental design.

there is no interaction, the effect of the combination must be precisely that of the active component on its own. If it is greater or less than this, the combination must be synergistic or antagonistic respectively.

Isoboles for heterergic interactions are shown in Fig. 13. Zero interaction is shown by an isobole parallel to the dose axis of the inactive agent, synergy by one diverging towards it but never meeting it, and antagonism by one diverging away from it. (This figure suggests that there is often an element of uncertainty in classifying a combination as heterergic, for it may not be possible to exclude the possibility that, at some dose higher than any tested, the supposedly inactive agent does, in fact, produce the effect of interest and therefore the isobole does eventually meet the dose axis of this agent).

An example possibly indicating a heterergic interaction is provided by the work of Williams (1979), who examined the effects of PGE_2 on bradykinin-induced plasma exudation in rabbit skin. Bradykinin alone produced substantial exudation, but PGE_2 in ten times the maximum dose tested in combinations had a negligible effect, so it will be assumed

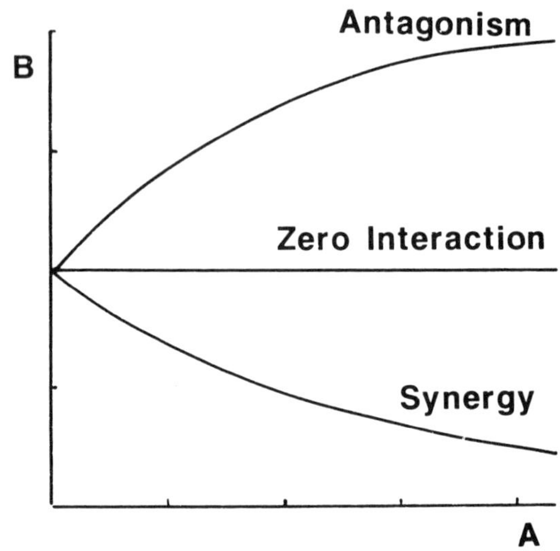

Fig. 13 Isoboles showing heterergic interactions. The specified effect is produced by B only. If A has no influence on the effect of B (zero interaction), the isobole runs parallel to the A axis. If A increases the effect of B, the dose of B required to produce the specified effect is reduced. The isobole is deflected towards the A axis, although it does not reach it, so it is concave-up, indicating synergy. If A reduces the effect of B, more B is needed to produce the effect, so the isobole is deflected away from the A axis.

that this combination of agents was heterergic in causing plasma exudation. (The possibility that very high doses of PGE_2 might cause significant exudation simply because of non-specific local toxicity cannot be excluded). Fig. 14 shows that the isobole for 90 μl exudate volume must pass between the points indicating 125 μl and 0 μl volume, and for 50 μl must pass between those indicating 90 μl and 0 μl and 125 μl and 0μl, so both must be deflected towards the PGE_2 axis, indicating synergy.

4 Isoboles may be inconsistent or dissimilar

While an isobole may be consistent in the sense that all combinations with the effect indicated by the isobole are synergistic, zero-interactive or antagonistic, this is not necessarily the case. Isoboles may cross the zero-interaction line so that some combinations with the specified effect are synergistic, some antagonistic and one (or more) zero-interactive (Fig. 4). Moreover, isoboles for different levels or types of effect produced by the same set of agents are not necessarily of similar shapes; some

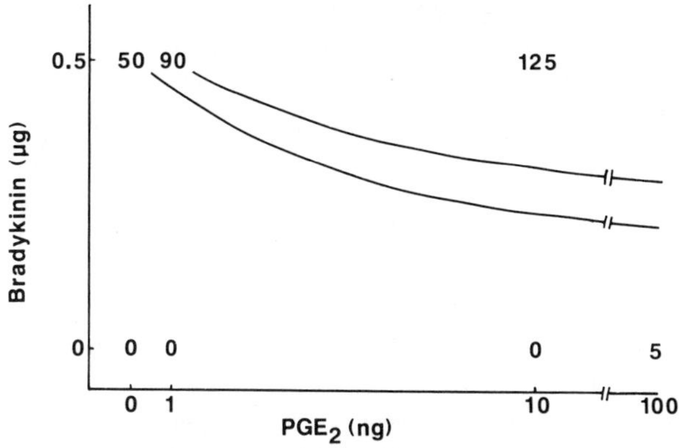

Fig. 14 Production by bradykinin and PGE_2 of plasma exudation in rabbit skin (Williams, 1979, Fig. 2). Results are volumes of plasma exudate after intradermal injection of agents. PGE_2 alone has a negligible effect, but it increases the effect of bradykinin. Isoboles for 50 and 90 μl exudate are deflected towards the PGE_2 dose-axis, but do not meet it, even at a dose of 100 μg, so the combination may be assumed to be heterergic. The isoboles are concave-up, indicating synergy.

combinations may show synergy and others antagonism (Chen and Ensor, 1953; Gessner and Cabana, 1970; Loewe, 1955a,b; Wallin *et al.*, 1970). It is evident that the classification of a particular combination of agents as synergistic, zero-interactive or antagonistic refers to that particular combination, and this does not imply anything about other combinations of the same agents.

5 *Pharmacokinetics and drug interactions*

The *in vivo* effect of a drug combination may be greatly influenced by pharmacokinetic factors (Berenbaum, 1987), as shown in Fig. 15. Suppose drugs A and B, after administration of 10 mg kg^{-1} of each, have levels at the site of action as shown in Fig. 15(a), and the isobole for some desired therapeutic effect (or some undesired toxic effect) is either synergistic or antagonistic as shown in Fig. 15(b). The joint levels of the two drugs at the site of action are shown by the arrowed path in Fig. 15(b). When the agents are synergistic, levels producing the effect under consideration will be present at the site of action for several hours after administration. On the other hand, if the isobole for the effect shows antagonism effective levels will not be reached at any time. Thus, pharmacokinetic factors may amplify drug interactions.

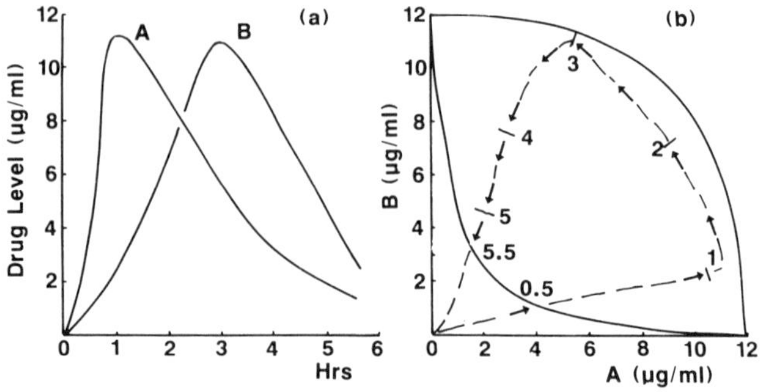

Fig. 15 Pharmacokinetic factors may interact with isobole shape to modify therapeutic (or other) effects. (a) Changes with time after administration in levels of drugs A and B at the site of action.

(b) The arrowed path, constructed with data from (a), shows how the joint levels of A and B at the site of action change with time after administration. Two possible isoboles describing the pharmacological interaction between A and B to produce some specified effect are shown. If the concave-up (synergistic) isobole pertains, drug levels at or above those required to produce the effect are present from 0.5–5.5 hours after administration. If the concave-down, antagonistic isobole prevails, the required levels are not reached at any time.

There are related therapeutic implications in inconsistency of isoboles, for this means that the effect of a combination may be affected by pharmacokinetic factors. When an isobole consistently shows either synergy or antagonism throughout its course, then this type of interaction will be produced consistently *in vivo* irrespective of changing ratios of drug levels brought about by pharmacological factors. Inconsistency of isoboles means that, for some period after drug administration, synergy may be replaced by antagonism and vice versa. Clearly, in searching for drug combinations that show synergy in producing their therapeutic effect, it would be preferable to use sets of agents that generate consistent rather than inconsistent isoboles. An efficient procedure for searching for sets of agents that generate consistently synergistic isoboles has been outlined (Berenbaum *et al.*, 1983).

C The zero interaction equation and the interaction index

The equation for the straight line isobole in Fig. 2 is

$$\frac{d_a}{D_a} + \frac{d_b}{D_b} = 1 \qquad (2)$$

where d_a and d_b are the doses of agents A and B in the combination and D_a and D_b are the doses of A and B that on their own have the same effect as the combination.

When synergy is present, smaller doses than expected are required in the combination to produce the observed effect, although the doses of the agents that on their own produce the effect are unchanged, so d_a and d_b are reduced while D_a and D_b are unaltered, giving

$$\frac{d_a}{D_a} + \frac{d_b}{D_b} < 1 \tag{3}$$

On the other hand, when antagonism is present, d_a and d_b are higher than expected (D_a and D_b being unchanged), so

$$\frac{d_a}{D_a} + \frac{d_b}{D_b} > 1 \tag{4}$$

(The two latter expressions are inequalities, not equations, but this term will be used here for convenience.)

Equations (2)–(4) are readily generalized to combinations of any number of agents (Berenbaum, 1977, 1981, 1985, 1989) and become

$$\sum_{i=1}^{n} \frac{d_i}{D_i} \begin{cases} < 1 \quad \text{(synergy)} & (5) \\ = 1 \quad \text{(zero interaction)} & (6) \\ > 1 \quad \text{(antagonism)} & (7) \end{cases}$$

For $n = 3$, the zero interaction isobole is a flat plane in three dimensions, and synergy and antagonism are shown by concave-up and concave-down surfaces (Berenbaum, 1977, 1978, 1981; Yu *et al.*, 1980; Crane and Milne, 1985).

The summation series in equations (5)–(7) is an interaction index, which specifies the nature of the interaction (whether synergistic, zero-interactive or antagonistic) and quantifies it.

The interaction index for a combination may be readily calculated when the doses of the agents that on their own produce the effect of the combination have been determined, either by titration to a specified end-point, as in the work of Olsson (1972) and Fuller *et al.* (1986) cited above, or by reference to more or less complete dose-response curves, as in the work of Undem and Adams (1988).

For example, Olsson (1972) found that the LD50 of theophylline for mice was 500 mg kg^{-1} and that of (−)-noradrenaline was 28 mg kg^{-1}. A combination of 100 mg kg^{-1} theophylline and 121 mg kg^{-1} (−)-noradrenaline had the same effect, so the appropriate equation is $121/28 + 100/500 = 4.52$, indicating marked antagonism (see Fig. 8).

In the experiments of Fuller *et al.* (1986), a combination of 0.2 PD35 of PGD_2 and 0.4 PD35 of histamine had the same effect as a PD35 of either agent alone, so the equation is simply $0.2 + 0.4 = 0.6$, which indicates synergy (Fig. 10).

In the experiments of Undem and Adams (1988), the three combinations analysed in Table 1 produced respectively 42%, 50% and 60% maximum contraction. The dose–response curves in Fig. 9a show that these effects would have been produced by 2.2, 5 and 13 × 10^{-8} M LTE_4 respectively and by 11.5, 18 and 30 × 10^{-7} M histamine. Thus the appropriate

Table 1

Expected effect (% maximum)	D_L (10^{-8} M)	D_H (10^{-7} M)	Sum (equation 2) d_L (10^{-8} M) = 1 d_H (10^{-7} M) = 1	 1 3	 1 10	Observed effect (% maximum)
33	0.95	6.8	1.20			
34	1.05	7.2	1.09			
35	1.15	7.5	1.00			42
36	1.25	8.0	0.93	1.18		
37	1.40	8.5	0.83	1.07		
38	1.50	9.0		1.00		50
39	1.70	9.5		0.90		
40	1.80	10.0				
.	.	.				
44	2.75	12.5			1.16	
45	2.90	13.0			1.11	
46	3.10	14.0			1.04	
46.5	3.20	14.5			1.00	60
47	3.40	15.0			0.96	
48	3.90	16.0			0.88	

Calculation of the expected effect of combinations of LTE_4 (L) and histamine (H) on contraction of guinea pig tracheal segments (experiments of Undem and Adams, 1988—see text). D_L and D_H are respectively the concentrations of LTE_4 and histamine that have the effects shown in column 1. The combinations consist of 1 × 10^{-8} M LTE_4 (d_L) and 1, 3 or 10 × 10^{-7} M histamine (d_H). The sum in equation 2 is given by $d_L/D_L + d_H/D_H$, and zero interaction is indicated by a sum of 1.00. The observed effects of the combinations (column 7) are to be compared with the effects expected if there were zero interaction (column 1). The observed effects of all three combinations exceeded expectation, showing that they were synergistic.

equations are 1/2.2 + 1/11.5 = 0.54; 1/5 + 3/18 = 0.37; and 1/13 + 10/30 = 0.41, all of which indicate synergy (Fig. 9(b)).

When the doses of the individual agents isoeffective with the combination are not known, but upper or lower limits can be set on them, it is possible to calculate lower or upper limits for the interaction index, which may show that it is necessarily less than or greater than 1, as follows.

For example, in the study by Archer *et al.* (1984) illustrated in Fig. 6, the dose of PGE_2 that produced a wheal volume of 70 μl must have exceeded 1 μg and that of PAF must have exceeded 60 ng. Therefore, the interaction index was necessarily less than 0.5/1 + 30/60, i.e. <1. This shows that the combination was synergistic, although the exact value of the interaction index could not be determined.

In the study by Elwood and Abboud (1982), the low-dose combination contained 50 μg fenoterol and 20 μg ipratropium bromide. For all effects shown in Fig. 7, isoeffective doses were greater than or equal to 200 μg fenoterol and greater than 40 μg ipratropium, so the interaction index was less than 50/200 + 20/40, i.e. <0.75.

Attempts to calculate an interaction index using the results obtained by 2 × 2 or 2 × *n* experimental designs confirm that such designs cannot detect synergy or zero interaction. In Fig. 11, which illustrates the investigation by Campbell *et al.* (1977), the doses in the combination were about 0.17 mg isoprenaline and 250 mg aminophylline. The effect of the combination exceeded those of each of these doses given individually, so the isoeffective doses of the individual agents must have exceeded 0.17 and 250 mg respectively. These lower limits show that the interaction index must have been less than 0.17/0.17 + 250/250, i.e. less than 2, but they set no other bounds on it, so it might have been <1, 1 or >1, and the nature of the interaction remains indeterminate.

However, when antagonism is so marked that a combination (d_a, d_b) is actually less effective than one of its constituents alone, say d_a (see Fig. 8), then d_a exceeds D_a, and so $d_a/D_a > 1$, and the interaction index necessarily exceeds 1.

Calculation of the interaction index for heterergic combinations presents no problems. Consider the combination of 1 ng PGE_2 and 0.5 μg bradykinin shown in Fig. 14 (Williams, 1979). The isoeffective doses of PGE_2 and bradykinin must have exceeded 100 ng and 0.5 μg respectively, so the index was less than 1/100 + 0.5/1, or <0.51, indicating synergy.

When it is certain that an agent (say agent A) does not produce the effect of the combination, no matter how high the dose, its isoeffective dose D_a may notionally be set at infinity, so d_a/D_a can be assumed to be zero. Then, if the effect of the combination is respectively equal to, less than or greater than the effect of d_b alone, it follows that D_b is respectively equal to, less than or greater than d_b and the index must be respectively equal to, less than or greater than 1, indicating zero interaction, synergy or antagonism as the case may be.

V CALCULATION OF THE EXPECTED EFFECT OF A COMBINATION

A The numerical method

Equation (2) enables calculation of the expected effect of a combination, i.e. that expected from the dose–response curves of the agents when no pharmacological interaction is present. The method entails finding D_a and/or D_b, where d_a and d_b are given. As D_a and D_b are isoeffective with the combination if it is zero-interactive, the expected effect of the combination is simply the effect of either of these, and may be obtained directly from their respective dose–response curves.

The only information available about D_a and D_b is (a) they are isoeffective with each other and with the combination and (b) the values of D_a and D_b must satisfy equation (2) with the given values of d_a and d_b.

The procedure is simple and may be demonstrated with the data of Undem and Adams (1988) referred to above for combinations of LTE_4 (L) and histamine (H). Values of D_L and D_H for a range of possible expected effects read off the dose–response curves in Fig. 9(a) are tabulated (Table 1). Then the sum in equation (2) is calculated using these values and the values of d_L and d_H for the combination to determine values of D_L and D_H that satisfy equation (2). The effect of a zero-interactive combination is then the effect of D_L and D_H. For example, for the combination of 1×10^{-8} M LTE_4 and 10×10^{-7} M histamine, the required values are $D_L = 3.2 \times 10^{-8}$ and $D_H = 14.5 \times 10^{-7}$, for $1/3.2 + 10/14.5 = 1.0$. Thus, if the combination had been zero-interactive, its effect would have been that of 3.2×10^{-8} M LTE_4 or of 14.5×10^{-7} M histamine, i.e. 46.5% of maximal contraction. The observed contraction was 60% of maximal, so the combination was synergistic.

Fig. 16 confirms that the expected effects calculated for all three combinations were indeed zero-interactive, because the isoboles are linear, whereas the isoboles for the observed effects shown in Fig. 9(b) are concave-up, indicating synergy.

It should be noted that this procedure requires only quantitative information about the dose–response curves. It does not require any

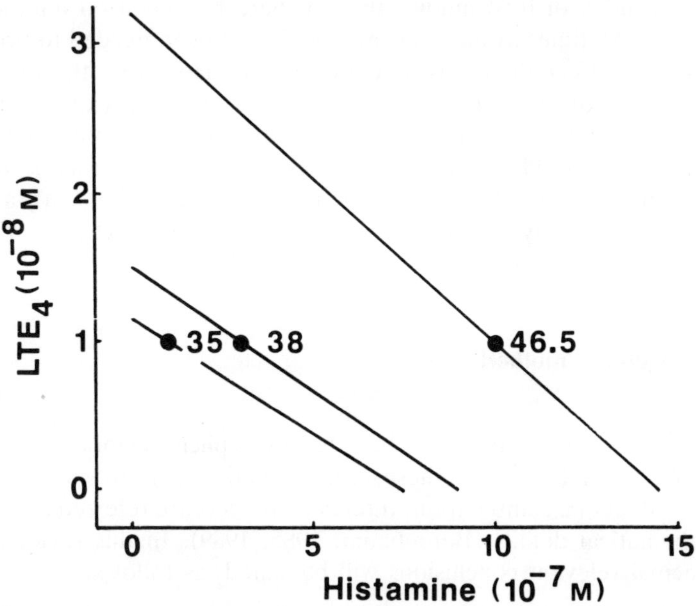

Fig. 16 Isoboles for expected effects calculated using equation (2) are linear. The expected effects of combinations of 1, 3 and 10 × 10^{-7} M histamine and 10^{-8} M LTE_4 on contraction of guinea-pig tracheal segments (Undem and Adams, 1988, Fig. 1A) are calculated in Table 1, which also gives the concentrations, D_H and D_L, of the individual agents that produce these expected effects. The isoboles joining the points representing the combinations with those representing D_H and D_L are straight lines.

account to be taken of the types of the curves, nor of whether they are similar or dissimilar (in fact, Fig. 9(a) shows that they are dissimilar).

Extending this procedure to incorporate combinations of any number of agents is simple. For example, for a combination of four agents, one would use the four-term expansion of equation (2) and find, from the four dose–response curves, the isoeffective doses of the four agents that satisfied the equation. Examples of the procedure for combinations of two, three and four agents are given elsewhere (Berenbaum, 1985, 1988, 1989).

It should be emphasized that, for full quantitation of the interaction shown by a combination, both the interaction index and the expected (zero interaction) effect are required, as they give different sorts of information. For example, for the synergistic combination of 10^{-8} M LTE_4 and 10^{-7} M histamine shown in Figs. 9(a) and 9(b) and in Table 1, the interaction index of 0.54 implies that, if there had been no interaction, $(0.54)^{-1} = 1.85$ times as much agent would have been needed to produce the observed effect than was actually needed. However, the observed effect was 1.2 times, not 1.85 times, greater than the expected (zero interaction) effect. The relationship between the interaction index and the ratio of observed to expected effects depends on the slope of the dose–response curves. When the slope is shallow, as in Fig. 9(a), a large increase in doses may only entail a small increase in effect and, when it is steep, the reverse is true.

B The algebraic method

When dose–response curves can be fitted by explicit algebraic functions, it is often possible to use these, with equation (2), to calculate the expected effect of a combination. Interested readers are referred elsewhere for mathematical details (Berenbaum, 1985, 1989). In this review, only the principal relevant conclusions will be stated, as follows.

1 Sigmoid dose–response curves

Typically, the agents used in treating asthma and the mediators involved in its pathogenesis have dose–response curves that are sigmoid with log dose (or occasionally linear or log-linear with log dose). The most plausible explanation for sigmoid curves is the way in which these agents combine with their receptors is governed by the law of mass action, which generates such curves, and that the "transistor function" (Black and Leff, 1983) representing the complex processes intervening between action on receptors and the end-effects that are measured, does not usually change the curves in fundamental respects.

Sigmoid curves are conveniently described by the median effect equation of Chou and Talalay (1977, 1981, 1984).

$$\left[\frac{E(d)}{1-E(d)}\right]^{1/m} = \frac{d}{M} \qquad (8)$$

where $E(d)$ is the fractional effect of dose d, i.e. effect as a fraction of the maximum, M is the median effective dose, i.e. which produces a 50% effect, and m is a constant, which specifies the order of sigmoidicity of the curve, and is believed to indicate the minimum number of molecular binding sites of the agents. A convenient method for determining m is obtained by rearranging of equation 8 to give

$$\log\left(\frac{E}{1-E}\right) = m(\log d - \log M) \tag{9}$$

which shows that a graph of $\log(E/(1-E))$ against log dose is a straight line of which m is the slope and M the intercept on the dose-axis.

Chou and Talalay (1977, 1981) showed that the effect of a zero-interactive combination (d_a,d_b) of two agents with sigmoid dose–response curves and the same value for m was given by

$$\left[\frac{E\,(d_a,d_b)}{1-E\,(d_a,d_b)}\right]^{1/m} = \left[\frac{E\,(d_a)}{1-E\,(d_a)}\right]^{1/m} + \left[\frac{E\,(d_b)}{1-E\,(d_b)}\right]^{1/m} = \frac{d_a}{M_a} + \frac{d_b}{M_b} \tag{10}$$

and re-arranging this equation gives

$$E(d_a,d_b) = \frac{\left(\dfrac{d_a}{M_a} + \dfrac{d_b}{M_b}\right)^{1/m}}{1 + \left(\dfrac{d_a}{M_a} + \dfrac{d_b}{M_b}\right)^{1/m}} \tag{11}$$

For combinations of zero-interactive agents with sigmoid curves but with unequal sigmoidicities, $m_a \neq m_b$, the effect of a zero-interactive combination may be calculated by first finding the isoeffective dose of one of the agents, say A, from equation (12).

$$D_a\left[1 - \left(\frac{D_a}{M_a}\right)^{-m_a/m_b} \frac{d_b}{M_b}\right] - d_a = 0 \tag{12}$$

D_a is the only unknown in this equation and it can be found by iteration. The effect of the combination is the effect of D_a, found by substituting D_a for d and m_a for m in the equation. An alternative expression has been proposed by Syracuse and Greco (1986), viz:

$$\frac{d_a}{M_a\left(\dfrac{E}{E_{max} - E}\right)^{1/m_a}} + \frac{d_b}{M_b\left(\dfrac{E}{E_{max} - E}\right)^{1/m_b}} = 1 \tag{13}$$

where E is the fractional effect of the combination and E_{max} is the maximum effect obtainable in the system. E is obtained by iteration from equation (13).

Equations (11)–(13) are rather complex and, in many cases, it would be preferable to use the simple numerical method of Table 1 to determine the expected effect of a combination, as this avoids the need to fit explicit particular functions to data that are not always so obliging as to fit a simple equation.

Calculation of the expected effect of a combination when dose–response curves are linear with log dose, or log-linear with log dose is described elsewhere (Berenbaum, 1989).

2 *Linear dose–response curves*

Only with a linear dose–response curve will the effect of a sham "combination" of one and the same agent be the sum of the effects of the individual doses and, by the same token, it is only with such curves that the effect of a zero-interactive combination is, generally, the sum of the effects of its constituents (Berenbaum, 1985). This is easily demonstrated.

With a linear dose–response curve, the effect of a drug is proportional to dose, i.e. effect of $d_a = k_a d_a$ and effect of $d_b = k_b d_b$, where k_a and k_b are constants (they are the slopes of the dose–response curves).

As D_a and D_b are isoeffective, $k_a D_a = k_b D_b$ so,

$$D_b = \frac{k_a}{k_b} D_a$$

Substitution of this into equation (2) for zero interaction and a little re-arranging gives

$$D_a = d_a + \frac{k_b}{k_a} d_b$$

The effect of the combination is

$$k_a D_a = k_a \left(d_a + \frac{k_b}{k_a} d_b \right) = k_a d_a + k_b d_b$$

i.e., the effect of a zero-interactive combination of agents with linear dose–response curves is the sum of the effects of its constituents. Therefore, use of the summative criterion and analysis of variance are correct for combinations of agents that have linear dose–response curves.

However, linear dose–response curves are not at all typical of the agents used in treating asthma or of the mediators involved. The great majority of dose–response curves for these agents are sigmoid. Such curves approximate to linearity only in the low dose–low effect range, for here all curves become statistically indistinguishable from straight lines (Crump *et al.*, 1976; Guess and Crump, 1978; Guess *et al.*, 1977; Peto, 1978). Take, for example, equation (8) with $m = 1$ and $M = 100$. Here, effect is linear with dose with an error of less than 1% over the dose range 0–0.7 (and fractional effect range 0–0.07), and diverges significantly from linearity only at higher levels. However, such minute effects would rarely be of interest, and linear dose–response curves are, therefore, largely irrelevant to the subject of this review, and the use of the summative criterion for zero interaction (and of analysis of variance) in the asthma literature is incorrect and leads to false conclusions. This usage should be abandoned.

VI THERAPEUTIC SYNERGY

The foregoing has been concerned with interactions between agents in regard to single effects. However, at the level of the whole cell or individual all agents have multiple effects. Some of these are adverse and limit treatment and, therefore, the phenomena produced by such multiple effects require consideration and analysis.

The problem may be introduced by two concrete examples.

(1) Wolfe *et al.* (1978) gave various doses of aminophylline or terbutaline or combinations of these to stable asthmatic patients and measured the effects over a period of 7 hours. Peak increases (%) in FEV_1 and the incidence of adverse effects are shown in Fig. 17. The isobole for the

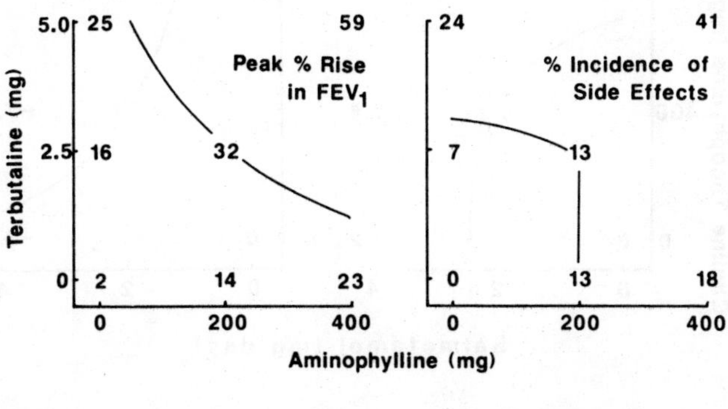

Fig. 17 Generation of therapeutic synergy in asthmatic patients with a combination of aminophylline and terbutaline (Wolfe *et al.*, 1978, Fig. 1 and Table 3).

effect of the combination of 200 mg aminophylline and 2.5 mg terbutaline on FEV_1 is concave-up, indicating synergy, whereas that for production of adverse effects is concave-down, indicating antagonism. Now, suppose it is decided that the maximum tolerable toxicity is the occurrence of adverse effects in 13% of patients. With aminophylline alone, this is produced at a dose of 200 mg, where peak improvement in FEV_1 is 14%. With terbutaline alone, this level of toxicity is produced at a dose of about 3 mg (found by interpolation on a logarithmic scale), where the increase in FEV_1 would be about 18% (by interpolation). Thus, the best that can be achieved with either drug alone, within the specified constraint on adverse effects, is an 18% increase in FEV_1 with terbutaline. However, the combination of 200 mg aminophylline and 2.5 mg terbutaline also reaches this limiting toxicity, but produces a 32% increase in FEV_1. Thus, a combination of both agents allows a better therapeutic result to be obtained than use of either drug on its own.

(2) The reverse state of affairs may be illustrated by the study of Dyson and Campbell (1977), who gave each of their patients choline theophylline, salmefamol and placebo, alone or in combination, and assessed the therapeutic effect by mean rise (%) in peak flow (PF) and toxicity by a tremor index (the greater the tremor, the lower the index). Results are shown in Fig. 18. Here, the isobole for the effect of the combination of

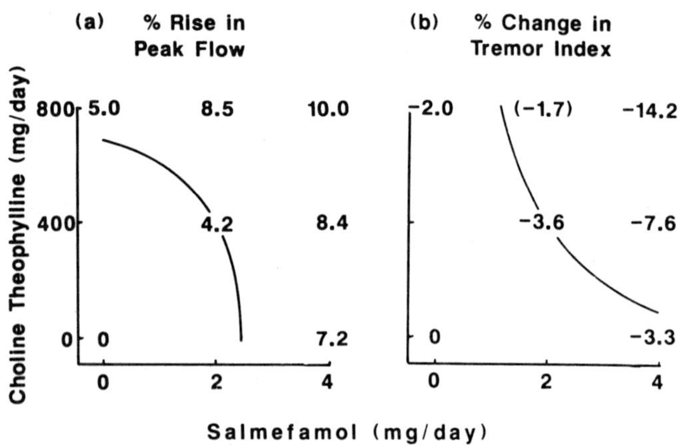

Fig. 18 Effects of combinations of salmefamol and choline theophylline on (a) peak expiratory flow, (b) Tremor index—the greater the tremor, the lower the index (Dyson and Campbell, 1977, Tables 2 and 4).

2 mg per day salmefamol and 400 mg per day theophylline in PF shows antagonism, while the isobole for the effect on tremor shows synergy.

Now suppose a maximum acceptable toxicity is a change in tremor index of −3.6%. With salmefamol alone, this is produced at some dosage greater than 4 mg per day, at which dosage the rise in PF is over 7.2%. With theophylline alone, this level of tremor is produced at a dose greater than 800 mg per day, when the increase in PF is over 5%. Thus, within this toxicity limit, a PF of over 7.2% can be obtained with salmefamol alone. The combination of 2 mg per day salmefamol with 400 mg per day theophylline also produces the specified level of tremor, but the increase in PF with this is only 4.2%. Thus, in this case it appears preferable to use a single drug rather than a combination of the two.

These points may be examined more systematically if a comprehensive set of isoboles is drawn which, at present, may be done only for hypothetical cases. Suppose combinations of A and B are synergistic with regard to some desired therapeutic effect, such as bronchodilatation, with concave-up isoboles for various levels of this effect (Fig. 19) and that they are antagonistic with regard to some toxic effect, such as tachycardia,

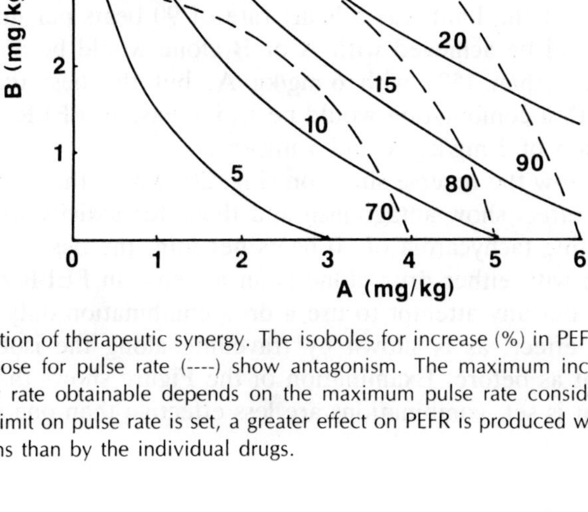

Fig. 19 Generation of therapeutic synergy. The isoboles for increase (%) in PEFR (——) show synergy and those for pulse rate (----) show antagonism. The maximum increase in peak expiratory flow rate obtainable depends on the maximum pulse rate considered tolerable but, whatever limit on pulse rate is set, a greater effect on PEFR is produced within this limit by combinations than by the individual drugs.

indicated by the concave-down isoboles for various levels of this effect. Attempts to improve the therapeutic effect by increasing the dose of A or B alone are constrained by toxicity, and the maximum bronchodilator effect obtained depends on what level of tachycardia is considered acceptable, i.e. on what constraint is set on this effect.

When interactions for therapeutic and toxic effects have the relation to each other as shown in this Figure, it may be possible with combinations to achieve a therapeutic effect that is not achievable with either agent alone. For example, if the maximum acceptable heart rate is set at 80 beats per min then, with A alone, this limit is reached at a dose of 5 mg/kg, which produces an increase in peak expiratory flow rate (PEFR) of 10%. For drug B, this limiting heart rate is reached at 4 mg/kg, which gives a 5% increase in PEFR. Thus, the best result that can be obtained with either drug alone within this toxicity limit is an increase in PEFR of 10% with 5 mg/kg A. However, if in Fig. 19 we start at the optimum dose for A and travel along the isobole representing the toxicity limit (thus keeping toxicity constant), we find that the combinations along the isobole produce an increased therapeutic effect until a maximum is reached with the combination of 3 mg/kg A and 3 mg/kg B, which increases PEFR by 20%. Travelling further along the isobole now locates combinations with decreasing therapeutic effect until we arrive at the optimum dose of B alone, where the increase in PEFR is 5%. Thus, although the best that can be achieved with one agent alone within the toxicity limit is an increase in PEFR of 10%, the greatest increase that can be achieved by a combination within this limit is 20%. Of course, this degree of bronchodilatation might be achievable by A or B alone, but only at the cost of exceeding the specified toxicity limit.

Similar considerations would apply if a different toxicity limit were set. For instance, if the limit was a heart rate of 90 beats per min, then the best that could be achieved with A or B alone would be an increase in PEFR of less than 15% with 6 mg/kg A, but the best that could be achieved with a combination would be an increase in PEFR of 25% with a combination of 3 mg/kg A and 4 mg/kg B.

Consider now the reverse situation (Fig. 20) where the isoboles for the therapeutic effect show antagonism and those for toxicity show synergy. With a limiting tachycardia of 80 beats per min, the best effect that can be obtained with either drug alone is an increase in PEFR of 25% with 5 mg/kg A, but any attempt to use a drug combination only reduces the therapeutic effect, as is shown by travelling along the isobole for the toxicity limit as before. Examination of the Figure shows that, whatever toxicity limit is set, combinations are less effective than one of the drugs on its own.

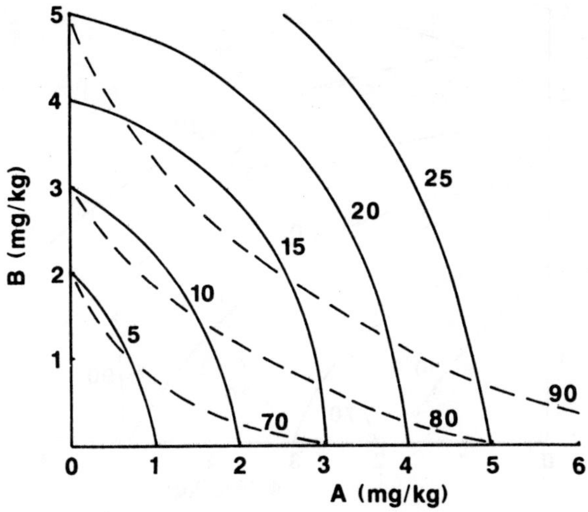

Fig. 20 When isoboles for the therapeutic effect (——) show antagonism and those for toxicity (----) show synergy, the greatest therapeutic effect achievable within a specified toxicity limit is produced by a single drug, and combinations are disadvantageous.

One last example is shown in Fig. 21, where the isoboles for both therapeutic and toxic effects show antagonism, but this is more marked for the latter. Here, the best that can be achieved with one drug alone, within a tachycardia constraint of 80 beats per min, is an increase in PEFR of 20%, at 3 mg/kg of B. Again, combinations are advantageous. For instance, a combination of 3 mg/kg A and 4 mg/kg B, which produces the same toxicity, increases PEFR by 30%.

In Figs. 19–21, for simplicity, only one toxicity constraint was set but, in practice, constraints might have to be specified for a number of different adverse effects, and this raises no special difficulties.

Therapeutic synergy, as Fig. 21 shows, can be present even when no individual effect shows synergy; in fact, it may be present when no individual effect shows any pharmacological interaction (Berenbaum, 1981, Fig. 30). This form of therapeutic synergy is a phenomenon arising out of the differences in the types and degrees of interaction for the desired and undesired effects, i.e. the differences in the shapes of the isoboles for these effects. If these differences did not exist, no therapeutic gain or loss would be obtained by using combinations rather than single agents. Given the complexity of biological phenomena and the varying susceptibility to different agents shown by different tissues and cell types, such differences are almost certain to be present for any set of agents.

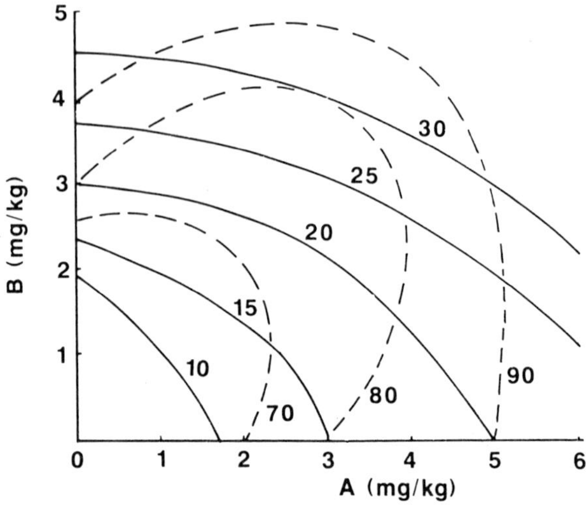

Fig. 21 Therapeutic synergy may be generated even when no individual effect shows synergy. Here, both effects on PEFR (——) and on pulse rate (----) show antagonism. Whatever limit on pulse rate is considered acceptable, combinations produce a greater effect on PEFR within this limit than the single drugs.

Thus, we can virtually be assured that, for any set of drugs, there will be an optimum "combination" (which may sometimes be one of the drugs on its own), and the search for such optima is a prime task of therapeutics.

It should be pointed out that toxicity is not the only constraint on therapy. In the management of asthma, as in other conditions where self-administration plays an important part of treatment and patient non-compliance a major limitation of effective treatment (Billing *et al.*, 1982; Eney and Goldstein, 1976), complexity of treatment may itself be a powerful constraint. Thus, constraints might well be set on the number of puffs with an inhaler and/or on the intervals between self-administration of different drugs.

VII THERAPEUTIC OPTIMIZATION

A The problem of multivariate regimens

As the foregoing discussion of therapeutic synergy shows, the problem of finding the best possible regimen with a given set of drugs is essentially a problem in optimization under constraints, i.e. one of finding the combination of all the relevant variables (drug dose, dose intervals, dose frequency, etc.) that produces the maximum therapeutic effect without transgressing one or more specified limits (e.g. heart rate, tremor, measures of treatment complexity, etc.). The problem is generally approached by way of formal clinical trials in which two (or more) different regimens are compared for therapeutic effect and toxicity. If one regimen has a significantly better therapeutic effect than the other(s) and is not more toxic, then it is clearly to be preferred. Unfortunately, regimens that are more effective therapeutically are often also more toxic (Baardsgaard *et al.*, 1985; Billing *et al.*, 1982; Campbell *et al.*, 1977; Shapiro *et al.*, 1981; Sims *et al.*, 1978; Svedmyr and Svedmyr, 1982; Weinberger and Bronsky, 1974; Weinberger *et al.*, 1975; Wolfe *et al.*, 1978), so the matter is not resolved by taking only the therapeutic effect into account, but also by deciding whether the benefit of increased therapeutic effect outweighs the cost in extra toxicity. However, an even greater problem arises once such a decision is made, for the multivariate nature of most therapeutic regimens makes it difficult to decide on the next step.

Combination therapy in asthma typically comprises two or three drugs, each of which may vary in dose, number of doses, intervals between doses and so on. For example, one of the regimens used by Rossing *et al.* (1981) for treating acute asthmatic episodes comprised ephedrine given subcutaneously every 20 minutes for three doses, an intravenous loading dose of aminophylline and then an aminophylline intravenous infusion. Thus, there were five independent variables in this regimen (dose, frequency and number of doses of ephedrine, dose of aminophylline load and dose-rate of aminophylline infusion). Again, Weinberger *et al.* (1975) gave varying doses of theophylline, ephedrine and hydroxyzine, each 6-hourly for a week. Thus, with a fixed duration of treatment, there were 9 independent variables in this study and, if duration of treatment with each drug had also been varied, there would have been 27 variables.

A typical regimen in asthma may involve many variables, each of which may materially influence the therapeutic outcome. Thus if, in a formal clinical trial comparing two such regimens (i.e. two particular arrangements of these variables), it was found that one regimen was therapeutically superior to the other, the question would arise as to how these possibly numerous variables should be altered so as to achieve a still better result.

It is sometimes supposed that the problem might be tackled by finding the optimum level of each variable in turn, in the expectation that the best therapeutic effect will be produced by a combination of each at its optimum level. However, this approach is ruled out when optimum drug levels are determined by toxicity constraints. In Fig. 20, for example, the optimum level of A within the specified constraint is 5 mg/kg, thus, if this dosage is kept fixed and any dose of B added then a toxicity above the specified limit is produced. The same problem would arise if the optimum level of B alone were first found and attempts made to add A to this.

Two approaches may be used to find the optimum combination of several variables. These are response surface methods and direct search methods.

B Response surface methods

Here, a predetermined number of different combinations of predetermined composition is examined, distributed over what are believed to be the appropriate ranges of the variables. The observed therapeutic effects of the combinations are then fitted by an algebraic function (most often a second-order polynomial) and the same exercise is performed for the toxic effects. Standard mathematical methods then enable us to calculate what combination of the variables will give the maximum of the therapeutic effect function, keeping within the bounds imposed by the toxicity constraints.

There is no requirement that the differences between the effects of the different combinations be statistically significant, as it is the overall shape of the response surface that is of interest, and, accordingly, only a few individuals may be needed to test each combination. Wampler *et al.* (1987) used groups of two only in a cancer chemotherapy experiment. Response surface methods have been used extensively, especially in exploring combinations of cancer chemotherapeutic agents and in toxicology (Carter, 1985; Carter and Wampler, 1986; Carter *et al.*, 1983; Myers, 1971; Wampler *et al.*, 1987). However, these methods have a serious drawback which is that the number of combinations that must be tested to fit a second-order surface rises more or less exponentially with the number of variables. One highly economical experimental design (Box and Wilson, 1951) requires testing $2^n + 2n + 1$ combinations for n variables, so that a regimen of 6 variables would entail testing 77 combinations, one of 9 variables would require 531, and so on. Such numbers are not feasible in a clinical context and, in practice, response surface methods have so far been limited to experiments with only 2 or 3 variables.

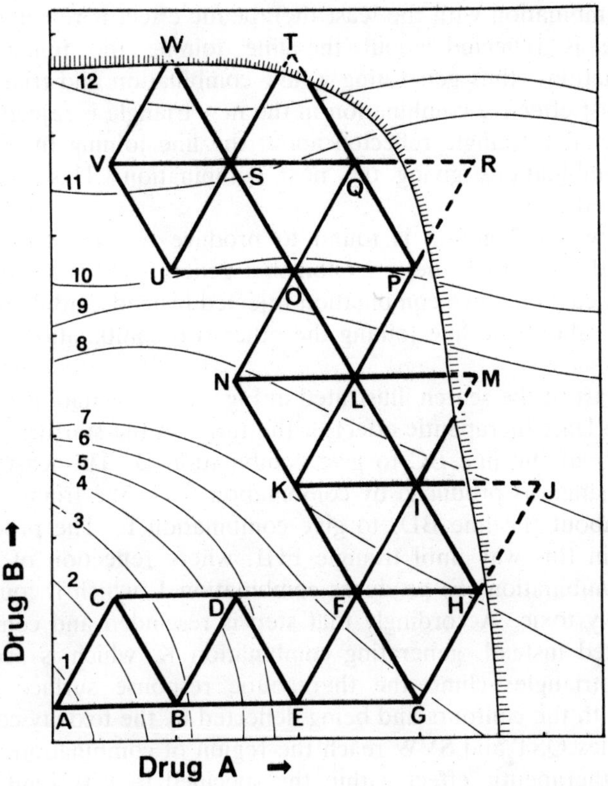

Fig. 22 Direct search of a therapeutic response surface, subject to a toxicity constraint. Isoboles for the therapeutic effect are indicated by (——) and the constraint by (ɯɯɯɯ). The search procedure is that of Spendley *et al.* (1962).

C Direct search methods

The alternative to a predetermined coverage of the response surface is a step-by-step search. Illustrated in Fig. 22 is a problem in finding the optimum combination of two drugs, only the dose being varied (Spendley *et al.*, 1962). Initially, the investigator is unaware of the shape of the surface. The search is initiated by measuring the effects of three combinations (represented by the vertices of triangle ABC). The rules of the search are as follows:

(1) The combination with the least therapeutic effect is rejected and the triangle is reflected about the line joining the remaining two combinations, thus generating a new combination and triangle.
(2) The least effective combination in the new triangle is rejected in turn and the new triangle reflected about the line joining the remaining two combinations giving the next combination. This sequence is continued.
(3) If a new combination is found to produce toxicity exceeding the specified limit, then the reflection that generated it is rescinded, the second least-effective combination rejected instead, and the reflection is made about the line joining the other two combinations.

At the start of the search illustrated in Fig. 22, combination A is found to have the least therapeutic effect of the three so the starting triangle is reflected about the line BC to give combination D. The least effect in this new triangle is produced by combination C, so the triangle is again reflected, about the line BD, to give combination E. The procedure is continued in this way until triangle FHI, where reflection of the least effective combination (F) produces combination J, which is found to be unacceptably toxic. Accordingly that step is rescinded and combination H is rejected instead, generating combination K, which is acceptable. Thus, the triangles climb the therapeutic response surface changing direction with the contours and being deflected by the toxicity constraint, until triangles QST and SVW reach the region of combinations with the maximum therapeutic effect within the specified toxicity limit. At this point, with the rules specified above, the search ends because reflection from the final triangle (SVW) recreates a combination (T) already tested. However, if the size of the triangles is reduced, the search could be made to continue if desired so as to approach the optimum more closely.

This method is readily generalized for combinations of any number of variables but it has drawbacks, mainly that it is relatively inflexible in the direction and size of moves and so it often comes to a premature halt before the optimum has been reached. Accordingly, the method has been modified to make the moves more adaptable to the surface and to toxicity constraints (Nelder and Mead, 1964; Box, 1965; Berenbaum, 1989).

Direct search methods are economical as only one combination is examined at a time. As with response surface methods, there is no need for the differences in the effects of successive combinations to be statistically significant, so small numbers of individuals may be used to test each combination, and it appears (surprisingly) that performance may improve as the number of variables increases (Spendley *et al.*, 1962).

Direct search methods are also highly flexible because, as they are made one step at a time, the procedure may be changed at any stage without sacrificing the information gained up to that point, so a new variable (such as an additional drug) may be added after the search is under way. Such adaptability would be important in a clinical setting, where pressure may arise to change the terms of a trial after it has begun.

Direct search methods may be particularly worth investigating in the treatment of asthma, where it is possible (and indeed customary in many trials) to investigate the effects of different combinations in rapid succession in the same patient. This would raise the possibility of individually optimized regimens.

ACKNOWLEDGEMENTS

I am indebted to the Cancer Research Campaign for support.

REFERENCES

Advenier, C., Naline, E, Matran, R., Toty, L. and Bakdach, H. (1988). Interaction between fenoterol, ipratropium, and acetylcholine on human isolated bronchus. *J. Allergy Clin. Immunol.* **82,** 40–46.

Anderson, G., Jariwalla, A.G., Turnbull, P. and Veale, J. (1981). The effects of fenoterol, ipratropium bromide and their combination in asthma and chronic bronchitis. *ICRS Medical Sci.* **9,** 251.

Archer, C.B., Frohlich, W., Page, C.P., Paul, W., Morley, J. and McDonald, D.M. (1984). Synergistic interactions between prostaglandins and PAF-acether in experimental animals and man. *Prostaglandins* **27,** 495–501.

Archer, C.B., Page, C.P., Juhlin, L., Morley, J. and MacDonald, D.M. (1987). Delayed-onset synergism between leukotriene B4 and prostaglandin E2 in human skin. *Prostaglandins* **73,** 799–805.

Ardlie, N.G., Bell, L.K. and McGuiness, J.A. (1987). Synergistic potentiation by epinephrine of collagen or thrombin-induced calcium mobilization in human platelets. *Thromb. Res.* **46,** 519–526.

Baardsgaard, O., Oberg, B., Thomsen, L., Kitgaard, N. and Simonsen, E. (1985). Bronchodilator effects of terbutaline and theophylline alone and in combination in patients with chronic obstructive lung disease. *Allergol. et Immunopathol.* **13,** 471–474.

Bachelet, M., Adolfs, M.J.P., Masliah, J., Bereziet, G., Vargaftig, B.B. and Bonta, I.L. (1988). Interaction between PAF-acether and drugs that stimulate cyclic AMP in guinea-pig alveolar macrophages. *Eur. J. Pharmacol.* **149,** 73–78.

Baraban, J.M., Gould, R.J., Peroutka, S.J. and Snyder, S.H. (1985). Phorbol ester effects on neurotransmission: interaction with neurotransmitters and calcium in smooth muscle. *Proc. Natl. Acad. Sci.* **82,** 604–607.

Barnes, N.C., Watson, A., Koulouris, N., Piper, P.J. and Costello, J. (1984). Effect of preinhalation of leukotriene D4 on sensitivity to inhaled prostaglandin F2α. *Thorax* **39,** 697.

Barnes, P.J., Chung, K.F. and Page, C.P. (1988). Inflammatory mediators and asthma. *Pharmacol. Rev.* **40,** 49–84.

Basran, G.S., Morley, J., Paul, W. and Turner-Warwick, M. (1982). Evidence in man for synergistic interactions between putative mediators of acute inflammation and asthma. *Lancet* **1,** 935–937.

Beck, R., Robertson, C.F., Galdes-Sebalt, M. and Levinson, H. (1985). Combined salbutamol and ipratropium bromide by inhalation in the treatment of severe acute asthma. *J. Pediatrics* **107,** 605–608.

Berenbaum, M.C. (1977). Synergy, additivism and antagonism in immunosuppression. A critical review. *Clin. Exp. Immunol.* **28,** 1–18.

Berenbaum, M.C. (1978). A method for testing for synergy with any number of agents. *J. Infect. Dis.* **137,** 122–130.

Berenbaum, M.C. (1981). Criteria for analysing interactions between biologically active agents. *Adv. Cancer Res.* **35,** 269–335.

Berenbaum, M.C. (1985). The expected effect of a combination of agents: the general solution. *J. Theor. Biol.* **114,** 413–431.

Berenbaum, M.C. (1987). Minor synergy and antagonism may be clinically important. *J. Antimicrob. Chemother.* **19,** 271–273.

Berenbaum, M.C. (1988). Isobolographic, algebraic and search methods in the analysis of multi-agent synergy. *J. Am. Coll. Toxicol.* **7,** 17–28.

Berenbaum, M.C. (1989). What is synergy? *Pharmacol. Rev.* (in press).

Berenbaum, M.C., Cope, W.A., and Bundick, R.V. (1976). Synergistic effect of cortisol and prostaglandin E_2 on the PHA response. Relation to immunosuppression induced by trauma. *Clin. Exp. Immunol.* **26,** 534–541.

Berenbaum, M.C., Yu, V.L. and Felegie, T.P. (1983). Synergy with double and triple antibiotic combinations compared. *J. Antimicrob. Chemother.* **12,** 555–563.

Bertelli, A., Bianchi, C. and Beani, L. (1973). Interaction between β-adrenergic stimulant and phosphodiesterase inhibiting drugs on the bronchial muscle. *Experientia* **29,** 300–302.

Bich-Thuy, L.T. and Fauci, A.S. (1986). Recombinant interleukin 2 and gamma-interferon act synergistically on distinct steps of *in vitro* terminal B cell maturation. *J. Clin. Invest.* **77,** 1173–1179.

Billing, B., Dahlqvist, R., Garle, M., Hornblad, Y. and Ripe, E. (1982). Separate and combined use of terbutaline and theophylline in asthmatics. *Eur. J. Resp. Dis.* **63,** 399–409.

Black, J.W. and Leff, P. (1983). Operational models of pharmacological agonism. *Proc. Roy. Soc. B.* **220,** 141–162.

Blumenthal, I. (1980). A comparative trial of slow-release aminophylline, salbutamol and a half-dose combination in the prevention of childhood asthma. *Int. J. Med. Res.* **8,** 400–403.

Bongrani, S., Schiantarelli, P., Papatti, M. and Folco, G.C. (1981). Evidence of overadditive interaction between fenoterol and ipratropium bromide in the counteraction of cholinomimetic-induced tracheobronchial contractions. *Arzneimittelforschung* **31,** 970–973.

Box, G.E.P. and Wilson, K.W. (1951). On the experimental attainment of optimum conditions. *J. Roy. Stat. Soc. Series B* **13,** 1–45.

Box, M.J. (1965). A new method for constrained optimization and a comparison with other methods. *Computer J.* **8,** 42–52.

Britton, J.R., Burney, P.G.J., Chinn, S., Papacosta, A.O. and Tattersfield, A.E. (1988). The relation between change in airway reactivity and change in respiratory symptoms and medication in a community study. *Am. Rev. Resp. Dis.* **138,** 530–534.

Brooks, S.M., Werk, E.E., Ackerman, S.J., Sullivan, I. and Thrasher, K. (1972). Adverse effects of phenobarbital on corticosteroid metabolism in patients with bronchial asthma. *New Eng. J. Med.* **286,** 1125–1128.

Bruderman, I., Cohen-Aronovski, R. and Smorzik, J. (1983). A comparative study of various combinations of ipratropium bromide and metaproterenol in allergic asthmatic patients. *Chest* **83,** 208–210.

Bryant, D.H. (1985). Nebulized ipratropium bromide in the treatment of acute asthma. *Chest* **88,** 24–29.

Campbell, I.A. (1979). The additive and/or synergistic effects of combined sympathomimetic and methylxanthine therapy. *Current Med. Res. Opinion* **6,** Supp. 6, 85–91.

Campbell, I.A., Middleton, W.G., McHardy, G.J.R., Shotter, M.V., McKenzie, R. and Kay, A.B. (1977). Interaction between isoprenaline and aminophylline in asthma. *Thorax* **32,** 424–428.

Carter, W.H. Jr. (1985). Response surface methodology and the design of clinical trials for the evaluation of cancer chemotherapy. *Cancer Treat. Rep.* **69,** 1049–1051.

Carter, W.H. Jr. and Wampler, G.L. (1986). Review of the application of response surface methodology in the combination therapy of cancer. *Cancer Treat. Rep.* **70,** 133–140.

Carter, W.H. Jr., Wampler, G.L., Crews, S.L. and Howells, R. (1977). On determining the levels of treatment to optimize the probability of a favorable response. *Cancer Treat. Rep.* **61,** 849–853.

Carter, W.H. Jr., Wampler, G.L., Stablein, D.M. and Campbell, E.D. (1982). Drug activity and therapeutic synergism in cancer treatment. *Cancer Res.* **42,** 2963–2971.

Carter, W.H. Jr., Wampler, G.L. and Stablein, D.M. (1983). *Response Analysis of Survival Data in Cancer Chemotherapy.* Marcel Dekker, New York.

Cartwright, A. and Smith, C. (1988). *Elderly People, Their Medicines and Their Doctors.* Routledge, London.

Chen, G. and Ensor, C.R. (1953). The combined anticonvulsant activity and toxicity of dilantin and N-methyl-5-phenylsuccinamide. *J. Lab. Clin. Med.* **41,** 78–83.

Chou, T-C. and Talalay, P. (1977). A simple generalized equation for the analysis of multiple inhibitions of Michaelis–Menten kinetic systems. *J. Biol. Chem.* **252,** 6438–6447.

Chou, T-C. and Talalay, P. (1981). Generalized equations for the analysis of Michaelis–Menten and higher-order kinetic systems with two or more mutually exclusive and non-exclusive inhibitors. *Eur. J. Biochem.* **115,** 207–216.

Chou, T-C. and Talalay, P. (1984). Quantitative analysis of dose-effect relationships: the combined effects of multiple drugs or enzyme inhibitors. *Adv. Enzyme Reg.* **22,** 27–55.

Chou, T-C. and Talalay, P. (1987). Applications of the Median-Effect Principle for the assessment of low-dose risk of carcinogens and for the quantitation of synergism and antagonism of chemotherapeutic agents. In *New Avenues in Developmental Cancer Chemotherapy* (Eds K.R. Harrap and T.A. Connors), pp. 37–64. Academic Press, New York.

Crane, L.R. and Milne, D.A. (1985). Comparative activities of combinations of acyclovir, vidarabine or its 5′-monophosphate, and cloned human interferons against herpes simplex virus type 2 in human and mouse fibroblast cultures. *Antiviral Res.* **5,** 325–333.

Crump, K.S., Hoel, D.G., Langley, C.H. and Peto, R. (1976). Fundamental carcinogenic processes and their implications for low-dose risk assessment. *Cancer Res.* **36,** 2973–2979.

Dale, M.M. and Penfield, A. (1984). Synergism between phorbol ester and A23187 in superoxide production by neutrophils. *FEBS Letters* **175,** 170–172.

De Chauffoy de Courcelles, D., Roevens, P., van Belle, H. and De Clerk, F. (1987). The synergistic effect of serotonin and epinephrine on the human platelet at the level of signal transduction. *FEBS Letters* **219,** 283–288.

De Maeyer, E. and De Maeyer-Guignard, J. (1988). *Interferons and Other Regulatory Cytokines*. John Wiley, New York.

Douglas, N.J., Davidson, I., Sudlow, M.F. and Flenley, D.C. (1979). Bronchodilatation and the site of airway resistance in severe chronic bronchitis. *Thorax* **34,** 51–56.

Dyson, A.J. and Campbell, I.A. (1977). Interaction between choline theophylline and salmefamol in patients with reversible airways obstruction. *Br. J. Clin. Pharmacol.* **4,** 677–682.

Elion, G.B., Singer, S. and Hitchings, G.H. (1954). Antagonists of nucleic acid derivatives. VIII. Synergism in combinations of biochemically related antimetabolites. *J. Biol. Chem.* **208,** 477–488.

Elwood, R.K. and Abboud, R.T. (1982). The short-term bronchodilator effects of fenoterol and ipratropium in asthma. *J. Allergy Clin. Immunol.* **69,** 467–473.

Eney, R.D. and Goldstein, E.O. (1976). Compliance of chronic asthmatics with oral administration of theophylline as measured by serum and salivary levels. *Pediatrics* **57,** 513–517.

Ennist, D.L., Elkins, K.L., Cheng, S.C. and Howard, M. (1987). Activity of a partially purified human BCFG on murine assays for B cell stimulatory factors. II. Synergy between two distinct BCGF II-like factors in promoting B cell differentiation. *J. Immunol.* **139,** 1525–1531.

Evans, W.V., Monie, R.D.H., Crimmins, J. and Seaton, A. (1980). Aminophylline, salbutamol and combined intravenous infusions in acute severe asthma. *Br. J. Dis. Chest.* **74,** 385–389.

Fernandez-Botran, R., Sanders, V.M., Mosmann, T.R. and Vitetta, E.S. (1988). Lymphokine-mediated regulation of the proliferative response of clones of T helper 1 and T helper 2 cells. *J. Exp. Med.* **168,** 543–558.

Fraser, T.R. (1870–1871). An experimental research on the antagonism between the actions of physostigma and atropia. *Proc. Roy. Soc. Edin.* **7,** 506–511.

Fraser, T.R. (1872). The antagonism between the actions of active substances. *Br. Med. J.* **2,** 485–487.

Fujimura, M., Azuma, H., Uotani, K., Mifune, J-I., Tanaka, T. and Matsuda, T. (1986). Additive effects of isoproterenol-phenyephrine aerosol following ipratropium bromide on airway obstruction in older patients with intrinsic asthma and chronic bronchitis. *Jap. J. Med.* **25,** 122–126.

Fuller, R.W., Dixon, C.M.S., Dollery, C.T. and Barnes, P.J. (1986). Prostaglandin D_2 potentiates airway responsiveness to histamine and methacholine. *Am. Rev. Resp. Dis.* **133,** 252–254.

Gessner, P.K. and Cabana, B.E. (1970). A study of the interactions of the hypnotic effects and of the toxic effects of chloral hydrate and ethanol. *J. Pharmacol. Exp. Ther.* **174,** 247–259.

Gilchrist, W.J., Lee, Y.C., Tam, H.C., MacDonald, J.B. and Williams, B.O. (1987). Prospective study of drug reporting by general practitioners for an elderly population referred to a geriatric service. *Br. Med. J.* **294,** 289–290.

Grandordy, B.M., Thomas, V., de Lauture, D. and Marsac, J. (1988). Cumulative dose–response effects of salbutamol and ipratropium bromide in chronic asthma. *Eur. Resp. J.* **1,** 532–535.

Grant, J.A. and Scrutton, M.C. (1980). Positive interaction between agonists in the aggregation response of human blood platelets: interaction between ADP, adrenaline and vasopressin. *Br. J. Haematol.* **44,** 109–125.

Guess, H.A. and Crump, K. (1978). Best-estimate low-dose extrapolation of carcinogenicity data. *Environ. Health Perspect.* **22,** 149–152.

Guess, H.A., Crump, K. and Peto, R. (1977). Uncertainty estimates for low-dose-rate extrapolations of animal carcinogenicity data. *Cancer Res.* **37,** 3475–3483.

Hahn, F., Bernauer, W., Mahlstedt, J., Resch-Bollhagen, S. and Beck, S. (1970). Synergistic effects of adrenaline and mepyramine on the anaphylactic reactions of the bronchi and pulmonary vessels in the guinea-pig heart-lung-preparation. *Naun-Schmeid. Arch. Pharmak.* **267,** 224–240.

Hanna, C.J. and Eyre, P. (1979). On the action of combined bronchodilators. *Agents and Actions* **9,** 301–309.

Hanna, C.J. and Roth, S.H. (1979). Combination bronchodilators: antagonism of airway smooth muscle contractions in vitro. *Agents and Actions* **9,** 18–21.

Haslam, R.J., Williams, K.A. and Davidson, M.M.L. (1985). Receptor–effector coupling in platelets: roles of guanine nucleotides. In *Mechanisms of Stimulus-Response Coupling in Platelets* (Eds J. Westwick, M.F. Scully, D.E. MacIntyre and V.V. Kakkar), pp. 160–173. Plenum Press, New York.

Hayashi, Y., Sumukawa, K., Tashiro, C. and Yoshiya, I. (1988). Synergistic interaction of α_1- and β-adrenoceptor agonists on induction arrhythmias during halothane anesthesia in dogs. *Anesthesiology* **68,** 902–907.

Heaton, R.W., Henderson, A.F., Dunlop, L.S. and Costello, J.F. (1984). The influence of pretreatment with prostaglandin $F_{2\alpha}$ on bronchial sensitivity to inhaled histamine and methacholine in normal subjects. *Br. J. Dis. Chest* **78,** 168–173.

Hellewell, P.G. and Williams, T.J. (1988). Interactions between eicosanoids and other mediators of inflammation. In *Eicosanoids in Inflammatory Conditions of the Lung, Skin and Joints* (Eds M. Church and C. Robinson), pp. 43–66. MTP Press, Lancaster.

Howarth, P.H., Stanforth, J.N. and Holgate, S.T. (1982). Bronchodilator efficacy of nebulized salbutamol and ipratropium bromide in chronic airflow obstruction. *Thorax* **37,** 789.

Hughes, J.A., Tobin, M.J., Bellamy, D. and Hutchinson, D.C.S. (1982). Effects of ipratropium bromide and fenoterol aerosols in pulmonary emphysema. *Thorax* **37,** 667.

Jackson, J.E., Powell, J.R., Wendell, M., Bentley, J. and Dorr, R. (1981). Cimetidine decreases theophylline clearance. *Am. Rev. Resp. Dis.* **123,** 615–617.

Kaibuchi, K., Takai, Y., Sawamura, M., Hoshijima, M., Fujikura, T. and Nishizuka, Y. (1983). Synergistic functions of protein phosphorylation and calcium mobilization in platelet activation. *J. Biol. Chem.* **258,** 6701–6704.

Kaliner, M.A., Orange, R.P., Koopman, W.J., Austen, K.F. and Laraia, P.J. (1971). Cyclic adenosine 3′-,5′-monophosphate in the human lung. *Biochim. Biophys. Acta* **252,** 160–164.

Kreisman, H., Frank, H., Wolkove, N. and Gent, M. (1981). Synergism between ipratropium and theophylline in asthma. *Thorax* **36,** 387–391.

Lefcoe, N.M., Toogood, J.H., Blennerhassett, G., Baskerville, J. and Paterson, N.A.M. (1982). The addition of an aerosol anticholinergic to an oral beta agonist plus theophylline in asthma and bronchitis. A double-blind single dose study. *Chest* **82**, 300–305.

Leff, A.R. (1988). Endogenous regulation of bronchomotor tone. *Am. Rev. Resp. Dis.* **137,** 1198–1216.

Leff, A.R. and Munoz, N.M. (1981). Cholinergic and *alpha* adrenergic augmentation of histamine-induced contraction of canine airway smooth muscle. *J. Pharmacol. Exp. Ther.* **218,** 582–587.

Leopold, D. and Handslip, P. (1979). Additive interaction of aminophylline and salbutamol in asthma: and *in vivo* study using dose–response curves. *J. Int. Med. Res.* **7,** Suppl. 1, 52–55.

Lichtenstein, L.M. and Margolis, S. (1968). Histamine release *in vitro*: inhibition by catecholamines and methylxanthines. *Science* **161,** 902–903.

Lightbody, I.M., Ingram, C.G., Legge, J.S. and Johnston, R.N. (1978). Ipratropium bromide, salbutamol and prednisolone in bronchial asthma and chronic bronchitis. *Br. J. Dis. Chest* **72,** 181–188.

Lindsay, D.A. (1988). Fixed dose combination therapy in the treatment of asthma—the case against it. In *Mechanisms in Asthma: Pharmacology, Physiology, and Management* (Eds C.L. Armour and J.L. Black), pp. 421–425. Alan R. Liss, New York.

Loewe, S. (1928). Die quantitativen Probleme der Pharmakologie. *Ergebn. Physiol.* **27,** 47–187.

Loewe, S. (1953). The problem of synergism and antagonism of combined drugs. *Arzneimittelforschung* **3,** 285–290.

Loewe, S. (1955a). Isobols of dose-effect relations in the combination of pentylenetetrazole and phenobarbital. *J. Pharmacol. Exp. Ther.* **114,** 185–191.

Loewe, S. (1955b). Isobols of dose-effect relations in the combination of nikethamide (coramine) and phenobarbital. *J. Pharmacol. Exp. Ther.* **115,** 6–15.

Loewe, S. (1957). Antagonisms and antagonists. *Pharmacol. Rev.* **9,** 237–243.

Loewe, S. and Muischnek, H. (1926). Über Kombinationswirkungen. I. Mitteilung: Hilfsmittel der Fragestellung. *Arch. Exp. Path. Pharmak.* **114,** 313–326.

Marlin, G.E., Berend, N., Harris, M.R., Hartnett, B.J.S. and Rutland, J. (1979a) Clinical studies of the relative potencies and the combined effects of theophylline and beta-adrenoceptor agonists, *Current Med. Res. Opinion* **6,** Supp. 6, 92–100.

Marlin, G.E., Berend, N. and Harrison, A.C. (1979b). Combined cholinergic antagonist and β_2-adrenoceptor agonist bronchodilator therapy by inhalation. *Aust. N.Z. J. Med.* **9,** 511–514.

Marquardt, D.L., Parker, C.N. and Sullivan, T.J. (1978). Potentiation of mast-cell mediator release by adenosine. *J. Immunol.* **120,** 871–878.

Marquis, J.F., Carruthers, S.G., Spence, D., Brownstone, Y.S. and Toogood, J.H. (1982). Phenytoin-theophylline interaction. *New Eng. J. Med.* **307,** 1189–1190.

Mazzoni, L., Morley, J., Page, C.P. and Sanjar, S. (1985). Induction of airway hyperreactivity by platelet activating factor in the guinea-pig. *J. Physiol.* **365,** 107P.

Mitchell, C.L. (1976). The design and analysis of experiments for the assessment of drug interactions. *Ann. N.Y. Acad. Sci.* **281,** 118–135.

Mitchell, H.W., Hau, H. and Denborough, M.A. (1979). *In vitro* action of combined salbutamol and theophylline on anaphylactic contractions, mediator release and cyclic 3′,5′-adenosine monophosphate in lung parenchyma. *Eur. J. Pharmacol.* **57,** 399–406.

Myers, D.J., Bigby, B.G., Calvayrac, P., Sheppard, D. and Boushey, H.A. (1986). Interaction of cromolyn and a muscarinic antagonist in inhibiting bronchial reactivity to sulfur dioxide and to eucapnic hyperpnoea alone. *Am. Rev. Resp. Dis.* **133,** 1154–1158.

Myers, R.H. (1971). *Response Surface Methodology*. Allyn and Bacon, Boston.

Nelder, J.A. and Mead, R. (1964). A simplex method for function minimization. *Computer J.* **7,** 308–313.

Nichols, A.C. (1948). Bactericidal action of streptomycin-penicillin mixtures *in vitro*. *Proc. Soc. Exp. Biol. Med.* **69,** 477–478.

Nishizuka, Y. (1984). The role of protein kinase C in cell surface signal transduction and tumour promotion. *Nature* **308,** 693–698.

Olsson, O.A. (1972). The interaction between theophylline and some adrenergic α- and β-receptor agonists evaluated as effect on the LD50 of mice. *Acta. Pharmacol. et Toxicol.* **31,** 49–53.

Peters, S.P., Schulman, E.S., Schleimer, R.P., MacGlashan, D.W., Jr., Newball, H.H. and Lichtenstein, L.M. (1982). Dispersed human lung mast cells. *Am. Rev. Resp. Dis.* **126,** 1034–1039.

Peto, R. (1978). Carcinogenic effects of chronic exposure to very low levels of toxic substances. *Environ. Health Perspect.* **22,** 155–159.

Pfeifer, H.J., Greenblatt, P. and Friedman, P. (1978). Effect of antibiotics on theophylline kinetics in humans. *Clin. Pharmacol. Ther.* **23,** 124–125.

Pierce, R.J., Allen, C.I. and Campbell, A.H. (1957). A comparative study of atropine methonitrate, salbutamol, and their combination in airways obstruction. *Thorax* **34,** 45–50.

Pöch, G. (1981). The confusion about additive combinations. *Trends Pharmacol. Sci.* **2,** 256–257.

Pöch, G. and Holzmann, S. (1980). Quantitative estimation of overadditive and underadditive drug effects by means of theoretical, additive dose-response curves. *J. Pharmacol. Methods* **4,** 179–188.

Pöch, G. and Zimmermann, I. (1988). Simple pA_2 estimation of partial agonists: comparison with the Kaumann–Blinks method. *J. Pharmacol. Methods* **19,** 47–56.

Raoof, S., Wollschlager, C. and Khan, I.A. (1987). Ciprofloxacin increases serum levels of theophylline. *Am. J. Med.* **82,** 115–118.

Rebuck, A.S., Gent, M. and Chapman, K.R. (1983). Anticholinergic and sympathomimetic combination therapy of asthma. *J. Allergy Clin. Immunol.* **71,** 317–323.

Reisman, J., Galdes-Sebalt, M., Kazim, F., Canny, G. and Levison, H. (1988). Frequent administration by inhalation of salbutamol and ipratropium bromide in the initial management of severe acute asthma in children. *J. Allergy Clin. Immunol.* **81,** 16–20.

Rieder, M.J. and Spino, M. (1988). The theophylline–erythromycin interaction. *J. Asthma* **25,** 195–204.

Rossing, T.H., Fanta, C.H. and McFadden, E.R. (1981). A controlled trial of the use of single versus combined-drug therapy in the treatment of acute episodes of asthma. *Am. Rev. Resp. Dis.* **123,** 190–194.

Shapiro, G.G., McPhillips, J.J., Smith, K., Furukawa, C.T., Pierson, W.E. and Bierman, C.W. (1981). Effectiveness of terbutaline and theophylline alone and in combination in exercise-induced bronchospasm. *Pediatrics* **67,** 508–513.

Shenfield, G.M. (1982). Combination bronchodilator therapy. *Drugs* **24,** 414–439.

Sims, J.A., doPico, G.A. and Reed, C.E. (1978). Bronchodilator effect of oral theophylline ephedrine combinations. *J. Allergy Clin. Immunol.* **62,** 15–21.

Spendley, W., Hext, G.R. and Himsworth, F.R. (1962). Sequential application of simplex designs in optimisation and evolutionary operation. *Technometrics* **4,** 441–461.

Steen, S.N. (1978). Therapeutic synergism. *Chest* **73,** 131–132.

Svedmyr, K. and Svedmyr, N. (1982). Does theophylline potentiate inhaled β_2-agonists? *Allergy* **37,** 101–110.

Syracuse, K.C. and Greco, W.R. (1986). Comparison between the method of Chou and Talalay and a new method for the assessment of the combined effects of drugs: a Monte Carlo simulation study. *Proc. Am. Stat. Assoc. Biopharmacol. Section,* 127–132.

Takagi, K., Hasegawa, T., Ogura, Y., Suzuki, R., Yamaki, K., Watanabe, T., Kitazawa, S. and Satake, T. (1988). Comparative studies on interaction between theophylline and quinolones. *J. Asthma* **25,** 63–71.

Taylor, W.F., Heimlich, E.M., Strick, L. and Busser, R. (1965). Ephedrine and theophylline in asthmatic children: quantitative observations on the combination and ephedrine tachyphylaxis. *Ann. Allergy* **23,** 437.

Trotman, C.J., Thomas, P., Broder, I., Mintz, S. and Silverman, F. (1978). Effect of oxytriphylline and terbutaline alone and in combination on pulmonary function and methacholine response of asthmatics. *Curr. Ther. Res.* **23,** 436–442.

Undem, B.J. and Adams, G.K., III. (1988). An analysis of the functional interactions of selected contractile agonists in the guinea pig isolated trachea. *J. Pharmacol. Exp. Ther.*

288, 47–53.

Vargaftig, B.B., Lefort, J., Wal, F., Chignard, M. and Medeiros, M.C. (1982). Non-steroidal anti-inflammatory drugs if combined with antihistamine and anti-serotonin agents interfere with the bronchial and platelet effects of "platelet-activating factor" (PAF-acether). *Eur. J. Pharmacol.* **82,** 121–130.

Wallin, R.F., Blackburn, W.H. and Napoli, M.D. (1970). Pharmacologic interactions of albutoin with other anticonvulsant drugs. *J. Pharmacol. Exp. Ther.* **174,** 276–282.

Wampler, G.L., Carter, W.H. Jr., Campbell, E.D. and Goldman, I.D. (1987). Demonstration of a schedule-dependent therapeutic synergism utilizing the interacting drugs methotrexate and teniposide in L1210 leukemia. *Cancer Treat. Rep.* **71,** 581–591.

Ware, J.A., Smith, M. and Salzman, E.W. (1987). Synergism of platelet-aggregating agents. Role of elevation of cytoplasmic calcium. *J. Clin. Invest.* **80,** 267–271.

Watson, J.W., Drazen, J.M. and Stimler-Gerard, N.P. (1988). Synergism between inflammatory mediators *in vivo*. Induction of airway hyperresponsiveness to C3a in the guinea pig. *Am. Rev. Resp. Dis.* **137,** 636–640.

Weinberger, M., Bronsky, E., Bensch, G.W., Bock, G.N. and Yecies, J.J. (1975). Interaction of ephedrine and theophylline. *Clin. Pharmacol. Ther.* **17,** 585–592.

Weinberger, M., Hudgle, D., Spector, S. and Chidsey, C. (1976). Effect of triacetyloleandomycin (TAO) on the metabolism of theophylline. *Clin. Pharmacol. Ther.* **19,** 118.

Weinberger, M.M. and Bronsky, E.A. (1974). Evaluation of oral bronchodilator therapy in asthmatic children. *J. Pediatrics* **84,** 421–427.

Weinberger, M.M., Smith, G., Milavetz, G. and Hendeles, L. (1981). Decreased theophylline clearance due to cimetidine. *New Eng. J. Med.* **304,** 672.

Wijnands, W.J.A., Van Herwaarden, C.L.A. and Vree, T.B. (1984). Enoxacin raises plasma theophylline concentration. *Lancet* **2,** 108–109.

Williams, T.J. (1979). Prostaglandin E_2, prostaglandin I_2, and the vascular changes of inflammation. *Br. J. Pharmacol.* **65,** 517–524.

Williams, T.J. and Morley, J. (1973). Prostaglandins as potentiators of increased vascular permeability in inflammation. *Nature* **246,** 215–217.

Williams, T.J. and Peck, M.J. (1977). Role of prostaglandin-mediated vasodilatation in inflammation. *Nature* **270,** 530–532.

Wolfe, J.D., Tashkin, D.P., Calvarese, B. and Simmons, M. (1978). Bronchodilator effects of terbutaline and aminophylline alone and in combination in asthmatic patients. *New Eng. J. Med.* **298,** 363–367.

Yu, V.L., Felegie, T.P., Yee, R.B., Pasculle, A.W. and Taylor, F.H. (1980). Synergistic interaction *in vitro* with use of three antibiotics simultaneously against *Pseudomonas maltophilia*. *J. Infect. Dis.* **142,** 602–607.

Zarowitz, B.J.M., Szefler, S.J. and Lasezkoy, G.M. (1981). Effect of erythromycin base on theophylline kinetics. *Clin. Pharmacol. Ther.* **29,** 601–605.

3

Inhibitors of the biosynthesis or actions of the leukotrienes

P.J. Gardiner

Bayer UK, Stoke Court, Stoke Poges, Slough, Bucks SL2 4LY, UK

I THE ROLE OF LEUKOTRIENES IN ASTHMA

Although the structures of the leukotrienes have only recently been resolved, their activity was identified half a century ago. (Feldberg and Kellaway, 1938; Kellaway and Trethewie, 1940). Antigen challenge of guinea-pig lungs was shown to produce a substance that in the presence of an antihistamine contracted the guinea-pig ileum. Brocklehurst (1960, 1962) characterized the pharmacological uniqueness of this substance, and called it Slow Reacting Substance of Anaphylaxis (SRS-A) due to the late onset and long lasting contractions it produced. Interest in SRS-A increased when it was shown to be released following antigen challenge of human lung and to be a potent long acting contractile agonist on human asthmatic airways both *in vitro* and *in vivo* (Schild *et al.*, 1951; Brocklehurst, 1960; Herxheimer and Stresemann, 1963). In view of the poor therapeutic value of antihistamines in asthma, many groups concluded that SRS-A was predominantly responsible for this disease and that new therapy, aimed specifically at this substance, would be highly effective.

Problems with sample availability and purity thwarted any attempt to resolve the structure of SRS-A. However, resolution was recently achieved by a number of groups after SRS-A was shown to comprise metabolites of arachidonic acid, specifically produced by a 5-lipoxygenase enzyme (Parker *et al.*, 1979; Borgeat and Samuelsson, 1979a–d; Murphy *et al.*,

ASTHMA REVIEWS VOLUME 2
ISBN 0-12-040922-4

1979; Morris *et al.*, 1978, 1980). These products were called the leukotrienes, the sulphur and peptide containing types, LTC_4 and LTD_4, and their metabolite LTE_4 mainly constitute SRE-A. A non-peptide, 5.12. diHETE or LTB_4, is also produced by the 5-lipoxygenase, but this leukotriene has no direct spasmogenic activity (Borgeat and Samuelsson, 1979d).

The sulphidopeptide leukotrienes were shown to act as potent spasmogenic agents on a range of tissues, but they were most potent on guinea-pig and human airways both *in vitro* and *in vivo* (Drazen *et al.*, 1980; Krell *et al.*, 1981; Dahlen *et al.*, 1980; Jones *et al.*, 1982; Gardiner and Cuthbert, 1988). Assays for leukotrienes were used to demonstrate the presence of these substances in plasma, sputum and bronchial lavage fluid of asthmatics and a clear correlation between the severity of asthma and the leukotriene plasma levels was shown (Isono *et al.*, 1985; Ishihara *et al.*, 1985; Schonfeld *et al.*, 1985; Zakrzewski *et al.*, 1985). Needless to say this additional circumstantial evidence with the leukotrienes strengthened the earlier suggestions that SRS-A was predominantly responsible for asthma. Consequently, investigations aimed at identifying new therapeutics to reduce the effects of SRS-A/leukotrienes were intensified. However, the importance of the leukotrienes in asthma has become a highly controversial question with many groups now believing that asthma is caused by many mediators and, therefore, antagonism of any one mediator will have no significant therapeutic value.

A low level of chronic pulmonary inflammation is now considered to be a significant component of asthma. If this is true then LTB_4, a pro-inflammatory agent, might be especially important in asthma. It seems likely, however, that as with bronchospasm, several mediators are responsible for the inflammation of asthma and, therefore, therapy aimed at a single mediator might be of little value. It is also possible that interactions between the various mediators is essential for the full expression of the pathophysiology of asthma. In the absence of extensive studies aimed at analysing such interactions it is tempting to speculate that there might be a single mediator that amplifies the effects of others and its antagonism might prove to be of outstanding therapeutic value. In any case, the controversy surrounding the leukotrienes will only be resolved when sufficiently potent new drugs with selective effects on leukotrienes are thoroughly evaluated in asthma.

At present the anti-leukotriene drugs being developed mainly fall into two types, firstly those which inhibit the biosynthesis of leukotrienes and secondly those which antagonise their actions.

II INHIBITION OF LEUKOTRIENE BIOSYNTHESIS

The drugs in this group can be further subdivided according to their point of intervention in the arachidonic acid cascade. It can be seen in Fig. 1 that the starting point in the biosynthesis of leukotrienes is the membrane phospholipids. Arachidonic acid predominantly exists in an esterified form bound to these phospholipids and it is released in its free form by the hydrolytic activity of phospholipase A_2 (PLA_2). The free arachidonic acid is then oxidized either to prostanoids by the active cyclooxygenase, which is present in virtually all cell membranes, or to leukotrienes via the 5-lipoxygenase enzyme present in the cytoplasm. The latter enzyme is thought to require a stimulus to the cell of a more severe nature before it is activated. On actuation it works in two stages, initially oxidizing the arachidonic acid to 5-hydroperoxy eicosatetraenoic (5HPETE) acid. This is then converted to the unstable epoxide LTA_4, which in turn is enzymatically converted either by LTA_4 hydrolase to LTB_4 or by glutathione-*S*-transferase to LTC_4. LTD_4 and LTE_4 are produced from LTC_4 by γ-glutamyl transpeptidase and aminopeptidase respectively.

On the left of Fig. 1 are theoretical points of intervention that might reduce the adverse effects of the leukotrienes. In brief, such intervention firstly involves the diversion or shunting of arachidonic acid away from 5-lipoxygenase by potentiation of the cyclooxygenase pathway. The validity of such shunting as a therapeutic approach depends on the use of the same arachidonic acid pool by both enzymic pathways. This is another subject of some controversy as it has been suggested that the arachidonic acid available for each of the enzymes is separately compartmentalized (Kuehl *et al.*, 1984). Moving down the pathway another approach involves shunting the 5HPETE predominantly to 5HETE by increasing the activity of glutathione peroxidase. A more selective approach that might alter the levels of LTB_4 or of the sulphidopeptide leukotrienes involves modification of the activity of LTA_4 hydrolase or LTC_4 synthase. Finally, the levels of leukotrienes could be reduced by increasing the rate of their metabolism. In practice, little or no effort is being paid to any of these areas.

On the right of Fig. 1 are the three main approaches being followed at present. Each of these will be discussed in greater depth below.

A Phospholipase inhibitors

The first approach involves inhibition of the release of arachidonic acid from membrane phospholipids. Most of the arachidonic acid is bound to

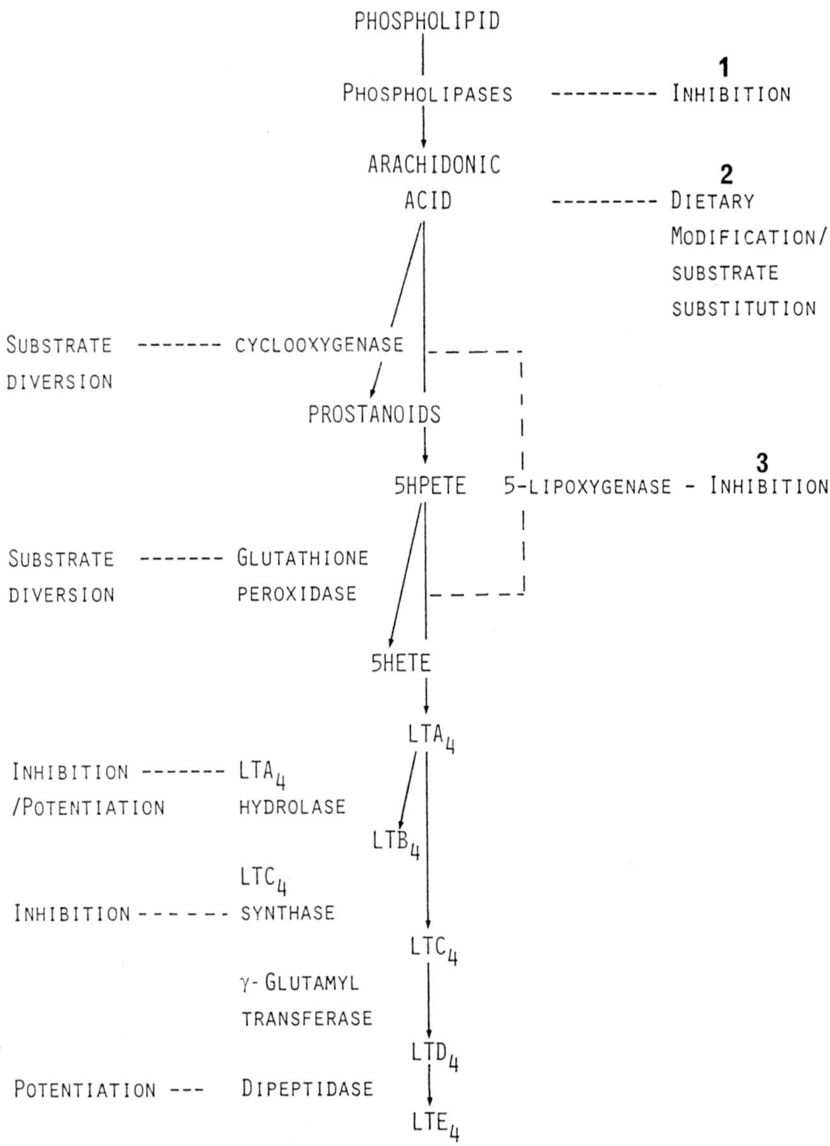

Fig. 1 Potential points of intervention to prevent the biosynthesis of leukotrienes. On the left are theoretical points of intervention, such as potentiation of cyclooxygenase activity to divert arachidonic acid to the cyclooxygenase pathway or potentiation of dipeptidase to increase leukotriene metabolism. On the right are three points of intervention that are being pursued, (1) inhibition of phospholipase to decrease substrate availability, (2) incorporation of alternative substrate(s) by dietary manipulation and (3) inhibition of the 5-lipoxygenase itself.

membrane phospholipids. The phospholipids can be considered as glyceryl structures with three carbon atoms referred to as α, β and α_1 (Fig. 2). Unsaturated fatty acids are predominantly esterified in the β position (Blackwell and Flower, 1983). The hydrolytic phospholipase enzymes act at specific points on the phospholipid and although four types (PLA_1, PLA_2, PLC and PLD) can lead to the liberation of free arachidonic acid, the phospholipase which acts directly and is thought to be predominantly responsible is PLA_2. It acts directly at the β position and in one step releases free arachidonic acid. A greater understanding of the phospholipases can be found in comprehensive reviews by Van den Bosch (1980), Waite (1985), Elsbach *et al.* (1979) and Irvine (1982). Numerous drugs have been shown to inhibit PLA_2, however, the majority have additional actions and it remains controversial whether PLA_2 inhibition is responsible for their therapeutic role. Such drugs can be subdivided into the following three different groups according to their mechanism of action.

1 Agents which directly interact with the enzyme

Glucocorticoids. Although these well known anti-inflammatory agents do not directly interact with the enzyme they do induce the synthesis and release of proteins that possess antiphospholipase activity (Blackwell and Flower, 1983). Following the interaction of steroids with their intracellular

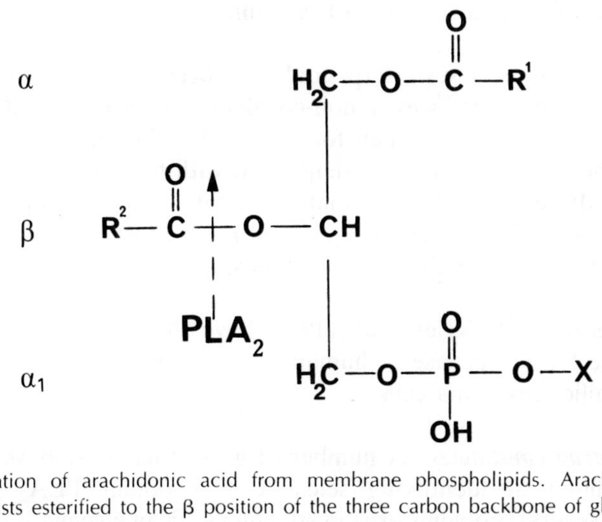

Fig. 2 Liberation of arachidonic acid from membrane phospholipids. Arachidonic acid normally exists esterified to the β position of the three carbon backbone of glycerol. PLA_2 a hydrolytic enzyme acts at this β position to liberate the fatty acid.

receptors a complex is formed that translocates to the nucleus where it interacts with chromatin. This interaction modulates the expression of specific genes leading to the synthesis of mRNA and then to the synthesis of proteins (lipocortin) with antiphospholipase activity (DiRosa *et al.*, 1984). The small amount of pure lipocortin available has meant that the exact mechanism of action is unclear, some speculate that it may interfere with the calcium binding site of PLA_2 or that it may interact with the substrate. One study of lipocortin inhibition of pancreatic PLA_2 *in vitro* has shown that a substrate inhibitor complex was formed and that no specific interaction with the enzyme occurred (Davidson *et al.*, 1987). It seems unlikely that lipocortin selectively inhibits PLA_2 as it has also been shown to inhibit bacterial PLC (Hirata, 1981). More recently cDNA for human lipocortin has been cloned and expressed in *E. Coli* (Wallner *et al.*, 1986). Two proteins with PLA_2 inhibitory activity have been purified from human placenta and have been designated lipocortins I and II (Huang *et al.*, 1986). Whether or not lipocortin is the sole mechanism for the beneficial effects of glucocorticoids in asthma remains unresolved.

Parabromophenacyl bromide (pBPB). This is a reactive organic reagent (Fig. 3) that forms a covalent bond with the histidine 48 of PLA_2 (Drenth *et al.*, 1976). The close proximity of this amino acid to the calcium binding site leads, following such an interaction, to decreased enzyme activity. However, pBPB will also covalently bind to any nucleophilic group and *in vivo* will alkylate thiol and amine groups of many proteins. Consequently it has little value as a selective PLA_2 inhibitor.

Manoalide. This is a sesterterpenoid that occurs naturally in sponges. The natural form produces a non-covalent complex with the enzyme, which is converted to the open form (Fig. 3). The amine groups of the PLA_2 lysine residue form a covalent bond with the open form (Chang *et al.*, 1987). It seems that on formation of this covalent bond manoalide changes the specificity of the PLA_2, inhibiting its effect on phosphatidylcholine but enhancing its activity towards phosphatidylethanolamine (Dennis, 1987).

More recently De Vries *et al.* (1988) have shown that manoalide also inhibits the 5-lipoxygenase of human polymorphonuclear leucocytes and rat basophilic leukaemia cells.

Synthetic drug candidates. A number of groups have established specific screens aimed at identifying selective and potent PLA_2 inhibitors. However, several problems exist in studying such an enzyme. Firstly PLA_2 has a higher affinity for aggregated than non-aggregated phospholipid, secondly classical Michaelis–Menten kinetics do not apply to the enzyme.

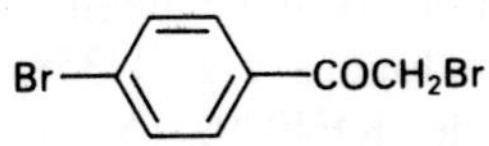

p-Bromophenacyl bromide

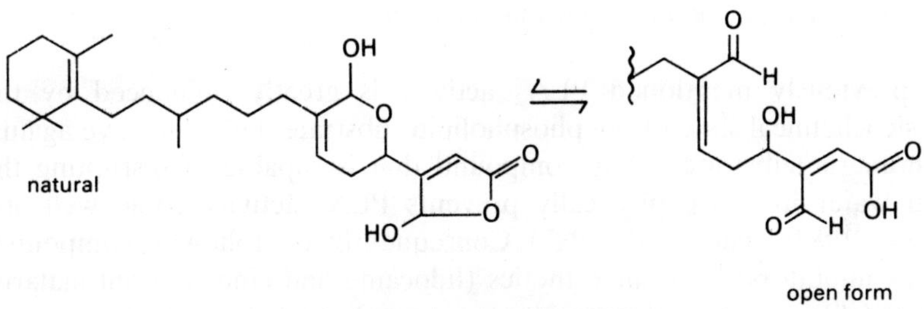

MANOALIDE (A SESTERTERPENOID)

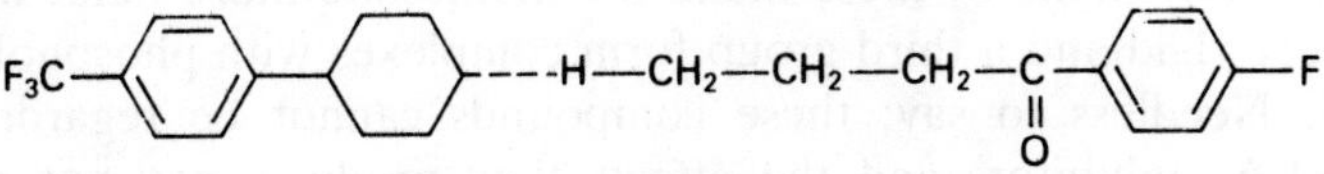

U3583

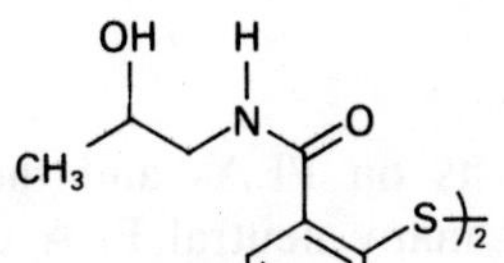

KF4939

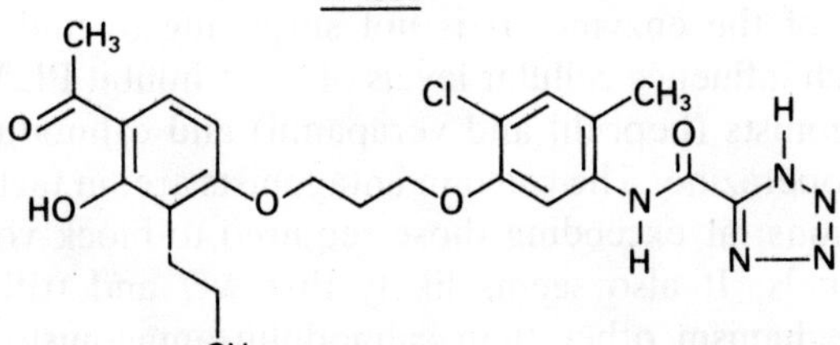

CGP35949B

Fig. 3 Structures of some PLA_2 inhibitors.

In addition, it can exist in either the inactivated or activated state and finally the enzyme exists in solution as monomers or dimers of varying stability (Chang *et al.*, 1987).

Nevertheless, several inhibitors have been identified these include a series of butyrophenone analogues e.g. U3583, (Wallach and Brown, 1981), a diphenyl disulphide KF4939, (Yamada *et al.*, 1985) and a hydroxyacetophenone CGP 35949B (Bray *et al.*, 1987). (Fig. 3). However, none of these compounds are very potent or selective inhibitors.

2 *Agents which interact with the substrate*

As previously mentioned PLA_2 activity is greatly influenced by the physicochemical state of the phospholipid substrate, being inactive against monomeric substrates. Any compound that is capable of disrupting the lipid water interface physically prevents PLA_2 activity (Blackwell and Flower, 1983; Chang *et al.*, 1987). Consequently, the following compounds act as inhibitors: local anaesthetics (lidocaine and cincaine) antimalarial agents (chloroquine and mepacrine), antipsychotic agents (chlorpromazine and promethazine), antibiotics (streptomycin) and organic solvents (chloroform) etc. Some of these make the membrane more fluid, others make it more rigid and a third group form complexes with phospholipids in general. Needless to say, these compounds cannot be regarded as selective PLA_2 inhibitors and the effects they produce may not result solely from PLA_2 inhibitory effects.

3 *Agents which act on* Ca^{2+}

A calcium binding site exists on PLA_2 and the presence of Ca^{2+} is essential for the activity of many neutral PLA enzymes (Chang *et al.*, 1987). Addition of Ca^{2+} increases enzyme activity, whereas Quin 2 a calcium chelator inhibits enzyme activity. The exact role of the calcium is uncertain, however, it has been suggested that it maintains the structural conformation of the enzyme. It is not surprising to find that a number of agents which influence cellular levels of Ca^{2+} inhibit PLA_2, for example calcium antagonists (bepridil and verapamil) and calmodulin antagonists w-7 and trifluoperazine. The calcium antagonists are, in fact, only effective at concentrations far exceeding those required to block voltage operated calcium channels. It also seems likely that w-7 and trifluoperazine act through a mechanism other than calmodulin antagonism as calmodulin does not activate purified PLA_2. It seems more likely that these agents are acting through the formation of complexes with the substrate rather than an effect on calcium.

It is clear that all existing PLA_2 inhibitors lack either desirable specificity or potency. In any case, inhibition of PLA_2 as a new therapeutic target has been questioned as phospholipases are involved in phospholipid remodelling that is critical to cellular integrity. However, if PLA_2 activities involved in basal phospholipid turnover are distinct from those activated upon cell stimulation this may not be a problem. Recent studies have indicated that intracellular PLA_2 activity exists in multiple forms with distinct properties (Billah, 1987). If this is indeed the case perhaps selective inhibitors could be developed.

B Alternative fatty acid substrates

The dietary origin of the arachidonic acid that occurs in cell membranes is either direct from arachidonic acid in meat or from linoleic acid and linolenic acid that occur in the seeds and leaves of plants. These fatty acids can be converted to arachidonic acid by chain elongation and desaturation (Willis, 1981).

The amount of arachidonic acid incorporated into the cell can be decreased by diet supplementation with cold-water oily fish. Such fish are rich in eicosatrienoic and eicosapentaenoic acids; both of these substrates are incorporated into tissue phospholipids in place of arachidonic acid and are a necessary adaption to temperatures at which the fat of animals from a temperate climate would solidify (Sinclair, 1952). In their free form they are converted by lipoxygenase to leukotrienes of the 3 and 5 series respectively (Fig. 4). It has been suggested that reduction of the naturally occurring 4 series leukotrienes by such dietary manipulation may be beneficial in asthma. However, unless the activity of such products is markedly less or qualitatively different to that of the 4 series leukotrienes then such dietary manipulation is of little value. In studies aimed at answering this question LTB_3 and LTB_4 were shown to have similar chemotactic and degranulating activity, whereas LTB_5 was markedly weaker in all test systems (Terano *et al.*, 1984; Evans *et al.*, 1985). This suggests that a diet rich in eicosapentaenoic acid leading to high levels of LTB_5 would be beneficial in inflammatory conditions. This seems to be borne out by some recent clinical studies, in which marked improvement occurred in patients either with rheumatoid arthritis or psoriasis when they were fed eicosapentaenoic acid rich diets (Table 1).

It has been suggested that airway hyperreactivity, which is so characteristic of asthma, is a result of a chronic low level of inflammation and that LTB_4, with its chemotactic/degranulating activity on polymorphonuclear leucocytes (PMN), might at least in part be responsible for

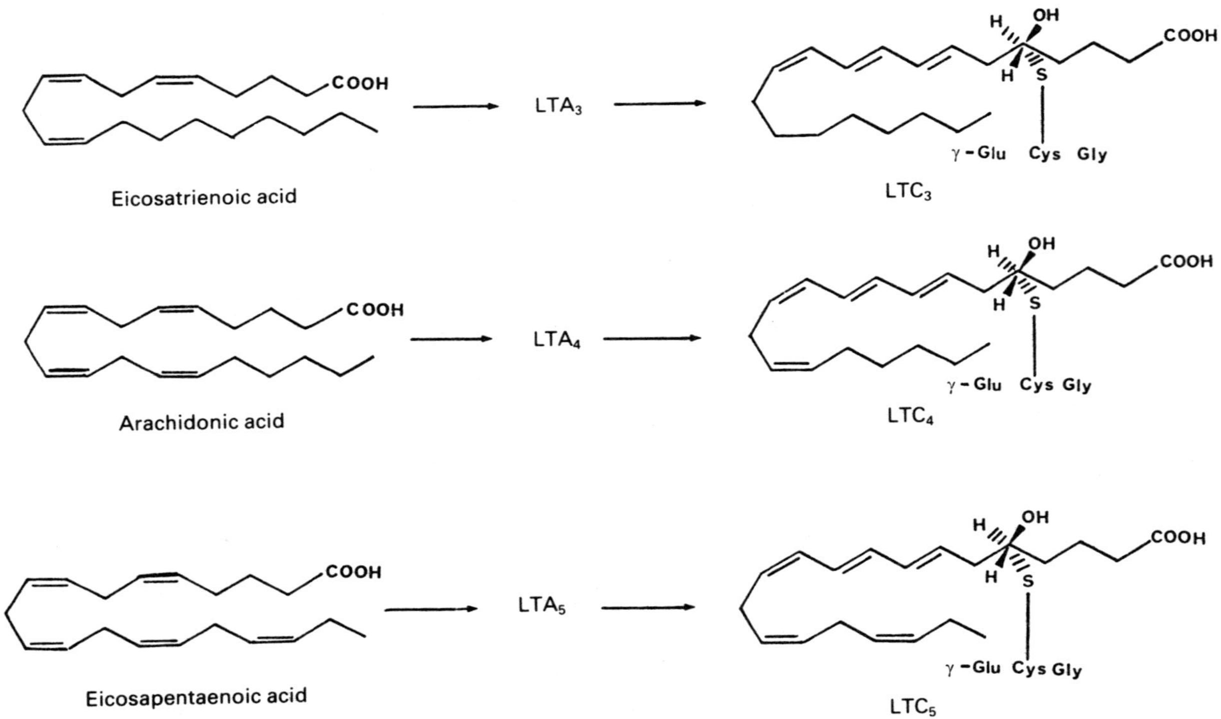

Fig. 4 Biosynthesis of 3, 4 and 5 series leukotrienes. Eicosa-trienoic and -pentaenoic acid are unsaturated fatty acids commonly found in cold-water fish. Both are converted by lipoxygenase to leukotrienes of the 3 or 5 series.

this. However, a recent study, in which asthmatics were fed diets rich in fish oil for 10 weeks, failed to show any beneficial effects despite a decreased production of LTB_4 by PMNs and suppression of PMN chemotaxis (Table 1).

The spasmogenic activity of the 3 and 5 series sulphidopeptide leukotrienes has also been evaluated (Hammerstrom, 1981; Dahlen *et al.*, 1983a). Both series were similar to or slightly less active than the 4 series as spasmogenics on the guinea-pig ileum and the guinea-pig lung strip. These results suggest that dietary manipulation leading to higher levels of such products would be unlikely to improve asthma. This conclusion received further support when it was shown that passively sensitized guinea-pigs given diets rich in fish oil, produced comparable bronchoconstrictor responses to control animals when challenged with antigen (Lee *et al.*, 1985). As already mentioned mild asthmatics showed no improvement in their symptoms or hyperreactivity when fed diets rich in fish oil. Consequently, although dietary manipulation can lead to the incorporation of alternative fatty acids into the cell membrane the therapeutic potential of such diets in asthma is somewhat disappointing, and may relate to the comparable spasmogenic activity of the 5 series sulphidopeptide leukotrienes. Alternatively, this may reflect inhibition of the synthesis of bronchodilator prostanoids, which is known to occur with eicosapentaenoic acid, such prostanoids may normally attenuate the asthmatic response.

Table 1 Clinical evaluation of dietary fatty acid manipulation in asthma and some inflammatory diseases. Patients took a dietary supplement of fish oil rich in eicosapentaenoic acid (EPA) for 6–12 weeks. In the study of mild asthma the neutrophil content of EPA increased 10-fold and LTB synthesis decreased by 50%. Neutrophil chemotaxis to FMLP and LTB_4 also decreased, but no improvement was observed.

Study	Disease	Comments
Kremer *et al.*, 1985	Rheumatoid arthritis	Improvement (fewer tender and stiff joints)
Bittiner *et al.*, 1988	Psoriasis	Improvement (less itching erythema and scaling)
Arm *et al.*, 1988	Mild asthma	Ineffective (decreased neutrophil chemotaxis)
Picado *et al.*, 1988	Aspirin induced asthma	Deleterious

C Agents which inhibit 5-lipoxygenase

Probably the greatest amount of effort has been directed towards the identification of inhibitors of the cytosolic enzyme 5-lipoxygenase. Selective inhibition of this enzyme should prevent leukotriene production without affecting the cyclooxygenase pathway. However, it has been suggested that such selective inhibition may make extra arachidonic acid available for oxidation by the cyclooxygenase pathway. This possibility remains speculative as it is also strongly argued, as previously mentioned, that the arachidonic acid used by 5-lipoxygenase and cyclooxygenase is separately compartmentalized and thus such shunting cannot occur (Kuehl *et al.*, 1984).

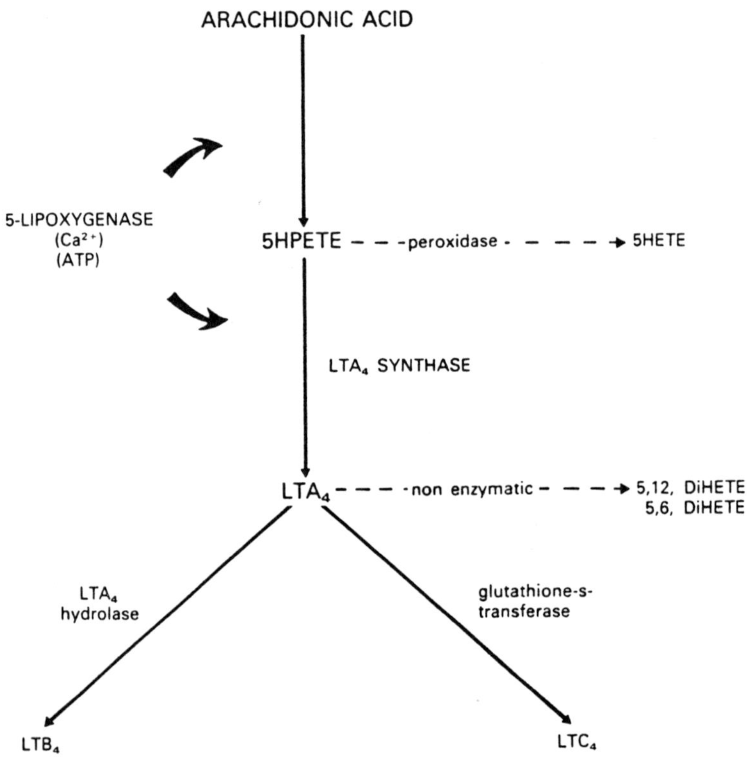

Fig. 5 Oxidation of arachidonic acid to LTA_4 by the 5-lipoxygenase. This enzyme is present predominantly in the cytoplasm of inflammatory cells e.g. PMN, eosinophils etc. and requires Ca^{2+}, ATP and cellular components for activation. It acts in two stages, firstly oxidizing arachidonic acid to 5-hydroperoxy eicostetraenoic acid (5HPETE) and then acts as a dehydrase to produce the unstable intermediate LTA_4. This is enzymatically converted to LTB_4 or LTC_4.

Arachidonic acid is oxidized to the unsaturated epoxide intermediate LTA_4 by a 5-lipoxygenase enzyme. This enzyme has dual activities, initially it oxidizes the arachidonic acid to 5HPETE and then acts as a dehydrase to produce LTA_4 (Samuelsson *et al.*, 1987) (Fig. 5). The enzyme requires Ca^{2+} and ATP and a number of cellular components for maximal activity. It seems likely that it exhibits a reversible Ca^{2+} dependent association with cellular membranes. On cell activation, and an increase in intracellular Ca^{2+}, the enzyme may form as an activated complex at the membrane surface.

A large number of 5-lipoxygenase inhibitors have been identified, however, their selectivity for this enzyme varies considerably. In an attempt to determine such selectivity, data have been collected from a number of studies in which inhibitory activity was evaluated on the 5-lipoxygenase and cyclooxygenase. In a further attempt to determine whether selectivity also exists within the lipoxygenases, activity on the 12-lipoxygenase has been included. One problem in comparing such activity, however, is the wide range of test systems and protocols used by the large numbers of groups working in this area. Differences exist in the species used, some groups use human cells whereas others use rat, guinea-pig or rabbit cells. The source and condition of the cells also differ, with some groups using PMNs from blood or the peritoneal cavity and others using RBL-1 or HL-60 cell lines. Whole cells, broken cells or the cell supernatant are used as the enzyme source. Differences also exist in the stimuli used to activate the enzyme, including the calcium ionophore, opsonized zymosan or in some cases no real stimulus is used at all as the cells are incubated with exogenous arachidonic acid. The substrates used include endogenous arachidonic acid or exogenous radiolabelled ^{14}C or ^{3}H arachidonic acid. Finally, the following wide range of methods have been used to determine the end product(s) 5HPETE, 5HETE or LTB_4: radioimmunoassay, TLC autoradiography, radiochromatography and HPLC and UV. Despite these numerous differences a table of inhibitory activities from a wide range of groups has been compiled and gives an approximate indication of relative selectivities and potencies (Table 2).

The pharmacokinetics of many of the compounds shown restricted their evaluation *in vivo*. Many of the *in vivo* studies reported have not included measurement of leukotriene production. Consequently negative results in an animal model of asthma could be due to the failure of the compound to achieve an effective inhibitory concentration, rather than an inability to inhibit the asthma-like reaction *per se*. On the other hand, some of these compounds are dual inhibitors of lipoxygenases and cyclooxygenase and caution should be exercised before attributing positive effects to inhibition on any one of these enzymes.

Table 2 Inhibitors of 5-lipoxygenase: (1) Antioxidants; (2) Substrate analogues; (3) Miscellaneous. The compounds are also grouped into structurally similar types. The IC_{50} values are taken from a number of groups, who invariably use different experimental protocols consequently such values only represent an approximate comparison of relative potencies. The cell types used were as follows: RBL, rat basophilic leukaemia cells; PP, porcine platelets; SSV and RSV, sheep and ram seminal vesicles; HPMN, human polymorphonuclear leukocytes; HP, human platelets; BP, bovine platelets; ME, mouse epidermis; GPPMN, guinea-pig polymorphonuclear leukocytes.

		IC_{50}μM (cell type used)			
Drug	Structure	5LO	12LO	CO	References
1. Antioxidants					
Phenidone	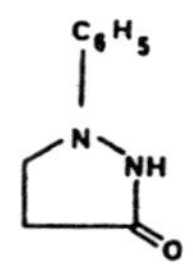	100 (RBL)	400 (PP)	60 (SSV)	Blackwell and Flower (1978)
BW755C	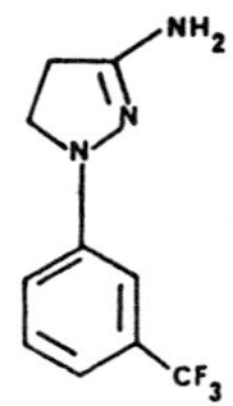	5 (HPMN)	7 (HPMN/ HP)	5 (HPMN)	Higgs *et al.* (1979) Salmon (1986)
Nafazatrom	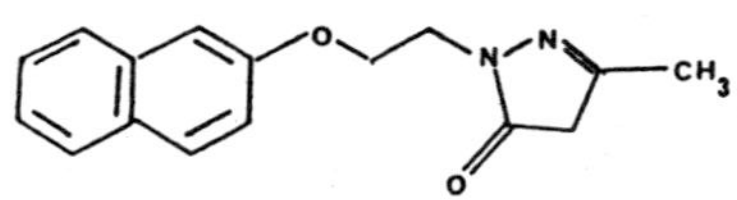	2 (HPMN)	>100 (HPMN/ HP)	>100 (HPMN/ HP)	Fischer *et al.* (1983) Salmon (1986)

NDGA	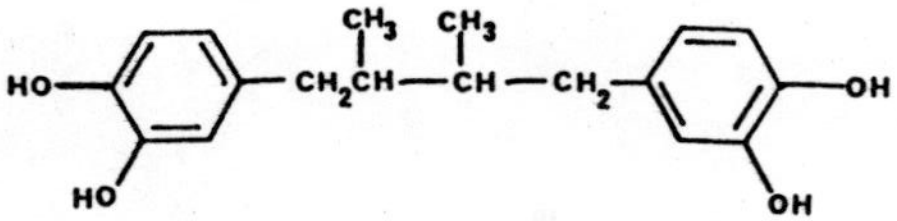	0.5 (HPMN)	30 (HPMN/HP)	8 (HPMN)	Salmon (1986)
Quercetin (Flavinoids; Baicalein, Esulin)	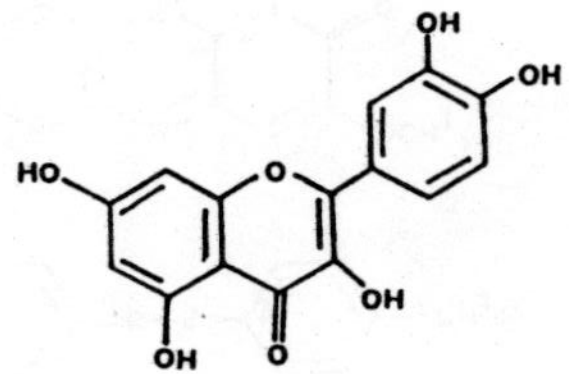	0.2 (RBL)	5 (HP)	>100 (SSV)	Hope *et al*. (1983)
(Linolenoyldopamine) R = $C_{17}H_{29}$	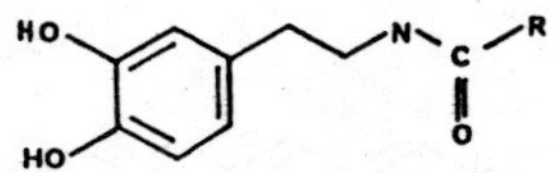	0.003 (RBL)	—	5–20 (SSV)	Iwakami *et al*. (1986)
KF8940 (Hydroxyquinoline)	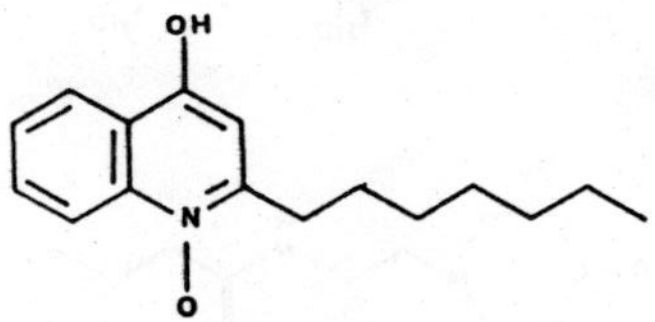	0.2 (RBL)	40 (BP)	200 (BP)	Kitamura *et al*. (1986)
AA861 (Benzoquinone)	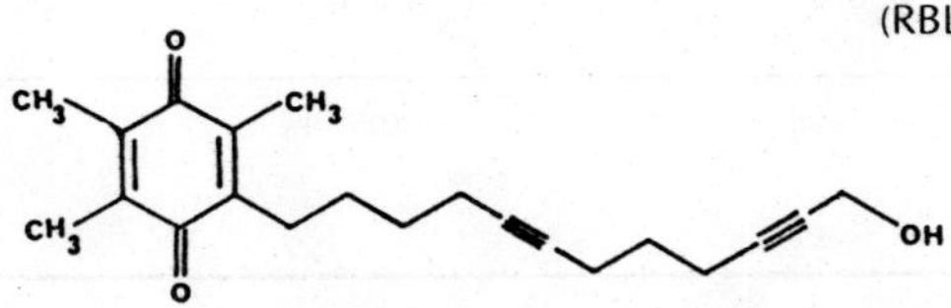	1 (RBL)	>100 (BP)	>100 (BP)	Kitamura *et al*. (1986)
			2 (ME)		Nakadate *et al*. (1985)

Table 2 *Continued*

Drug	Structure	IC_{50} μM (cell type used) 5LO	12LO	CO	References
TMK-688 (Caffeic acid)	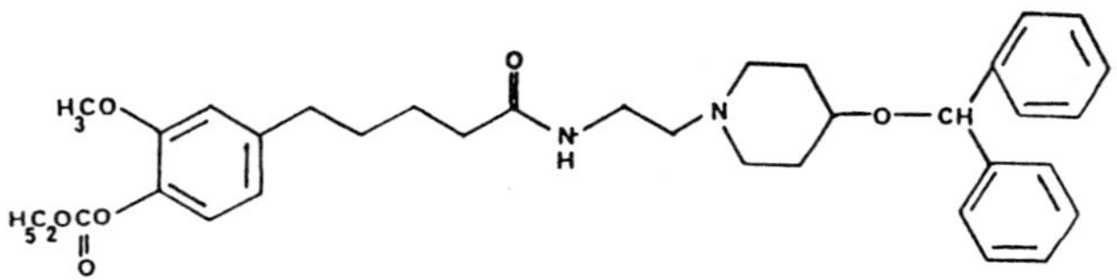	2 (RBL)	30 (BP)	200 (BP)	Kitamura *et al.* (1986)
Vit A (Retinol)	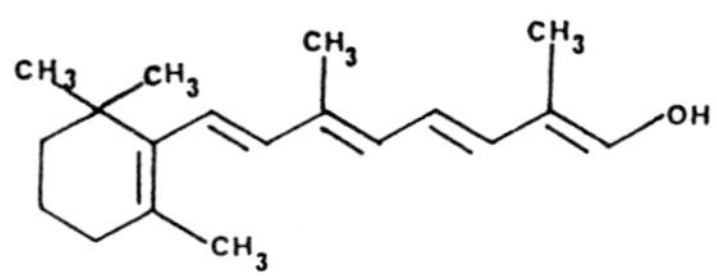	18 (HPMN)	—	>100 (HPMN)	Salmon (1986)
Diphenyl Disulphides	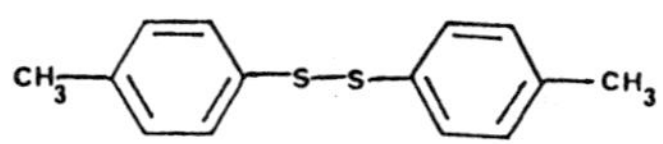	0.8 (RBL)	—	>500 (SSV)	Egan *et al.* (1983)
L651392 Phenothiazines	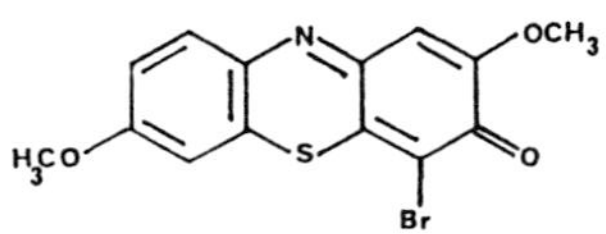	0.08 (RBL) + NADH	>1 (HP/PPMN)	>1 (RSV)	Guindon *et al.* (1987)

2. Substrate Analogues

ONO-Lp-221	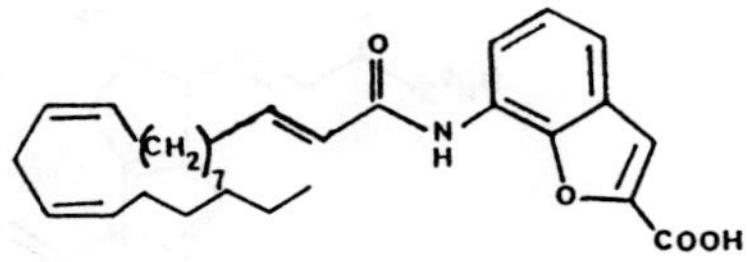	2 (GPPMN)	1000 (RBL)	240 (SSV)	Toda *et al.* (1987)
5,8,11,14 ETYA	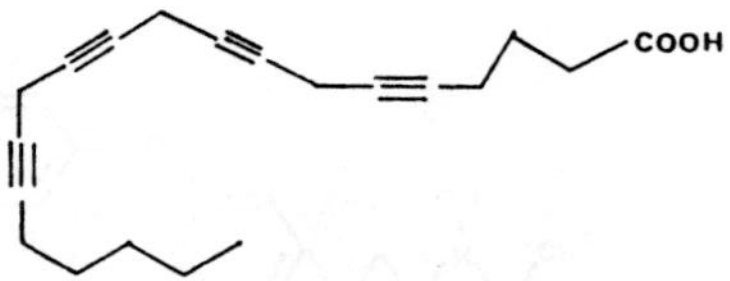	2 (HPMN)	0.05 (HPMN/ HP)	0.6 (HPMN)	Salmon (1986)
5,6 Dehydroarachidonic Acid	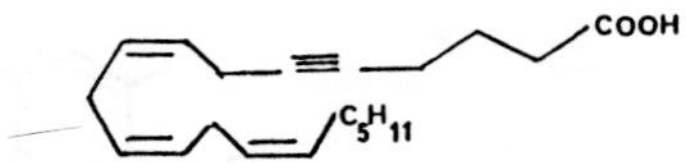	0.5 (Irreversible) RBL	—	Inactive	Corey and Munroe (1982)
15HETE	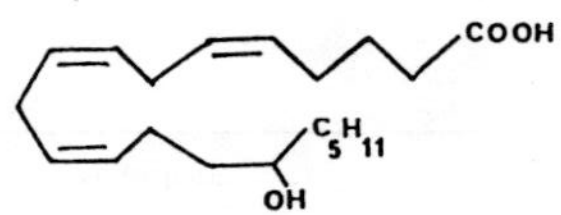	6 (RPMN)	8 (HP)	>25 (HP)	Vanderhoek *et al.* (1980a,b)
REV5901	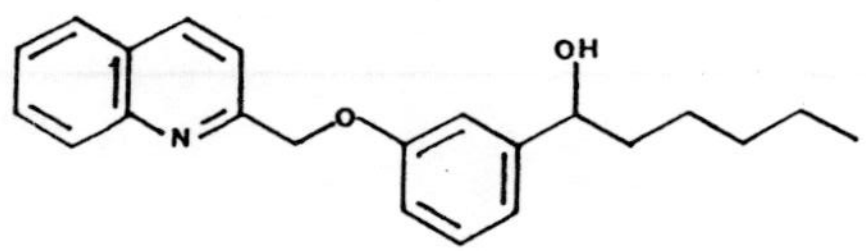	0.2–80 (RPMN/ RBL)	>100 (RP)	>200 (SSV)	Coutts *et al.* (1985)

Table 2 *Continued*

Drug	Structure	IC_{50} μM (cell type used)			References
		5LO	12LO	CO	
3. Miscellaneous					
Abbot	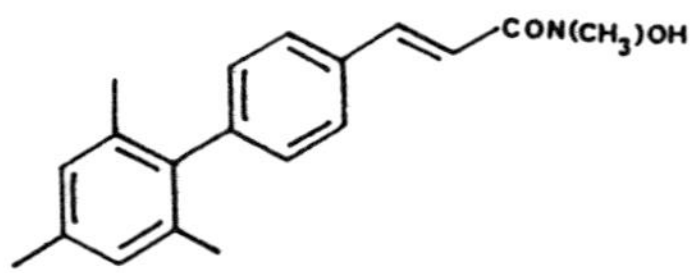	0.02 4 (RBL)	— 4 (HP)	— 100 (SSV)	Summers *et al.* (1987a)
BWA4C	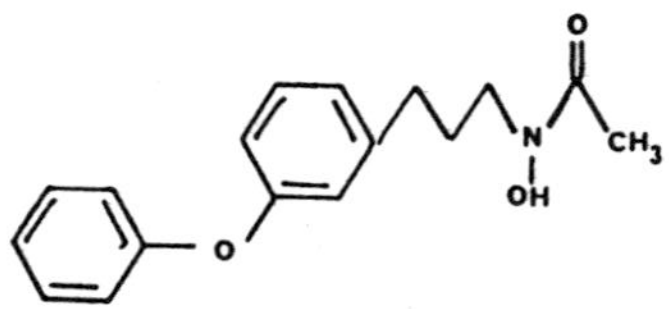	0.1 (HPMN)	—	3 (HPMN)	Tateson *et al.* (1988)
Piriprost	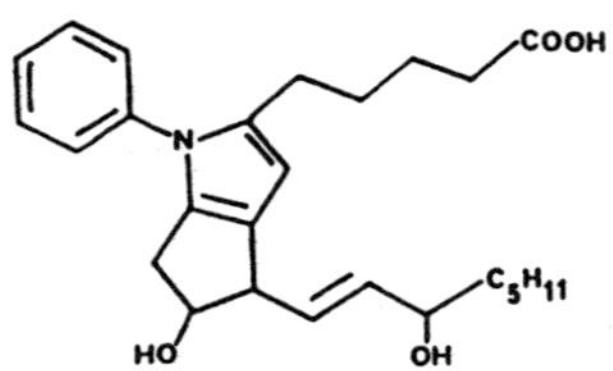	4 (HPMN)	>100 (HP)	>>100 (SSV/HP)	Sun and McGuire (1983)

Verapamil	—	2 (RBL)	—	—	Levine (1983)
FPL55712	See Fig. 7	20 (RBL)	—	>100	Casey *et al.* (1983)
Benoxyprofen	—	10–>100 (GPPMN/ HPMN)	>300 (HP)		Harvey *et al.* (1983), Masters and McMillan (1984)
Manoalide	See Fig. 3	0.3 (RBL)	>100 (HP/ME)	—	De Vries *et al.* (1988)

At present the 5-lipoxygenase inhibitors can be divided into 3 types, firstly antioxidants, secondly substrate analogues and finally a general or miscellaneous group.

1 *Antioxidants*

In vitro—Although a large number of chemical antioxidants also inhibit 5-lipoxygenase it seems unlikely that the two activities are linked in a simple way. If they were linked so then phenol, a typical antioxidant that inhibits most lipoxygenases, would also inhibit the 5-lipoxygenase. In fact, phenol does not inhibit the 5-lipoxygenase even at high concentrations (Egan *et al.*, 1983). As the number of compounds in the group is large they are also grouped by chemical structure.

BW755C and nafazatrom are structural derivatives of phenidone. No selectivity for the 5-lipoxygenase is present in this series, as all three compounds have comparable inhibitory potencies for the 5- and 12-lipoxygenases. Phenidone and BW755C also inhibit cyclooxygenase at the same or slightly lower concentrations, whereas nafazatrom is reported to be either inactive or to act as a stimulant of cyclooxygenase. A second group of three active compounds are catechols. They are much more potent than the phenidone derivatives as 5-lipoxygenase inhibitors and they seem to have greater selectivity for this enzyme relative to both the 12-lipoxygenase and cyclooxygenase.

AA861 is a benzoquinone that has been reported to have a high level of selectivity for the 5-lipoxygenase with at least 100-fold higher concentrations required to inhibit the 12-lipoxygenase and cyclooxygenase (Yoshimoto *et al.*, 1982). However, Nakadata *et al.* (1985), using a different enzyme source, showed that AA861 was a potent inhibitor of 12-lipoxygenase although it was again relatively weak against cyclooxygenase. Unfortunately these workers were unable to determine activity against 5-lipoxygenase in the same cell system as used for 12-lipoxygenase. It seems unlikely that such anomalous effects apply only to AA861 so caution should be used when interpreting such selectivity values.

The remaining antioxidant 5-lipoxygenase inhibitors are mixed structural types. Diphenyl disulphide has little or no activity on the soluble cyclooxygenase enzyme from RBL-1 cells. However, when tested against zymozan-induced leukotriene and prostanoid synthesis in intact murine peritoneal macrophages, it was equipotent against both enzymes; although the 5-lipoxygenase inhibitor potency of the compounds was reduced in comparison with the RBL-1 cells (Egan *et al.*, 1983). This suggested to this group that:

"in the whole cell system the diphenyl disulphide may not infuse to the 5-lipoxygenase enzyme but may be consumed by reacting with membrane sulfhydryl groups".

In vivo—BW755C is probably the most widely tested compound in animal models of asthma. This is unfortunate from the point of view of determining the role of 5-lipoxygenase in disease as it is a dual inhibitor of lipoxygenase and cyclooxygenase. Two studies that are representative of many involved the evaluation of BW755C against ovalbumin challenge of sensitized guinea-pigs and ozone-induced airway hyperreactivity in dogs (Andersson, 1982; Fabbri *et al.*, 1985). It significantly reduced the antigen responses in the guinea-pigs and blocked ozone-induced hyperreactivity in the dogs. Neither study, however, measured lipoxygenase or cyclooxygenase product levels and it is difficult to draw firm conclusions on the mechanism by which BW755C had its effects or the significance of 5-lipoxygenase products in the models used. AA861 also provided significant protection against ovalbumin-induced bronchoconstriction in sensitized guinea-pigs (Ashida *et al.*, 1983).

2 Substrate analogues

A number of research groups have produced structural analogues of arachidonic acid following early indications that such compounds could inhibit lipoxygenases (Vanderhoek *et al.*, 1980a,b; Corey and Parker, 1982; Sok *et al.*, 1982). Probably the most noteworthy of such analogues is REV5901 the structure of which is based upon 15HETE (Table 2). Although REV5901 has a higher potency in intact PMNs it is relatively weak against 5-lipoxygenase from cell free systems (Coutts *et al.*, 1985). This was thought to be due to the high uptake of this compound by cells and its low aqueous solubility. In addition to its lipoxygenase inhibitory activity it has been suggested that REV5901 is a leukotriene antagonist (Van Inwegan *et al.*, 1987).

3 Miscellaneous

It is not surprising that this is a structurally diverse group (Table 2). The intense interest in the 5-lipoxygenase pathway led to the evaluation of a wide range of new compounds. In addition, compounds active in other systems were evaluated for 5-lipoxygenase inhibitory activity and some, such as the leukotriene antagonist FPL55712 and the calcium antagonist verapamil, were shown to inhibit the enzyme albeit at high concentrations (Casey *et al.*, 1983; Levine, 1983).

In vitro—The most notable compounds in this category are the hydroxamic acids. The 5-lipoxygenase is thought to contain a catalytically important iron atom. It was postulated that this iron atom interacts in the vicinity of the C_5 of arachidonic acid where oxidation occurs. As hydroxamic acids are known to form strong complexes with a variety of transition metals it is not surprising to find that they inhibit the 5-lipoxygenase (Summers *et al.*, 1987a). Corey demonstrated that a hydroxamate bearing the first 10 carbons of the arachidonic acid and capped by a phenyl ring inhibits 5-lipoxygenase (Corey *et al.*, 1984). However, such compounds are chemically unstable and would probably be degraded rapidly *in vivo*. More recently two groups have identified potent and stable hydroxamates (Summers *et al.*, 1987b; Tateson *et al.*, 1988). The Abbott compound is the more potent of the two but it seems from similar compounds in this series that the hydroxamates have relatively low selectivities, as they are either equipotent or at best only 10–30 times weaker than 12-lipoxygenase or cyclooxygenase inhibitors.

In vivo—One of the main advantages of the hydroxamates relative to most of the other lipoxygenase inhibitors is that they are active *in vivo* (Summers *et al.*, 1987b; Payne *et al.*, 1988). BWA4C given orally to anaesthetized guinea-pigs markedly reduced the component of anaphylactic bronchoconstriction, shown to be leukotriene dependent. The inhibition persisted for three hours. Although endogenous leukotriene levels were not monitored in the study the model used had been thoroughly characterized and it seems likely that the inhibition does reflect a selective lipoxygenase effect.

Table 3 Selectivity of action of the most potent 5-lipoxygenase inhibitors. The inhibitory potencies and the selectivity ratios are taken from studies using different protocols consequently they only provide an approximate idea of activity. The higher the selectivity ratio the more specific the compound appears to be for the 5-lipoxygenase.

Compound	5LO potency (μM)	Selectivity ratio 5LO/12LO	5LO/CO
Linolenoyldopamine	0.003	—	1600
Abbot-hydroxamic acid	0.02	1	>25*
L651392	0.08	—	—
BWA4C	0.1	—	30
Quercetin	0.2	25	>500
KF8940	0.2	200	1000

*These values are extrapolated from a similar compound reported in the same study.

In Table 3 a summary of the existing 5-lipoxygenase inhibitors is given in order of decreasing potency. In addition to its highest potency as a 5-lipoxygenase inhibitor it can be seen that linolenoyldopamine is also the most selective compound with respect to potency against cyclooxygenase. However, no data exist on the activity of this compound *in vivo* and it seems possible that such a compound will have additional effects through adreno/dopamine receptors although no reports exist.

In general most of the lipoxygenase inhibitors that have been tested, to date, have good activity in animal models of asthma. This suggests that leukotrienes play a significant part in the acute bronchoconstrictor response to antigen challenge, although the absence of any concomitant assays of endogenous leukotriene levels warrants caution in the interpretation of the studies.

4 Clinical studies

Despite the immense effort devoted to the search for 5-lipoxygenase inhibitors relatively few have, as yet, been evaluated clinically in the field of allergy/asthma. (Table 4.)

In only two of these studies (nafazatrom and L652343) were endogenous leukotriene levels monitored to demonstrate if the drugs were inhibiting leukotriene biosynthesis. Both drugs were ineffective probably because of the low bioavailability and low potency for nafazatrom and L-652343 respectively. As yet only benoxyprofen, a weak dual inhibitor of lipoxygenase and cyclooxygenase, has been shown to have beneficial effects in asthma (Morley *et al.*, 1982). However, indomethacin had comparable effects in such a study suggesting that the lipoxygenase inhibitory activity of benoxyprofen was either of little additional value or, as seems more likely throughout this and all of the other clinical studies reported to date, that the lipoxygenase pathway was unaffected. Consequently, the conclusions of some of these studies on leukotriene involvement in allergy/asthma are questionable. The role of leukotrienes in these disease states can only be determined when a selective lipoxygenase inhibitor is evaluated concomitantly for efficacy and inhibition of endogenous leukotriene production.

III LEUKOTRIENE ANTAGONISTS

As described previously, a large amount of effort has been devoted to the pharmacology of SRS-A and the leukotrienes. Leukotrienes can be

Table 4 Clinical evaluation of lipoxygenase inhibitors in asthma and psoriasis. Inhibition of endogenous leukotriene production was only evaluated in the nafazatrom and L652343 studies. Two of the compounds (Piripost and REV5901) despite being ineffective caused side-effects of airway irritation/coughing and nausea respectively in some patients.

Drug	Route of administration and dose	Test	Comments	References
Benoxyprofen	Oral, 600mg	Allergen-induced early/late airway reactions	Indomethacin also effective suggests no lipoxygenase inhibition	Morley *et al.* (1982)
Piriprost	Inhaled, 1 mg	Allergen/exercise challenge	Ineffective (local irritant)	Mann *et al.* (1986)
AA861	Oral, 1.1 g (over 4 days)	ACh hyperreactivity	Ineffective	Fujimura *et al.* (1986)
Nafazatrom	Oral, 2 × 3 g	Allergen challenge	Ineffective (poor bioavailability)	Dollery *et al.* (1987)
L-652343	Oral, 750 mg	Psoriasis	Ineffective (no inhibition of endogenous LTD_4 levels)	Barr *et al.* (1988)
REV 5901	Oral, 1 g	LTD_4/histamine bronchoconstriction	Ineffective (nausea)	Evans *et al.* (1988a)

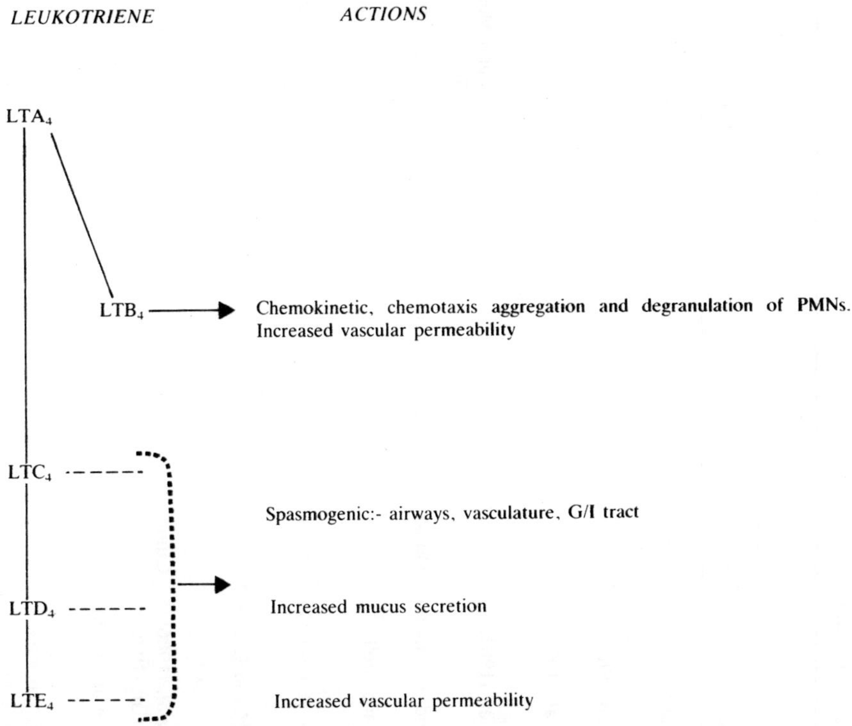

Fig. 6 Pathophysiological actions of leukotrienes. The leukotrienes can be divided into two types on both a structural and functional basis. LTB_4 is generally regarded as a pro-inflammatory agent with no direct spasmogenic activity whereas all three sulphidopeptide leukotrienes LTC_4, LTD_4 and LTE_4 are direct spasmogenic agents.

divided into two groups both on a structural and functional basis (Fig. 6). The first group are the sulphidopeptide leukotrienes LTC_4, LTD_4 and LTE_4. All three are spasmogenic agents that act directly on airway, vascular and other smooth muscles (Drazen *et al.*, 1980). In contrast the 5,12-diHETE leukotriene B_4 (LTB_4) has no sulphidopeptide group and has no direct spasmogenic activity. As previously mentioned this leukotriene is generally regarded as a pro-inflammatory mediator. The two groups of leukotrienes do have some similar actions. Firstly, they both have indirect spasmogenic activity induced by the stimulation of cyclooxygenase and/or phospholipase A_2, which leads to the synthesis/release of prostanoids (Dahlen *et al.*, 1983b). Secondly, both groups have been shown to increase vascular permeability another pro-inflammatory

Table 5 Pharmacological activity of hydroxyacetophenone analogues *in vitro* and *in vivo*.

	In vitro				*In vivo*			
Compound	Tissue	Leukotriene	Potency	References	Model	Leukotriene	Potency	References
FPL55712	Guinea-pig trachea	C_4	Inactive	Snyder and Krell (1984)	Guinea-pig	$C_4/D_4/E_4$	0.1–10 mg/kg i.v.	Jones and Mason (1985)
	Guinea-pig lung	D_4	pK_B 5.8–6.2	Snyder and Krell (1984)				
		C_4	Inactive	Krell *et al.* (1981)			Inactive orally	Jones and Mason (1985)
		D_4	pK_B 6.2–7	Krell *et al.* (1981)			IC_{50} 3–5 mg/ml aerosol	Jones and Mason (1985)
	Rat/rabbit lung strip and ferret trachea	C_4/D_4	Inactive	Piper and Samhoun (1981) Snyder and Krell (1986)	Monkey	C_4/D_4	Inactive i.v. Aerosol 10 mg/ml	Krell *et al.* (1986)
	Human bronchial muscle	C_4/D_4	pK_B 5.8–6.3	Buckner *et al.* (1986)	Sheep	D_4	Aerosol 10 mg/ml	Abraham *et al.* (1985)
	Human lung strip	C_4/D_4	pK_B 5	Gardiner and Cuthbert (1988)				
LY171883	Guinea-pig trachea	C_4 D_4	Inactive pK_B 6.4	Hand *et al.* (1986) Hand *et al.* (1986)	Guinea-pig	D_4	Oral 3–30 mg/kg	Fleisch *et al.* (1985)
	Guinea-pig lung strip	D_4 (No indo)	pK_B 6.5	Fleisch *et al.* (1985)				
	Human lung strip	D_4	pK_B 5.5	Cuthbert (personal communication)				

RO 23-3544	—	—	—	—	Guinea-pig	$B_4/C_4/D_4/E_4$	16–500 μg/ml	O'Donnell *et al.* (1987)
WY44329	Guinea-pig trachea	C_4 D_4	Inactive pK_B 6.5	Hand *et al.* (1986)	Guinea-pig	C_4/D_4	0.1 mg/kg i.v. orally inactive	Kreft *et al.* (1986)
L649923	Guinea-pig trachea	C_4	Inactive	Charette and Jones (1987)	Guinea-pig	D_4	5–10 mg/kg i.d.	Jones *et al.* (1986a)
		D_4/E_4	pA_2 7.2	Jones *et al.* (1986a)				
L648051	Guinea-pig trachea	C_4	Inactive	Charette and Jones (1987)	Guinea-pig	D_4	Inactive orally	Jones *et al.* (1986b)
		D_4/E_4	pA_2 7.3	Jones *et al.* (1986b)		C_4/D_4	ID_{50} 0.5 μg/kg i.v.	Jones *et al.* (1986b)
YM16638	Guinea-pig trachea	D_4/E_4	pK_B 7.1	Tomioka *et al.* (1988a)	—	—	—	—
	Guinea-pig lung	B_4	$IC_{50} 10^{-5}$M/L	Tomioka *et al.* (1988a)				
	Sheep trachea	C_4 D_4	Inactive pK_B 7.5	Tomioka *et al.* (1988b) Tomioka *et al.* (1988b)				
	Human bronchial muscle	$C_4/D_4/E_4$	pK_B 6.7–7.6	Tomioka *et al.* (1988a)				

effect thought to lead to oedema (Bray *et al.*, 1981; Hua *et al.*, 1985). As yet it is uncertain whether the two groups of leukotrienes induce indirect spasmogenic actions or increase vascular permeability by similar receptors/mechanisms. In contrast, the spasmogenic effects of the sulphidopeptide leukotrienes are strongly believed to act via specific receptor(s) that differ from the receptor(s) responsible for the pro-inflammatory actions of LTB_4 (Fleisch *et al.*, 1986).

A Antagonists of the sulphidopeptide leukotrienes

A wide range of sulphidopeptide leukotriene antagonists have been identified. They can be divided into the following four groups on the basis of their structures.

1 Hydroxyacetophenone analogues

In 1973, FPL55712 was shown to antagonize the spasmogenic activity of SRS-A (Augstein *et al.*, 1973). Shortly after the discovery of the structures of the leukotrienes, FPL55712 was shown to antagonize some of their actions. It competitively antagonizes one or more of the sulphidopeptides on the guinea-pig trachea and human bronchial muscle and is also effective against these leukotrienes in the guinea-pig *in vivo*, when given intravenously or by aerosol (Snyder and Krell, 1984; Buckner *et al.*, 1986; Hamel *et al.*, 1982; O'Donnel and Welton, 1984). This led to the development of a wide range of hydroxyacetophenones (Fig. 7). In general, all of these compounds have similar profiles of activity with respect to the leukotriene actions they antagonize but they differ in their potency, most active route of administration and/or duration of action. For example, FPL 55712 is only active by the intravenous and aerosol routes of administration whereas LY171883 is orally active (Table 5).

2 Leukotriene analogues

One approach frequently used to develop antagonists is to modify the structure of the endogenous agonist until partial agonism and eventually antagonism is achieved. However, relatively few reports exist on this approach with the leukotrienes, possibly because unlike the analogues of histamine or noradrenaline the synthesis of leukotrienes is complex, time consuming and expensive. In addition such structures are generally unstable.

Some limited studies have been reported in this area and some degree

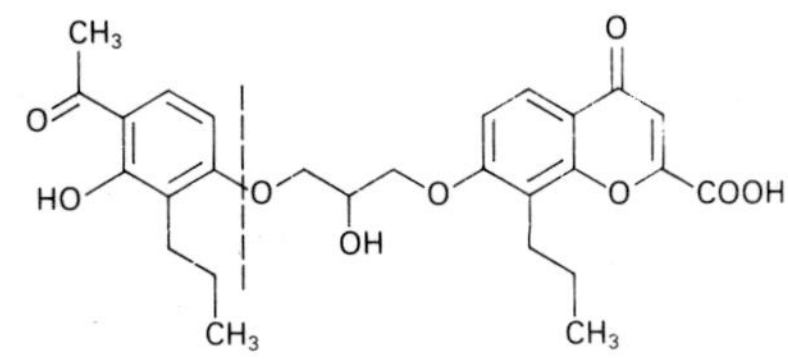

FPL55712

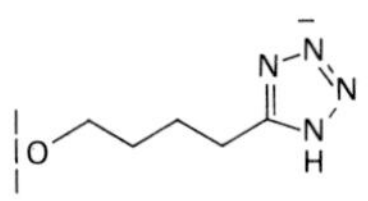

LY171883

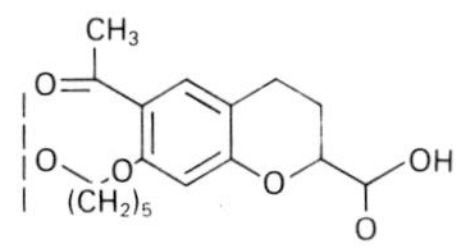

RO233544

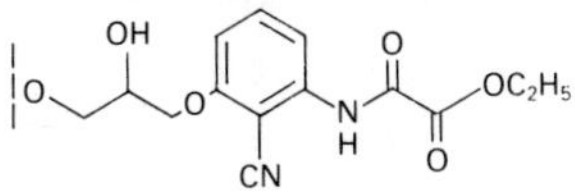

WY44329

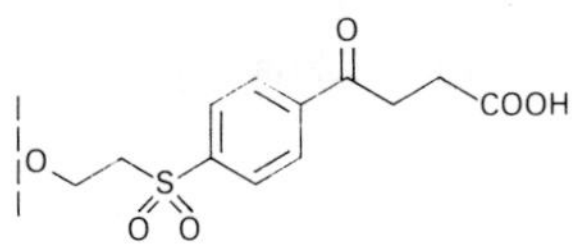

L649923

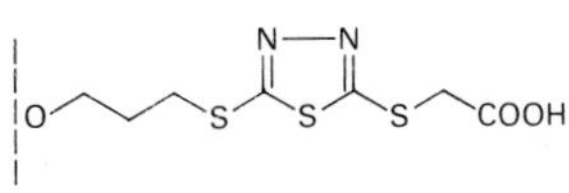

YM16638

Fig. 7 Sulphidopeptide leukotriene antagonists 1. Hydroxyacetophenone derivatives. FPL55712 was originally identified as an SRS-A and subsequently a leukotriene antagonist. This led to the synthesis of numerous additional hydroxyacetophenone analogues of which a representative few are shown here.

of success has been achieved with SKF104353. A good review of the programme of work which led to this compound is given by Perchonock *et al.* (1987). Briefly, the major compounds in the synthetic pathway are as follows (Fig. 8): SKF101132 is an analogue of LTD_4, which was the first pure leukotriene antagonist in this series, its main structural change was a shortened head chain and a saturated lipid tail. This was followed

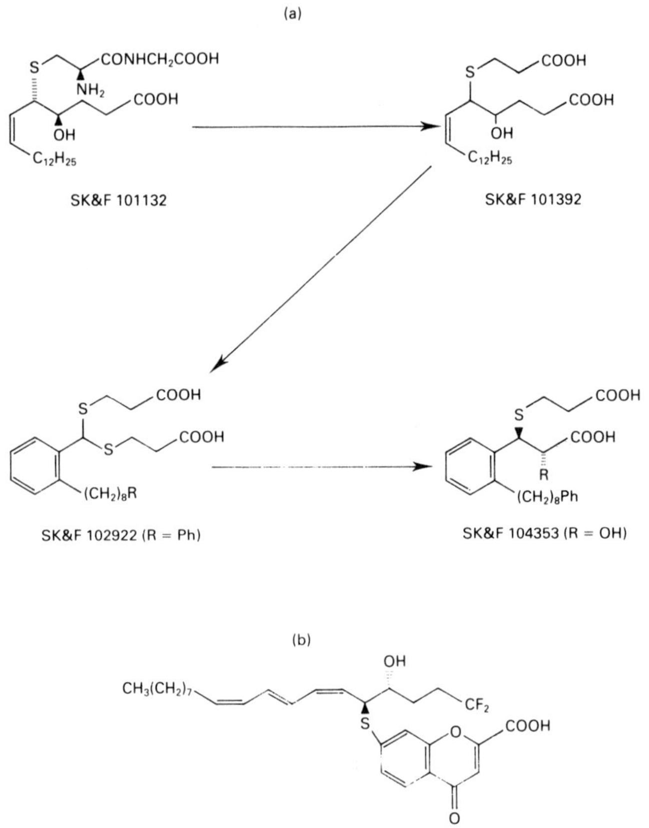

Fig. 8 Sulphidopeptide leukotriene antagonist 2. Leukotriene analogues. (a) This is a summary of the pathway of leukotriene analogue synthesis which eventually led to SKF104353. (b) This is one of the more recent analogues reported to antagonize LTD_4-induced bronchoconstriction in the anaesthetized guinea-pig (Sprecher *et al.*, 1988).

by a simplification of the peptide group which led to a ten-fold increase in antagonist potency (SKF101392). Metabolic stability of the molecule was enhanced by modification of the lipophilic tail (SKF102922). Finally, following further shortening of the head region the compound SKF104353 was developed and this has been shown to act as a potent antagonist of some leukotriene responses (Table 6). It generally has a higher potency than the hydroxyacetophenones. It is noteworthy, however, that the profile of antagonism of this leukotriene analogue is similar to that of the hydroxyacetophenones in that responses which are resistant to the latter (e.g. LTC_4 contractile effects on guinea-pig trachea) are also resistant to SKF104353.

SKF104353 has also been evaluated against Schultz–Dale responses using the guinea-pig trachea and human bronchial muscle (Hay *et al.*, 1987). It partially suppressed the secondary prolonged phase of the contractile response to antigen challenge. In combination with H_1 antagonists it markedly reduced the antigen-induced contraction on the guinea-pig trachea and abolished such responses on the human bronchial muscle.

More recently a further series of leukotriene analogues have been reported to act as antagonists of LTD_4-induced bronchoconstriction in the guinea-pig ((Sprecher *et al.*, 1988) Fig. 8). The two major structural changes of these analogues are replacement of the carboxymethylene group of the eicosanoid backbone by a trifluoromethyl group and replacement of the dipeptide sulphur side chain by other acidic residues. Although little detail was given with regards *in vitro* activity, selectivity, stability or optimum route of administration their potency when administered as aerosols seems impressive. The best compound has an IC_{50} of only 0.0007%. With so little experimental detail it is possible that this activity represents inhibition of indirect prostanoid mediated effects because we are not told whether the animals were pretreated with indomethacin. This possibility is made more likely by the fact that the compounds are reported to act as phospholipase A_2 inhibitors.

Table 6 Airway pharmacology of SKF104353.

Tissue/model	Leukotriene	Antagonist potency
Guinea-pig trachea	LTC_4	Inactive
	LTD_4	pA_2 8.6
	LTE_4	pK_B >8.9
Human bronchial muscle	$LTC_4/D_4/E_4$	pK_B 7.6–8.4
Human lung strip	LTC_4/D_4	*pK_B 6.4–7.2
Guinea-pig (anaesthetized spontaneously breathing)	LTD_4	Aerosol 10.2 μg inhibited bronchoconstriction of both large (airways resistance) and small (dynamic compliance) airways

*Personal communication from Cuthbert using ± SKF104353

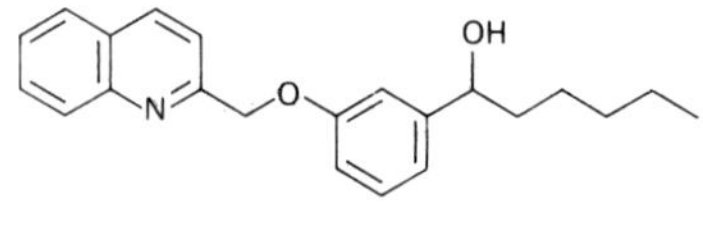

REV5901

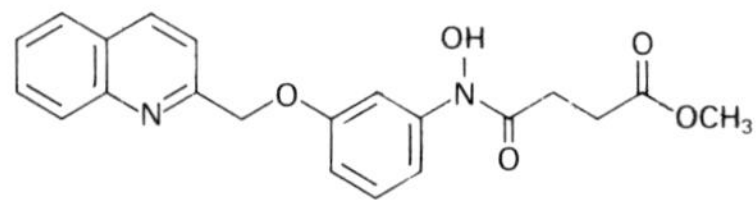

WY45911

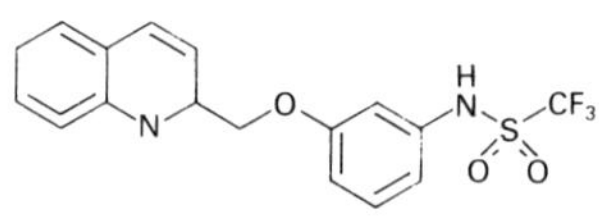

WY48257

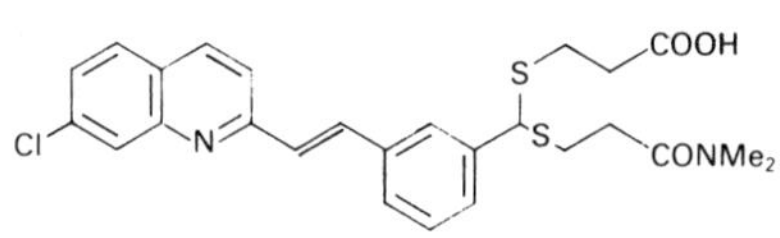

L660711

Fig. 9 Sulphidopeptide leukotriene antagonists 3. Quinoline derivatives.

3 *Quinolines*

This group of compounds probably originates from REV5901, which was initially identified as a lipoxygenase inhibitor. REV5901, however, was also described as an LTD_4 antagonist on the basis of its activity in the guinea-pig lung strip against LTD_4 and LTC_4 (in the absence of indomethacin) and in $^3HLTD_4$ ligand binding studies (Van Inwegan *et al.*, 1987).

A number of other quinolines have also been reported to act as leukotriene antagonists with the most recent being L660711. This compound seems to be a hybrid comprising a quinoline and the "head region" of the SK and F leukotriene analogues (Fig. 9). It can be seen that only the two most recent compounds in this series, WY48257 and L660711, are potent antagonists and both have been shown to be orally active (Table 7). L660711 was also evaluated against Schultz–Dale reactions on guinea-pig and human trachea. It blocked a small component of the guinea-pig contractile response, but produced complete blockage on the human tissue (Jones *et al.*, 1988). L660711 has also been evaluated against antigen-induced early and late airway responses in sheep (Abraham and Stevenson, 1988). Administered intravenously it was shown to block both types of response, but only the blockage of the late response was dose related.

4 *Miscellaneous*

A number of additional unrelated structures have also been reported to act as leukotriene antagonists (Fig. 10). Some of these, for example KC404, have numerous actions that cannot be related to leukotrienes, such as bronchodilatation (Nishimo *et al.*, 1983; Ohashi *et al.*, 1986).

Amongst the most notable of the miscellaneous group is the selective antagonist ICI198615 (Table 8). This compound is a hybrid structure of FPL55712 and LTC_4. It is one of the most potent and selective leukotriene antagonists *in vitro. In vivo* it is effective against bronchoconstriction induced by both LTD_4 and antigen in the guinea-pig. However, in the monkey, it is effective against LTD_4 but not against antigen (Patterson *et al.*, 1988). Whether this reflects a difference in the mediators that are involved in the antigen effects in the two species remains to be resolved.

At present a range of leukotriene antagonists are known and these have a wide variety of chemical structures. It is notable, that despite their structural differences and the differences that exist in potency, route of administration and duration of action, all antagonists are similar in their profile of interaction at leukotriene receptor(s). Despite an immense amount of effort no improvement in the "receptor profile" of the original compound, FPL55712 identified in 1973, seems to have been achieved. At present all of the known antagonists block LTD_4 contractile responses on the guinea-pig trachea, but none affect LTC_4 contractile effects on this tissue at least not when inhibitors of LTC_4 metabolism are present. Of course, these compounds do block both LTC_4 and LTD_4 on human bronchial muscle, but in our hands at least they tend to be much less active on human lung strip as well as being inactive on guinea-pig lung strip. In view of the limited profile of leukotriene antagonism of all the known compounds, the suggestion that any of them can provide an

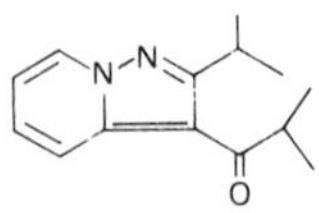

KC404

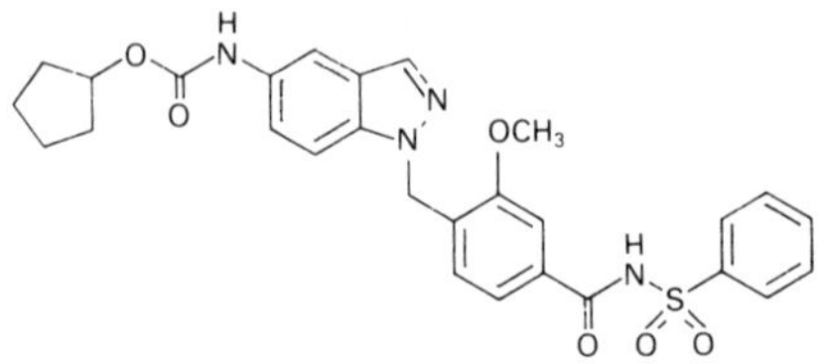

ICI198615

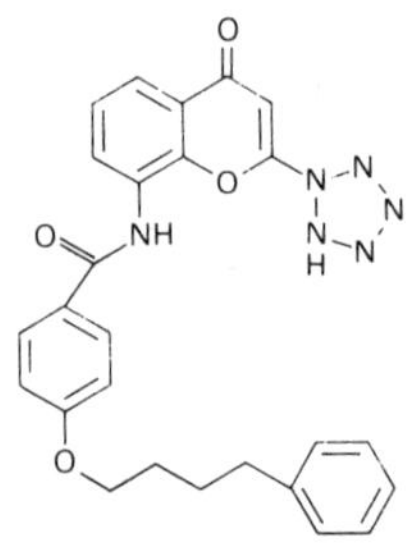

ONO RS-411/347/001

Fig. 10 Sulphidopeptide leukotriene antagonists 4. Miscellaneous.

unambiguous clinical test of the hypothesis regarding the aetiology of peptide leukotrienes in asthma seems misleading. Such a lack of ambiguity will only be achievable with compounds that block all leukotriene contractile receptors in the airways.

While on the subject of misleading suggestions it seems appropriate to correct another phrase commonly used in the literature relating to leukotriene receptors. Many antagonists are described as being "LTD_4 selective". This is misleading because of the ability of such substances to antagonize LTC_4-induced contractions of human bronchial muscle. At least four different types of leukotriene receptor may exist (Gardiner, 1989) and it seems rather misleading to designate any of them as an

Table 7 Airway pharmacology of quinoline analogues.

Compound	Tissue/model	Leukotriene	Antagonist potency	References
REV5901	Guinea-pig trachea	C_4	Inactive	Hand *et al.* (1986)
		D_4	pK_B 5.4	Hand *et al.* (1986)
	Guinea-pig lung strip	$C_4/D_4/E_4$	pK_B 5.5	Van Inwegan *et al.* (1987)
	Guinea-pig ventilated	D_4	i.d. 30 mg/kg 74% inhibition	Van Inwegan *et al.* (1987)
WY45911	Guinea-pig trachea	D_4	pK_B 5.3	Musser *et al.* (1986)
		C_4	Inactive	Chang *et al.* (1988)
	Guinea-pig ventilated	D_4	ID_{50} 3.3 mg/kg i.d.	
WY48252	Guinea-pig trachea	C_4	Inactive	Hand *et al.* (1987)
	Guinea-pig ventilated	D_4	ID_{50} 0.1 mg/kg i.g.	Hand *et al.* (1987)
L660711	Guinea-pig trachea	C_4	Inactive	Jones *et al.* (1988)
		D_4/E_4	pK_B 9.3	Jones *et al.* (1988)
	Human trachea	D_4	pA_2 8.5	Charette *et al.* (1988)
	Guinea-pig ventilated	$C_4/D_4/E_4$	i.v. 1–3 μg/kg	Masson *et al.* (1988)
		D_4	i.d. 500 μg/kg	
		D_4	aerosol 3 μg/kg	

Table 8 Airway pharmacology of a range of miscellaneous leukotriene antagonists.

Compound	Tissue/model	Leukotriene	Antagonist potency	References
KC404	Guinea-pig lung strip	C_4	Inactive	Ohashi *et al.* (1986)
		D_4	pA_2 7.4	Ohashi *et al.* (1986)
	Guinea-pig trachea	D_4	pA_2 6.5	Ohashi *et al.* (1986)
ONO347-411	Guinea-pig trachea	D_4	pK_B 7.5–8.4	Obata *et al.* (1985)
	Guinea-pig *in vivo*	$C_4/D_4/E_4$	ID_{50} 0.7–4.4 μg/kg i.v. ID_{50} 0.6–30 mg/kg p.o.	Obata *et al.* (1985)
ICI198615	Guinea-pig trachea	C_4	Inactive	Snyder *et al.* (1987)
		D_4/E_4	pK_B 9.3–10.3	
	Guinea-pig lung strip	D_4	pA_2 9.5	Snyder *et al.* (1987)
		C_4/D_4 (+ Indomethacin)	pK_B 5.3–5.7	Cuthbert (personal communication)
	Human bronchiole	C_4/D_4	pK_B 9.8	Snyder *et al.* (1987)
	Human lung strip	C_4	pK_B 6.5	Cuthbert (personal communication)
		D_4	pK_B 7.2	

"LTD_4" or an "LTC_4" receptor. Most antagonists appear to be effective against the leukotriene receptor(s) activated by LTD_4 and LTE_4 on guinea-pig trachea and against a second type or subtype of receptor activated by LTC_4, LTD_4 and LTE_4 on human bronchial muscle. However, the existing antagonists appear to be ineffective on the remaining two receptor types/subtypes. One found on the guinea-pig trachea activated by LTC_4 and the other found on human, rat and rabbit lung-strips activated by LTC_4 and LTD_4. More studies must be performed to resolve the leukotriene receptor types and subtypes.

5 *Clinical studies*

The hydroxyacetophenones were the first generation of leukotriene antagonists to be developed, and as such have been fairly extensively evaluated in the clinic (Table 9). The outcome of these studies were, however, rather disappointing. Of those compounds that were evaluated as antagonists of inhaled exogenous leukotrienes in man, none produced very significant antagonism. It was not surprising then to find that when the same compounds were evaluated against either allergen challenge or asthma itself none had significant beneficial effects. More recently the leukotriene analogue SKF104353 has been evaluated by inhalation against LTD_4 and histamine-induced bronchoconstriction in normals and mild asthmatics (Evans *et al.*, 1988c; Joos *et al.*, 1988). Although SKF104353 is approximately ten times more potent in animal studies than most hydroxyacetophenones, the study by Joos suggests that it produces less antagonism of LTD_4 induced bronchoconstriction than the hydroxyaceto-phenone L649923 in mild asthmatics. The results of the two studies with SKF104353 seem to differ, but this may be due to differences in procedure, dose administered or the patients studied (i.e. one study used normals and the other used mild asthmatics).

No clinical data is as yet available on the ICI antagonist.

B Antagonists of LTB_4

Although LTB_4 has no direct spasmogenic activity in the airways it has been proposed as a mediator of the inflammatory component of asthma. It is known to draw leucocytes into the airways, to promote adherence of these migrating cells to tissues and to induce the release of destructive hydrolytic enzymes (Ford-Hutchinson *et al.*, 1980; Smith *et al.*, 1980; O'Flaherty *et al.*, 1981).

Table 9 Clinical evaluation of sulphidopeptide leukotriene antagonists.

Compound	Clinical study	References	Comments
FPL55712 (aerosol)	vs. LTC_4 in normals	Holroyde *et al.* (1981)	n = 2 slight antagonism observed in one volunteer
	Mild asthmatics	Lee *et al.* (1981)	Slight improvement
LY171883 (oral)	Mild asthmatics	Cloud *et al.* (1987)	Reduction in bronchodilators required over 6 weeks
	vs. LTD_4 in normals	Phillips *et al.* (1987)	Four–six-fold shift LTD_4 dose–response curve
L649923 (oral)	vs. LTD_4 in normals	Barnes *et al.* (1987)	Weak antagonism—four-fold shift LTD_4 dose–response curve
	Antigen challenge asthmatics	Britton *et al.* (1987)	Little/no effect, gastrointestinal side effects
L648051 (aerosol)	vs. LTD_4 in mild asthmatics	Evans *et al.* (1988b)	Partial antagonism (no data supplied); no bronchodilatation
SKF104353	vs. LTD_4 in mild asthmatics	Joos *et al.* (1988)	Controversial—weak antagonism
	vs. LTD_4 in normals	Evans *et al.* (1988c)	Approximate two-fold shift single dose LTD_4
ICI204219	Not reported		
ONO RS-001	Not reported		

Less interest seems to have been paid to the development of LTB_4 antagonists, perhaps because of difficulties in the evaluation of such compounds. Unlike the spasmogenic leukotrienes it is difficult to assess pA_2/pK_B values for antagonism of chemo-taxis/kinesis or degranulation. Nevertheless, some antagonists have been reported (Fig. 11). Most of these compounds have been evaluated *in vitro* against LTB_4 and some, such as SM9064 and LY223982, seem to be potent antagonists (Table 10). SM9064 has been evaluated *in vivo* but this was not against LTB_4 and not in a model of asthma. Instead this compound was evaluated in the Arthus reaction in mice and carrageenin-induced oedema in the rat.

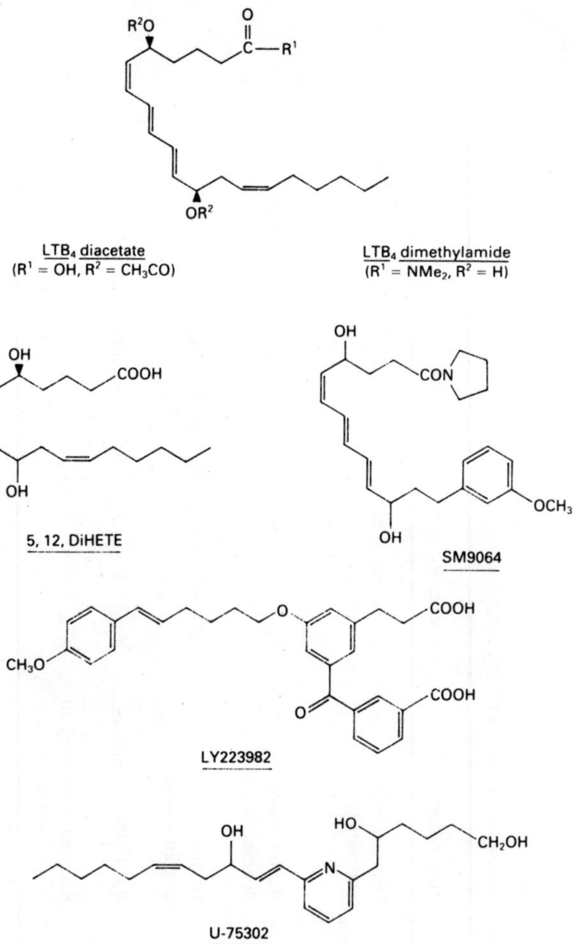

Fig. 11 LTB_4 antagonists.

The compound suppressed the Arthus response, but not surprisingly was inactive in the prostanoid dependent carrageenin test.

As yet no reports exist on the clinical evaluation of LTB_4 antagonists.

IV SUMMARY

At present only one group of inhibitors of phospholipase A_2, the glucocorticoids, is known to be effective in the treatment of asthma.

Table 10 Pharmacological activity of a range of LTB_4 antagonists.

Compound	Test system	Antagonist activity	References
LTB_4 diacetate	Human PMN chemotaxis	Competitive at equimolar concentrations to LTB_4	Goetzl and Pickett (1981)
LTB_4 dimethylamide	Rabbit PMN degranulation	K_D 2×10^{-7} M	Showell *et al.* (1982)
5,12 diHETE	Human PMN degranulation	42% Inhibition at 10^{-6} M	Feinmark *et al.* (1981)
SM9064	Rat PMN chemotaxis	IC_{50} 1.3×10^{-7} M	Namiki *et al.* (1986)
LY223982	Radiolabel binding to human PMN	IC_{50} 1.2×10^{-8} M	Gapinski *et al.* (1988)

However the glucocorticoids have numerous additional actions and, furthermore, the phospholipases influence the levels of prostanoid and PAF which like the leukotrienes, may have a significant role in asthma. Therefore, to conclude that phospholipase inhibition and reduction in leukotriene production are necessarily responsible for the beneficial actions of glucocorticoids would be short sighted. Although research is continuing with the aim of identifying more selective phospholipase (particularly PLA_2) inhibitors, new therapeutic candidates seem some way off.

The possibility of dietary manipulation of leukotriene synthesis and release seems unlikely to be useful in the treatment of asthma. Although leukotrienes of the 3 and 5 series are produced at the expense of the predominant naturally occurring 4 series, the spasmogenic activity of such compounds is as great or greater. Fish oil diets have been proven ineffective in a number of asthma studies and have even proven detrimental in aspirin sensitive asthmatics.

So far the areas of greatest interest with regard to the reduction of leukotriene effects, namely inhibition of the 5-lipoxygenase enzyme and antagonism of leukotriene actions have also proved disappointing in the treatment of asthma. In fact, as yet no 5-lipoxygenase inhibitor has been shown to inhibit the production of leukotrienes in the clinical situation. Similarly, the leukotriene antagonists that have been evaluated in man, have at best only produced a 2–10-fold reduction in the activity of exogenous leukotrienes and, subsequently, all of those reported have proved ineffective in asthma.

The role of leukotrienes in asthma is still uncertain. It will remain that way until selective inhibitors of either leukotriene biosynthesis or leukotriene activity are shown to be capable of reducing markedly the biosynthesis or the actions of leukotrienes in man. Then, and only then, can we expect to begin to understand the significance of the leukotrienes in this disease.

ACKNOWLEDGEMENTS

I am extremely grateful to Mrs M. Raynham for her patience in preparing this review and to Dr W.A. Taylor for his valuable constructive comments.

REFERENCES

Abraham, W.M. and Stevenson, J.S. (1988). A new leukotriene D_4 antagonist L-660711 blocks allergen-induced late responses in allergic sheep. *FASEB. J.* **2,** A1057.

Abraham, W.M., Russi, E., Wanner, A., Delehurst, J.C., Yerger, L.D. and Chapman, G.A. (1985). Production of early and late pulmonary responses with inhaled leukotriene D_4 in allergic sheep. *Prostaglandins* **29,** 715–726.

Andersson, P. (1982). Effects of inhibitors of anaphylactic mediators in two models of bronchial anaphylaxis in anaesthetised guinea-pigs. *Br. J. Pharmacol.* **77,** 301–307.

Arm, J.P., Horton, C.E., Mencia-Huerta, J.M., House, F., Eiser, N.M., Clark, T.J.H., Spur, B.W. and Lee, T.H. (1988). Effect of dietary supplementation with fish oil lipids on mild asthma. *Thorax* **43,** 84–92.

Ashida, Y., Saijo, T., Kuriki, H., Makino, H., Terao, S. and Maki, Y. (1983). Pharmacological profile of AA-861, a 5-lipoxygenase inhibitor. *Prostaglandins* **26,** 955–972.

Augstein, J., Farmer, J.B., Lee, T.B., Sheard, P. and Tattersall, M.L. (1973). Selective inhibitor of slow reacting substances of anaphylaxis. *Nature New Biol.* **245,** 215–217.

Barnes, N., Piper, P.J. and Costello, J. (1987). The effect of an oral leukotriene antagonist L-649923 in histamine and leukotriene D_4-induced bronchoconstriction in normal man. *J. Allergy Clin. Immunol.* **79,** 816–821.

Barr, R.M., Black, K., Dowd, P.M., Koro, O., Mistry, K., Isaacs, J.L. and Greaves, M.W. (1988). The *in vitro* 5-lipoxygenase and cyclo-oxygenase inhibitor L-652343 does not inhibit 5-lipoxygenase *in vivo* in human skin. *Br. J. Clin. Pharmacol.* **25,** 23–26.

Billah, M.M. (1987). Regulation of phospholipase A_2. *Ann. Reports Med. Chem.* **22,** 223–233.

Bittiner, S.B., Cartwright, I., Tucker, W.F.G. and Bleehen, S.S. (1988). A double-blind randomised placebo-controlled trial of fish oil in psoriasis. *Lancet* **i,** 378–380.

Blackwell, G.J. and Flower, R.J. (1978). 1 Phenyl-3-Pyrazolidone: An inhibitor of cyclooxygenase and lipoxygenase pathways in lung and platelets. *Prostaglandins* **16,** 417–425.

Blackwell, G.J. and Flower, R.J. (1983). Inhibition of phospholipase. *Br. Med. Bull.* **39,** 260–264.

Borgeat, P. and Samuelsson, B. (1979a). Transformation of arachidonic acid by rabbit polymorphonuclear leucocytes. *J. Biol. Chem.* **254,** 2643–2646.

Borgeat, P. and Samuelsson, B. (1979b). Arachidonic acid metabolism in polymorphonuclear leucocytes: Effects of ionophore A23187. *Proc. Natl Acad. Sci. USA* **76,** 2148–2152.

Borgeat, P. and Samuelsson, B. (1979c). Arachidonic acid metabolism in polymorphonuclear leucocytes. Unstable intermediate in formation of dihydroxy acids. *Proc. Natl Acad. Sci. USA* **76,** 3213–3217.

Borgeat, P. and Samuelsson, B. (1979d). Metabolism of arachidonic acid in polymorphonuclear leucocytes. *J. Biol. Chem.* **254,** 7865–7869.

Bray, M.A., Cunningham, F.M., Ford-Hutchinson, T. and Smith, M.J.H. (1981). Leukotriene B_4: A mediator of vascular permeability. *Br. J. Pharmacol.* **72,** 483–486.

Bray, M.A., Beck, A., Wenk, P., Marki, F., Subramanian, N., Niederhauser, W., Kuhn, M. and Sallmann, A. (1987). CGP 35949: A potent leukotriene antagonist and inhibitor of phospholipase. Biological profile. *Adv. Prostaglandins, Thromboxane and Leukotriene Research* **17,** 526–531.

Britton, J.R., Hanley, S.P. and Tattersfield, A.E. (1987). The effect of an oral leukotriene D_4 antagonist L-649923 on the response to inhaled antigen in asthma. *J. Allergy Clin. Immunol.* **79,** 811–816.

Brocklehurst, W.E. (1960). The release of histamine and slow-reacting substance (SRS-A) during anaphylactic shock. *J. Physiol.* **151,** 416–435.

Brocklehurst, W.E. (1962). Slow reacting substance and related compounds. *Progr. Allergy* **6,** 540–560.

Buckner, C.K., Krell, R.D., Laravuso, R.B., Coursin, D.B., Bernstein, P.R. and Will, J.A. (1986). Pharmacological evidence that human intralobular airways do not contain different receptors that mediate contractions to leukotriene C_4 and leukotriene D_4. *J. Pharmacol. Exp. Ther.* **237,** 558–562.

Casey, F.B., Appleby, B.J. and Buck, D.C. (1983). Selective inhibition of the lipoxygenase metabolic pathway of arachidonic acid by the SRS-A antagonist, FPL55712. *Prostaglandins,* **25,** 1–11.

Chang, J., Musser, J.H. and McGregor, H. (1987). Phospholipase A_2: Function and pharmacological regulation. *Biochem. Pharmacol.* **36,** 2429–2436.

Chang, J., Musser, J.H. and Hand, J.M. (1988). Effect of a novel leukotriene D_4 antagonist with 5-lipoxygenase and cyclooxygenase inhibitory activity, WY-45,911 on leukotriene D_4 and antigen-induced bronchoconstriction in the guinea-pig. *Int. Archs. Allergy Appl. Immunol.* **86,** 48–54.

Charette, L. and Jones, T.R. (1987). Effects of L-serine borate on antagonism of leukotriene C_4-induced contractions of guinea-pig trachea. *Br. J. Pharmacol.* **91,** 179–188.

Charette, L., Jones, T.R., Champion, E., Masson, P., Ford-Hutchinson, A.W., Dehaver, R., Pong, S.S., Belley, M., Frennette, R., Gauthier, J.Y., Leger, S., Rokach, J., Williams, M., Young, R.N. and Zamboni, R. (1988). *In vitro* pharmacology of L-660771 a new LTD_4 receptor antagonist. *FASEB. J.* **2,** A1264.

Cloud, M., Enas, G., Kemp, J., Platts-Mills, T., Altman, L., Townley, R., Tinkleman, D., King, T., Middleton, E., Sheffer, A. and McFadden, E. (1987). Efficacy and safety of LY171883 in patients with mild chronic asthma. *J. Allergy Clin. Immunol.* **79,** 256.

Corey, E.J. and Munroe, J.E. (1982). Irreversible inhibition of prostaglandin and leukotriene biosynthesis from arachidonic acid by 11,12-dehydro and 5,6-dehydroarachidonic acids, respectively. *J. Am. Chem. Soc.* **104,** 1752–1754.

Corey, E.J. and Parker, H. (1982). Irreversible inhibitors of the enzymic oxidation of arachidonic acid to 15-(Hydroperoxy)-5, 8, 11 (2), 13 (E)-eicosatetraenoic acid (15-HPETE) by 14, 15-dehydroarachidonic acid. *J. Am. Chem. Soc.* **104,** 1750–1752.

Corey, E.J., Cashman, J.R., Kantner, S.R. and Wright, S.W.J. (1984). Rationally designed potent competitive inhibitors of leukotriene biosynthesis. *J. Am. Chem. Soc.* **106,** 1503–1504.

Coutts, S.M., Khandwala, A., Van Ingram, R.G., Chakraborty, V., Musser, J.B., Jariwala, N., Dally-Meade, V., Ingram, R., Pruss, T., Jones, H., Neiss, E. and Weinryb, I. (1985). Arylmethyl phenyl ethers: A new class of specific inhibitors of 5-lipoxygenase. In *Prostaglandins, Leukotrienes and Lipoxins* (Ed. J.M. Bailey), pp. 626–637. Plenum Publishing, New York.

Dahlen, S.E., Hedquist, P., Hammerstrom, S. and Samuelsson, B. (1980). Leukotrienes are potent constrictors of human bronchi. *Nature* **288,** 484–486.

Dahlen, S.E., Hedqvist, P. and Hammerstrom, S. (1983a). Contractile activities of several cysteine-containing leukotrienes in the guinea-pig lung strip. *Eur. J. Pharmacol.* **86,** 207–215.

Dahlen, S.E., Hedqvist, P, Westlund, P., Granstrom, E., Hammarstrom, S., Lindgren, J.A. and Radmark, O. (1983b). Mechanisms of leukotriene-induced contractions of guinea-pig airways: Leukotriene C_4 has a potent direct action whereas leukotriene B_4 acts indirectly. *Acta. Physiol. Scand.* **118,** 393–403.

Davidson, F.F., Dennis, E.A., Powell, M. and Glenney, J. (1987). Inhibition of Phospholipase A_2 by lipocortins: An effect of binding to phospholipids. *J. Biol. Chem.* **262,** 1698–1705.

Dennis, E.A. (1987). Regulation of Eicosanoid production: Role of phospholipases and inhibitors. *Bio/Technology* **5,** 1294–1300.

De Vries, G.W., Amdahl, L., Mobasser, A., Wenzel, M. and Wheeler, L.A. (1988). Preferential inhibition of 5-lipoxygenase activity by manoalide. *Biochem. Pharmacol.* **37,** 2899–2905.

DiRosa, M., Flower, R.J., Hirata, F., Parente, L. and Russo-Marie, F. (1984). Nomenclature Announcement. Anti-Phospholipase Proteins. *Prostaglandins* **28,** 441–442.

Dollery, C.T., Fuller, R.W., Maltley, N. and Taylor, G.W. (1987). The effect of nafazatrom on allergen-induced bronchospasm. *Br. J. Clin. Pharmacol.* **23,** 619P.

Drazen, J.M., Austen, K.F., Lewis, R.A., Clark, D.A., Gato, G., Marfat, A. and Corey, E.J. (1980). Comparative airway and vascular activities of leukotrienes C-1 and D *in vivo* and *in vitro*. *Proc. Natl Acad. Sci. USA* **77,** 4354–4358.

Drenth, J., Enzing, C.M., Halk, K.H. and Vessies, J.C.A. (1976). Structure of porcine pancreatic prephospholipase A_2. *Nature (London)* **264,** 373–377.

Egan, R.W., Tischler, A.N., Baptista, E.M., Ham, E.A., Soderman, D.D. and Gale, P.H. (1983). Specific inhibition and oxidative regulation of 5-lipoxygenase. In *Advances in Prostaglandin, Thromboxane and Leukotriene Research*. vol. 11. (Eds B. Samuelsson, R. Paoletti and P. Rawell), pp. 151–157. Raven Press, New York.

Elsbach, P., Weiss, J., Franson, R., Beckerdite-Quagliata, S., Schneider, A. and Harris, L. (1979). Separation and purification of a potent bactericidal/permeability increasing protein and a closely associated phospholipase A_2 from rabbit polymorphonuclear leucocytes. *J. Biol. Chem.* **254,** 11000–11009.

Evans, J., Zamboni, R., Nathaniel, D., Leveille, C. and Ford-Hutchinson, A.W. (1985). Characterisation of biological properties of synthetic and biological leukotriene B_3. *Prostaglandins* **30,** 981–988.

Evans, J.M., Barnes, N.C., Piper, P.J. and Costello, J.F. (1988a). The effect of REV5901 on histamine and leukotriene D_4 induced bronchoconstriction in man. *Br. J. Clin. Pharmacol.* **25,** 111P–112P.

Evans, J.M., Barnes, N.C., Piper, P.J. and Costello, J.F. (1988b). The effect of a single dose of inhaled L-648,051 in mild asthma. *Br. J. Clin. Pharmacol.* **25,** 112P–113P.

Evans, J.M., Barnes, N.C., Zakrzewski, J.T., Glenny, H.P., Piper, P.J. and Costello, J.F. (1988c). Effects of an inhaled leukotriene (LT) antagonist SK&F 104353-Z_2 on LTD_4 and histamine induced bronchoconstriction in normal man. *Br. Pharmacol. Soc.* Abstract P61 Ireland 6–8 July 1988.

Fabbri, L.M., Aizawa, H., O'Byrne, P.M., Bethel, R.A., Walters, E.H., Mottzman, M.J. and Nadd, J.A. (1985). An antiinflammatory drug (BW755C) inhibits airway hyperresponsiveness induced by ozone in dogs. *J. Allergy Clin. Immunol.* **76,** 162–166.

Feinmark, S.J., Lindgren, J.A., Claesson, H.E., Malmsten C. and Samuelsson, B. (1981). Stimulation of human leucocyte degranulation by leukotriene B_4 and its ω-oxidised metabolites. *FEBS Letters.* **136,** 141–144.

Feldberg, W. and Kellaway, C.M. (1938). Liberation of histamine and formation of lysociethin-like substances by cobra venom. *J. Physiol.* **94,** 187–226.

Fischer, S., Struppler, M. and Weber, P.C. (1983). *In vivo* and *in vitro* effects of Nafazatrom (Bay g6575) an antithrombotic compound on arachidonic acid metabolism in platelets and vascular tissue. *Biochem. Pharmacol.* **32,** 2231–2236.

Fleisch, J.H., Rinkema, L.E., Haisch, K.D., Swanson-Bean, D., Goodson, T., Ho, P.P.K. and Marshall, W.S. (1985). LY171883, 1-<2-Hydroxy-3-Propyl-4<4-(1H-Tetrasol-5-yl) Butoxy > Phenyl > Ethanone, an orally active leukotriene D_4 antagonist. *J. Pharmacol. Exp. Ther.* **233,** 148–157.

Fleisch, J.H., Rinkema, L.E., Whitesith, C.A. and Marshall, W.S. (1986). Pharmacologic antagonism of leukotriene mediated events. In *The Leukotrienes: Their Biological Significance* (Ed. P.J. Piper). Raven Press, New York.

Ford-Hutchinson, A.W., Bray, M.A., Doig, M.V., Shipley, M.E. and Smith, M.J.H. (1980). Leukotriene B, a potent chemokinetic and aggregating substance released from polymorphonuclear leukocytes. *Nature,* **286,** 264–265.

Fujimura, M., Sasaki, F., Nakatsumi, Y., Takabashi, Y., Hifumi, S., Taga, K., Mifune, J.I., Tanake, T. and Matsuda, T. (1986). Effects of a thromboxane synthetase inhibitor (OKY-046) and a lipoxygenase inhibitor (AA-861) on bronchial responsiveness to acetylcholine in arthmatic subjects. *Thorax* **41,** 955–959.

Gapinski, D.M., Mallet, B.E., Froelich, L.L., Boyd, R.J. and Jackson, W.T. (1988). LY223982: A potent and selective antagonist of leukotriene B_4 structure activity relationships for the inhibition of LTB_4 binding to human neutrophils. *FASEB. J.* **2,** A1110.

Gardiner, P.J. (1989). Eicosanoids and airway smooth muscle. In *Pharmacology and Therapeutics*. (In press).

Gardiner, P.J. and Cuthbert, N.J. (1988). Characterisation of the leukotriene receptor(s) on human isolated lung strips. *Agents and Actions* Suppl. **23,** 121–128.

Goetzel, E.J. and Pickett, W.C. (1981). Novel structural determinants of the human neutrophil chemotactic activity of leukotrienes. *J. Expt. Med.* **153,** 482–487.

Guindon, Y., Girard, Y., Maycock, A., Ford-Hutchinson, A.W., Atkinson, J.G., Belanger, P.C., Dallob, A., DeSousa, D., Dougherty, H., Egan, R., Goldenberg, M.M., Ham, E., Fortin, R., Hamel, P., Hamel, R., Lau, C.K., Leblanc, Y., McFarlane, C.S., Piechuta, H., Therien, M., Yoakim, C. and Rokach, J. (1987). L-651,392: A novel, potent and selective 5-lipoxygenase inhibitor. In *Advances in Prostaglandin, Thromboxane and Leukotriene Research,* Vol. 17, (Eds B. Samuelsson, R. Paoletti and P.W. Ramwell), pp. 554–557. Raven Press, New York.

Hamel, R., Masson, P., Ford-Hutchinson, A.W., Jones, T.R., Brunet, G. and Piechuta, H. (1982). Differing mechanisms for leukotriene D_4-induced bronchoconstriction in guinea-pigs following intravenous and aerosol administration. *Prostaglandins* **24,** 419–432.

Hammerstrom, S. (1981). Leukotriene C_3, D_3, C_5 and D_5 slow reacting substances derived from eicosatrienoic acid (n-9) and eicosapentaenoic acid (n-3). In *SRS-A and Leukotrienes* (Ed. P.J. Piper), pp. 235–251. John Wiley,

Hand, J.M., Schwalm, S.F., Kreft, A.F., Chang, J. and Lewis, A.J. (1986). Comparison of leukotriene (LT) antagonist properties of WY44329, FPL 55712, LY 171883 and REV 5901 on isolated guinea-pig trachea. *Am. Rev. Respir. Dis.* **133,** A94.

Hand, J.M., Musser, J.H., Kreft, A.F., Schuralm, S., Englebach, I., Auen, M., Skowronek, M. and Chang, J.Y. (1987). UY-48252 (1,1,1-trifluoro-N-[3-(2-quinolinylmethyoxy) phenyl] methanesulfonamide). A selective orally active leukotriene antagonist. *The Pharmacologist* **29,** 174.

Harvey, J., Parish, H., Ho, P.P.K., Boot, J.R. and Dawson, W. (1983). The preferential inhibition of 5-lipoxygenase product formation by benoxyprofen. *J. Pharm. Pharmacol.* **35,** 44–45.

Hay, D.W.P., Muccstell, R.M., Tucker, S.S., Vickery-Clarck, L.M., Wilson, K.A., Gleason, J.G., Hall, R.F., Wasserman, M.A. and Torphy, T.J. (1987). Pharmacologic profile of SK & F 104353: A novel, potent and selective peptidoleukotriene receptor antagonist in guinea-pig and human airways. *J. Pharmacol. Exp. Ther.* **243,** 474–481.

Herxheimer, H. and Stresemann, E. (1963). The effect of slow reacting substance (SRS-A) in guinea-pigs and in asthmatic patients. *J. Physiol.* **165,** 78–79P.

Higgs, G.A., Flower, R.J. and Vane, J.R. (1979). A new approach to anti-inflammatory drugs. *Biochem. Pharmacol.* **28,** 1959–1961.

Hirata, F. (1981). The regulation of lipomodulin, a phosolipase inhibitory protein in rabbit neutrophils by phosphosylation. *J. Biol. Chem.* **256,** 7730–7733.

Holroyde, M.C., Altounyan, R.E.C., Cole, M., Dixon, M. and Elliott, E.V. (1981). Bronchoconstriction produced in man by leukotrienes C and D. *Lancet* **2,** 17–18.

Hope, W.C., Welton, A.F., Fiedler-Nagy, F., Batula-Bernardo, C. and Coffey, J.W. (1983). *In vitro* inhibition of the biosynthesis of slow reacting substance of anaphylaxis (SRS-A) and lipoxygenase activity by quercetin. *Biochem. Pharmacol.* **32,** 367–371.

Hua, X.Y., Dahlen, S.E., Lundberg, J.M. and Hedqvist, P. (1985). Leukotrienes C_4, D_4 and E_4 cause widespread and extensive plasma extravasation in the guinea-pig. *Naunyn-Schmiedbergs Arch. Pharmacol.* **330,** 136–141.

Huang, K.S., Wallner, B.P., Mattaliano, R.J., Tizard, R., Burne, C., Frey, C., Hession, P., McGray, P., Sinclair, L.K., Chow, E.P., Browning, J.L., Ramachandran, K.L., Tang, J., Smart, J.E. and Pepinsky, R.B. (1986). Two human 35Kcl inhibitors of phospholipase A_2 are related to substrates of pp60 v-src and of the epidermal growth factor receptor/kinase. *Cell* **46,** 191–199.

Irvine, R.F. (1982). How is the level of free arachidonic acid controlled in mammalian cells. *Biochem. J.* **204,** 3–16.

Ishihara, Y., Uchida, Y. and Kitamura, S. (1985). Measurement of leukotrienes in peripheral venous blood from patients with bronchial asthma. *Clin. Res.* **33,** 466A.

Isono, T., Koshikara, Y., Murota, S.I., Fukùda, Y. and Furukawa, S. (1985). Measurement of immunoreactive leukotriene C_4 in blood of asthmatic children. *Biochem. Biophys. Res. Commun.* **130,** 486–492.

Iwakami, S., Shibuya, M., Tseng, C.F., Hanaoka, F. and Sankawa, U. (1986). Inhibition of arachidonate 5-lipoxygenase by phenolic compounds. *Chem. Pharm. Bull.* **34,** 3960–3963.

Jackson, W.T., Boyd, R.J., Forelich, L.L., Goodson, T., Bollinger, N.G., Herron, D.K., Mallett, B.E. and Gapinski, D.M. (1988). Inhibition of LTB_4 binding and aggregation of neutrophils by LY255283 and LY223982. *FASEB. J.* **2,** A1110.

Jones, T.R., Davis, C. and Daniel, E.E. (1982). Pharmacological study of the contractile activity of leukotriene C_4 and D_4 on isolated human airway smooth muscle. *Can. J. Physiol. Pharmacol.* **60,** 638–643.

Jones, T.R. and Mason, P. (1985). Comparative study of the pulmonary effects of intravenous leukotrienes and other bronchoconstrictors in anaesthetised guinea-pigs. *Prostaglandins* **29,** 799–817.

Jones, T.R., Young, R., Champion, E., Charette, L., Denis, D., Ford-Hutchinson, A.W., Frenette, R., Gauthier, J-Y., Guindon, Y., Kakushima, M., Masson, P., McFarlane, C., Piechuta, H., Rokach, J., Zamboni, R., DeHaven, R.N., Maycock, A. and Pong, S.S. (1986a). L-649.923, Sodium (BS*,yR*)-4-3(4-acetyl-3-hydroxy-2-propylphenoxy) propyl-thio)-y-hydroxy-beta-methylbenzenebutanoate, a selective, orally active leukotriene receptor antagonist. *Can. J. Physiol. Pharmacol.* **64,** 1068–1075.

Jones, T.R., Guindon, Y., Young, R., Champion, E., Charette, L., Denis, D., Ethier, D., Hamel, R., Ford-Hutchinson, A.W., Fortin, R., Letts, G., Masson, P., McFarlane, C., Piechuta, H., Rokach, J., Yoakin, C., DeHaven, R.N., Maycock, A. and Pong, S.S. (1986b). L-648,051, sodium 4-[3-(4-acetyl-3-hydroxy-2-propylphenoxy)-propylsulfonyl]-y-oxo-benzenebutanoate: a leukotriene D_4 receptor antagonist. *Can. J. Physiol. Pharmacol.* **64,** 1535–1542.

Jones, T.R., Belley, M., Champion, E., Charette, L., DeHaven, R., Ford-Hutchinson, A.W., Frenette, R., Gauthier, J.Y., Leger, S., McFarlane, C.S., Masson, P., Piechuta, H., Pong, S.S., Rochach, J., Williams, M., Young, R.N. and Zamboni, R. (1988). Pharmacology of L-660711 a potent selective orally active LTD_4 receptor antagonist. *Am. Rev. Respir. Dis.* **137,** 427.

Joos, G., Pauwels, R., Kips, J. and Van der Straeten, M. (1988). The effect of aerosolised SKF 104353-Z_2 on bronchoconstriction induced by inhaled leukotriene D_4 in asthmatics.

In *Abstracts of the 23rd Annual Meeting Societas European Physiologiae Clinicae Respiratoire*. Athens, Greece June 20–24, 92S;.

Kellaway, C.M. and Trethewie, E.R. (1940). The liberation of a slow-reacting smooth muscle-stimulating substance in anaphylaxis. *Quart. J. Exp. Physiol.* **30,** 121–145.

Kitamura, S., Hashizume, K., Lida, T., Miyashita, E., Shirahata, K. and Kase, H. (1986). Studies on lipoxygenase inhibitors II. KF8940 (2-n-Heptyl-4-hydroxyquinoline-n-oxide), a potent and selective inhibitor of 5-lipoxygenase, produced by pseudomonas anethanica. *J. Antibiotics.* **39,** 1160–1166.

Kreft, A.F., Klaubert, D.H., Bell, S.C., Pattison, T.W., Yardley, J.P., Carlson, R.P., Hand, J.M., Chang, J.Y. and Lewis, A.J. (1986). Novel 1, 3-Bis (aryloxy) propanes on leukotriene D_4 antagonists. *J. Med. Chem.* **29,** 1134–1138.

Krell, R.D., Osborn, R., Vickery, L., Falcone, K., O-Donnel, M., Gleason, J., Kinsig, C. and Bryan, D. (1981). Contraction of isolated airway smooth muscle by synthetic leukotrienes C_4 and D_4. *Prostaglandins* **22,** 387–409.

Krell, R.D., Williams, J.C. and Giles, R.E. (1986). Pharmacology of aerosol leukotriene C_4- and D_4-induced alteration of pulmonary mechanics in anaesthetised cynomologous monkeys. *Prostaglandins* **32,** 769–780.

Krell, R.D., Giles, R.E., Yee, Y.K. and Snyder, D.W. (1987). *In vivo* pharmacology of ICI198615: A novel potent and selective peptide leukotriene antagonist. *J. Pharmacol. Exp. Ther.* **243,** 557–564.

Kremer, J.M., Michalek, A.V., Lininger, L., Huyck, C., Bigauoette, J., Timchalk, M.A., Rynes, R.I., Ziemeinski, J. and Bartholomew, L.E. (1985). Effects of manipulation of dietary fatty acids on clinical manifestations of rheumatoid arthritis. *Lancet* **i,** 184–187.

Kuehl, F.A., Dougherty, H.W. and Ham, E.A. (1984). Interactions between prostaglandins and leukotrienes. *Biochem. Pharmacol.* **33,** 1–5.

Lee, T.H., Walpost, M.J., Wilkinson, A.H., Turner-Warwick, M. and Kay, A.B. (1981). Slow reacting substance of anaphylaxis antagonist. FPL55712 in chronic asthma. *Lancet* **2,** 304–305.

Lee, T.H., Austen, K.F., Leitch, A.G., Israel, E., Robinson, D.R., Lewis, R.A., Corey, E.J. and Drasen, J.M. (1985). The effects of a fish-oil enriched diet on pulmonary mechanics during anaphylaxis. *Am. Rev. Respir. Dis.* **132,** 1204–1209.

Levine, L. (1983). Inhibition of the A23187-stimulated leukotriene and prostaglandin biosynthesis of rat basophil leukaemia (RBL-1) cells by non-steroidal anti-inflammatory drugs, antioxidants and calcium channel blockers. *Biochem. Pharmacol.* **32,** 3023–3026.

Mann, J.S., Robinson, C., Sheridan, A.Q., Clement, P., Bach, M.K. and Holgate, S.T. (1986). Effect of inhaled Piriprost (U-60257) a novel leukotriene inhibitor on allergen and exercise induced bronchoconstriction in asthma. *Thorax* **41,** 746–752.

Masson, P., Jones, T.R., Charette, L., Champion, E., McFarlane, C.S., Piechutta, H., Ford-Hutchinson, A.W., Belley, M., DeHaven, R., Frenette, R., Gauthier, J.Y., Leger, S., Pong, S.S., Rokach, J., Williams, H., Young, R.N. and Zamboni, R. (1988). *In vivo* pharmacology of L-660,711 a potent and selective leukotriene antagonist. *FASEB. J.* **2,** A1265.

Masters, D.J. and McMillan, R.M. (1984). 5-lipoxygenase from human leukocytes. *Br. J. Pharmacol.* **81,** 70P.

Morley, J., Fairfax, A.J. and Hanson, J.M. (1982). The role of phospholipid metabolites in airway hyperreactivity. In *Perspectives in Asthma* (Ed. J. Morley), pp. 219–234. Academic Press, London and New York.

Morris, H.R. and Wishka, D.G. (1988). Synthesis of novel antagonists of leukotriene B_4. *Tetrahedron Letters* **29,** 143–146.

Morris, H.R., Taylor, G.W., Piper, P.J., Sirvis, P. and Tippins, J.R. (1978). Slow-reacting substance of anaphylaxis* Purification and characterisation. *FEBS Letters* **87,** 203–206.

Morris, H.R., Taylor, G.W., Rokach, J., Girard, Y., Piper, P.J., Tippens, J.R. and Samhous, M.N. (1980). Slow reacting substances of anaphylaxis, SRS-A assignment of stereochemistry. *Prostaglandins* **20,** 601–607.

Murphy, R.C., Hammarstrom, S. and Samuelsson, B. (1979). Leukotriene C: A slow reacting substance (SRS) from murine mastocytoma cells. *Proc. natl Acad. Sci. USA* **76,** 4275–4279.

Musser, J.H., Kubrak, D.M., Chang, J., Lewis, A.J. (1986). Synthesis of [nappthalenyl-methoxy)- and [(quinolinyl methoxy)phenyl]amino] oxoalkanoic acid esters. A novel series of leukotriene D_4 antagonists and 5-lipoxygenase inhibitors. *J. Med. Chem.* **29,** 1429–1435.

Nakadate, T., Yamamoto, S., Aizu, E. and Kato, R. (1985). Inhibition of mouse epidermal 12-lipoxygenase by 2, 3, 4-trimethyl-6-(12-hydroxy-5, 10-dodecadiynyl)-1, 4-benzoquinone (AA861). *J. Pharm. Pharmacol.* **37,** 71–73.

Namiki, M., Igarashi, Y., Sakamoto, K., Nakamura, T. and Koga, Y. (1986). Pharmacological profiles of a potential LTB_4 antagonist SM-9064. *Biochem. Biophys. Res. Commun.* **138,** 540–546.

Nishimo, K., Ohkubo, H., Ohashi, M., Hara, S., Kito, J. and Irikura, T. (1983). KC-404: A potential anti-allergic agent with antagonistic action against slow reacting substance of anaphylaxis. *Japan J. Pharmacol.* **33,** 267–278.

Obata, T., Katsube, N., Miyamoto, T., Toda, M., Okegawa, T., Nakai, H., Kosuge, S., Konno, M., Arai, Y. and Kawasaki, A. (1985). New antagonists of leukotrienes: ONO-RS-411 and ONO-RS-347. In *Advances in Prostaglandin in Thromboxane and Leukotriene Research*, vol. 15, (Eds O. Hayaishi and S. Yamamoto), pp. 229–231. Raven Press, New York.

O'Donnell, M. and Welton, A.F. (1984). Pharmacologic properties of FPL55712 administered by aerosol. *Agents and Actions* **14,** 43–48.

O'Donnell, M., Welton, A.F., Crowley, H., Brown, D., Garippa, R., Cohen, N., Weber, G., Banner, B. and Lapresti, R.J. (1987). Pharmacological profile of RO 23-3544, a new aerosol active leukotriene receptor antagonist. In *Advances in Prostaglandin Thromboxane and Leukotriene Research,* Vol. 17, (Eds B. Samuelsson, R. Paoletti and P.W. Ramwell), pp. 512–518. Raven Press, New York.

O'Flaherty, J.T., Wukle, R.L., Lees, C.J., Shewmake, T.B., McCall, C.E. and Thomas, M.J. (1981). Neutrophil degranulation action of 5,12 dihydroxy-6,8,10,14-eicosatetraenoic acid and 1-0-alkyl-2-0-acetyl-sn-glycero-3-phosphocholine. Comparison with other granulating agents. *Am. J. Pathol.* **105,** 254–269.

Ohashi, M., Kanoi, R., Nishino, K., Sato, T. and Takayanagi, I. (1986). Antagonistic effect of KC404, a new anti asthmatic agent on leukotriene D_4-induced contractile responses in isolated guinea pig smooth muscles. *Prostaglandins* **32,** 875–888.

Parker, C.W., Jakschik, B.A., Muber, M.G. and Falkenheim, S.F. (1979). Characterisation of slow reacting substance as a familoy of thiolipids derived from arachidonic acid. *Biochem. Biophys. Res. Commun.* **89,** 1186–1192.

Patterson, R., Harris, K.E. and Krell, R.D. (1988). Effect of leukotriene D_4 (LTD_4) antagonist on LTD_4 and Ascaris antigen-induced airway responses in rhesus monkeys. *Int. Archs. Allergy Appl. Immunol.* **86,** 440–445.

Payne, A.N., Garland, L.G., Lees, I.W. and Salmon, J.A. (1988). Selective inhibition of arachidonate 5-lipoxygenase by novel acetohydroxamic acids: effects on bronchial anaphylaxis in anaesthetised guinea-pig. *Br. J. Pharmacol.* **94,** 540–546.

Perchonock, C.D., Torphy, T.J. and Mong, S. (1987). Peptidoleukotrienes: Pathophysiology, receptor biology and receptor antagonists. *Drugs of the Future,* **12,** 871–889.

Phillips, G.D., Rafferty, P. and Holgate, S.T. (1987). LY171883 as an oral leukotriene D_4 antagonist in non-asthmatic subjects. *Thorax* **42,** 723P.

Picado, C., Castillo, J.A., Schinca, N., Pujades, M., Ordinas, A., Coronas, A. and Agusta-Vidal, A. (1988). Effects of a fish oil enriched diet on aspirin intolerant asthmatic patients: a pilot study. *Thorax* **43,** 93–97.

Piper, P.J. and Samhoun, M.N. (1981). The mechanism of action of leukotrienes C_4 and D_4 in guinea-pig isolated perfused lung and parenchymal strips of guinea-pig, rabbit and rat. *Prostaglandins* **21,** 793–803.

Salmon, J.A. (1986). Inhibition of prostaglandin, thromboxane and leukotriene biosynthesis. *Ad. Drug Res.* **15,** 111–167.

Samuelsson, B., Dahlen, S.E., Lindgren, J.A., Rouzer, C.A. and Serhan, C.N. (1987). Leukotrienes and lipoxins: Structures, biosynthesis and biological effects. *Science* **237,** 1171–1176.

Schild, M.O., Hawkins, D.F., Mongar, J.L. and Herxheimer, H. (1951). Reactions of isolated human asthmatic lung and bronchial tissue to specific antigen. *Lancet* **2,** 376–382.

Schonfeld, W., Kuller, M., Knoller, J., Konig, W., Muller, H. and Van der Hardt, H. (1985). Leukotrienes and their metabolism in plasma and bronchial fluids. *J. Allergy Clin. Immunol.* **75,** 126A.

Showell, H.J., Otterness, I.G., Marfal, A. and Corey, E.J. (1982). Inhibition of leukotriene B_4-induced neutrophil degranulation by leukotriene B_4-dimethylamide. *Biochem. Biophys. Res. Commun.* **106,** 741–747.

Sinclair, H.M. (1952). Essential fatty acids and their relation to pyridoxine. *Biochem. Soc. Symp.* **9,** 80–99.

Smith, M.J.H., Ford-Hutchinson, A.W. and Bray, M.A. (1980). Leukotriene B: a potential mediator of inflammation. *J. Pharm. Pharmacol.* **32,** 517–518.

Snyder, D.W. and Krell, R.D. (1984). Pharmacological evidence for a distinct leukotriene C_4 receptor in guinea-pig trachea. *J. Pharmacol. Exp. Ther.* **231,** 616–622.

Snyder, D.W. and Krell, R.D. (1986). Pharmacology of peptide leukotrienes on ferret isolated airway smooth muscle. *Prostaglandins* **32,** 189–200.

Snyder, D.W., Giles, R.E., Keith, R.A., Yee, Y.K. and Krell, R.D. (1987). *In vitro* pharmacology of ICI 198615: A novel potent and selective peptide leukotriene antagonist. *J. Pharmacol. Exp. Ther.* **243,** 548–556.

Sok, D.E., Han, C.Q., Pai, J.K. and Sih, C.J. (1982). Inhibition of leukotriene biosynthesis by acetylenic analogs. *Biochem. Biophys. Res. Commun.* **107,** 101–108.

Sprecher, A.V., Beck, A., Lung, R.W., Anderson, W., Bray, M.A. and Marki, F. (1988). Novel leukotriene (LT) antagonists structure activity relationships of analogues of LTD_4. In *Biology of the Leukotrienes Annals New York Academy of Sciences.* **524,** 438–441.

Summers, J.B., Mazdiyasni, H., Holms, J.H., Ratajczyc, J.D., Dyer, R.D. and Carter, G.W. (1987a). Hydroxamic acid inhibitors of 5-lipoxygenase. *J. Med. Chem.* **30,** 574–580.

Summers, J.B., Gunn, B.P., Mazdiyasni, H., Goetze, A.M., Young, P.R., Bouska, J.B., Dyer, R.D., Brooks, D.W. and Carter, G.W. (1987b). *In vivo* characterisation of hydroxamic acid inhibitors of 5-lipoxygenase. *J. Med. Chem.* **30,** 2121–2126.

Sun, F.F. and McGuire, J.C. (1983). Inhibition of human neutrophil arachidonate 5-lipoxygenase by 6, 9-deepoxy-6, 9-(Phenylimino)- 6, 8-prostaglandin I_1 (v-60257). *Prostaglandins* **26,** 211–221.

Tateson, J.E., Randall, R.W., Reynolds, C.H., Jackson, W.P., Bhattacherjee, P., Salmon, J.A. and Garland, L.G. (1988). Selective inhibition of arachidonate 5-lipoxygenase by novel acetohydroxamic acids: biochemical assessment *in vitro* and *ex vivo*. *Br. J. Pharmacol.* **94,** 528–539.

Terano, T., Salmon, J.A. and Moncada, S. (1984). Biosynthesis and biological activity of leukotriene B_5. *Prostaglandins* **27,** 217–232.

Toda, M., Nakai, H., Sakuyama, S., Arai, Y., Kaneko, S., Ohno, H. and Okegawa, T. (1987). Development of 5-lipoxygenase inhibitor. In *Advances in Prostaglandin and*

Thromboxane Research. Vol. 17 (Eds. B. Samuelsson, R. Paoletti and P.W. Ramwell), pp. 768–770). Raven Press, New York.

Tomioka, K., Yamada, T., Mase, T., Hara, H. and Murase, K. (1988a). Pharmacological properties of the orally active leukotriene antagonist [[5-(I 3-(4-acetyl-3-hydroxy-2-propylphenoxy)-propyl]thio]-1,3,4-thiadiasol-2-yl]thio] acetic acid. *Arzneim-Forsch/Drug Res.* **38,** 682–685.

Tomioka, K., Jackowski, J.T. and Abraham, W.M. (1988b). Characterisation of sulfidopeptide leukotriene responses in sheep tracheal smooth muscle *in vitro. Abstract American Thoracic Society,* Las Vegas, USA p.100.

Van den Bosch, H. (1980). Intracellular phospholipases A. *Biochem. Biophys. Acta.* **604,** 191–246.

Vanderhoek, J.Y., Bryant, R.W. and Bailey, J.M. (1980a). 15-Hydroxy-5,8,11,13-eicosatetraenoic acid. *J. Biol. Chem.* **255,** 5996–5998.

Vanderhoek, J.Y., Bryant, R.W. and Bailey, J.M. (1980b). Inhibition of leukotriene biosynthesis by the leukocyte product 15-hydroxy-5, 8, 11, 13-eicosatetraenoic acid. *J. Biol. Chem.* **255,** 10064–10066.

Van Inwegan, R.G., Khandwala, A., Gordon, R., Sonnino, P., Coutts, S. and Jolly, S. (1987). REV 5901: An orally effective peptidoleukotriene antagonist, detailed biochemical/pharmacological profile. *J. Pharmacol. Exp. Ther.* **241,** 117–124.

Waite, M. (1985). Approaches to the study of mammalian cellular phospholipase. *J. Lipid Res.* **26,** 1379–1388.

Wallner, B.P., Mattaliano, R.J., Hession, C., Cate, R.L., Tizard, R., Sinclair, L.K., Foeller, C., Chow, E.P.P., Browning, J.L., Ramachandron, K.L. and Pepinsky, R.B. (1986). Cloning and expression of human lipocortin, a phospholipase A_2 inhibitor with potential anti-inflammatory activity. *Nature* **320,** 77–81.

Wallach, D.P. and Brown, V.J.R. (1981). Studies on the arachidonic acid cascade—1. Inhibition of phospholipase A_2 *in vitro* and *in vivo* by several novel series of inhibitor compounds. *Biochem. Pharmacol.* **30,** 1315–1324.

Willis, A.L. (1981). Nutritional and pharmacological factors in eicosanoid biology. *Nutrition Review* **39,** 289–301.

Yamada, K., Kumada, Y. and Kubo, K. (1985). KF4939, a new anti-platelet agent, inhibits activation of phospholipase C and A_2 in rabbit platelets. *Japan. J. Pharmacol.* **39,** 108–111.

Yoshimoto, T., Yokoyami, C., Ochi, K., Yamamoto, S., Maki, Y., Ashida, Y., Terso, S. and Shiraishi, M. (1982). 2, 3, 5-Trimethyl-6-(12-hydroxy-5, 10-dodecadinyl)-1, 4-benzoguinone (AA861), a selective inhibitor of the 5-lipoxygenase reaction and the biosynthesis of slow-reacting substance of anaphylaxis. *Biochem. Biophys. Acta.* **713,** 470–473.

Zakrzewski, J.T., Barnes, N.C., Piper, P.J. and Costello, J.F. (1985). Quantitation of leukotrienes in asthmatic sputum. *Br. J. Clin. Pharmacol.* **19,** 549P–550P.

4

Measurement of lung mucociliary clearance in man

Demetri Pavia

Clinical Research Department, Medical Division, Boehringer Ingelheim, Ellesfield Avenue, Bracknell, Berks RG12 4YS, UK

I INTRODUCTION

The lungs possess several mechanisms with which they are able to defend themselves from inhaled materials, keeping the lungs clean and sterile even when they are exposed to a polluted atmosphere. The host defence mechanisms of the tracheobronchial tree are divided into non-specific and specific. Mucociliary clearance is one of the lungs' non-specific host defence mechanisms and is the result of beating cilia propelling the overlying secretions, carrying both trapped inhaled material as well as locally produced biological debris, towards the epiglottis (Pavia, 1984a).

A Cilia

The mucociliary clearance mechanism operates from the level of the terminal bronchioles, i.e. 16th airway generation on Weibel's (1963) model of the human lungs, to the larynx, where the conducting airways are lined with a ciliated mucus secreting epithelium. Ciliated cells are characterized by their long cytoplasmic projections and numerous microvilli. Cilia are cellular projections, containing fibrils—essential for

ASTHMA REVIEWS VOLUME 2
ISBN 0-12-040922-4

the bending action of the cilia—surrounded by cytoplasm and enclosed by the membrane of the cell (Sleigh, 1981).

Each ciliated cell has some 200 cilia with each cilium having a diameter of the order of 0.3 μm. The length of the cilia varies at different levels of the airways (Serafini and Michaelson, 1977); for example, they are longer in the trachea (5–7 μm) than in the 7th airway generation (2–3 μm). The cilia beat in the periciliary (sol) layer, the thickness of which is approximately equivalent to the length of the cilia. The biochemical constitution and physical properties of the periciliary layer are still unclear. *In vitro* the cilia beat with a frequency of 13 Hz; there is some evidence suggesting that cilia beat more slowly in the distal airways than in the proximal airways. The beat cycle of a cilium starts with a recovery stroke, during which the cilium moves clockwise to one side of the cell near the surface, and finishes with an effective stroke when the cilium is extended and penetrates the mucus layer by 0.5 μm or so. In any one beating cycle, approximately one third of the time is taken by the effective stroke and two thirds by the recovery stroke. The tips of the cilia have a crown of "claws" which penetrate into the overlying mucus and help to propel it cephalad (Lopez-Vidriero, 1984). ATP and ATPase are thought to be the major source of energy for the beating action of the cilia. In the human respiratory epithelium ciliary activity is independent of nervous control and mechanical stimulation. Ciliary activity appears to be spontaneous, arising from a small group of active cilia beating in a co-ordinated manner, probably due to viscochemical coupling. β adrenergenic and cholinergic agonists have cilio-excitory properties (Melville and Iravani, 1974). Although the direction of ciliary beat varies between groups of cells, the overall direction of beat cephalad is similar between regions.

B Mucus

Lung secretions originate from five main sources:

(a) the submucosal gland, which is present primarily in the cartilaginous airways and is the main source of lung secretions;

(b) the goblet cell;

(c) the Clara cell, found mainly in the respiratory bronchioles;

(d) the type II cell, found in the alveoli and responsible for the production of surfactant;

(e) tissue fluid transudate (Lopez-Vidriero, 1984; Jeffery, 1987).

One estimate of the daily quantity of secretion travelling up the airways of the healthy human lungs gives a value of 10 ml (Torelmalm, 1960), although the figure of 100 ml has been proposed from data on animal studies and extrapolating to man. In patients with airways disease (e.g. bronchietasis, chronic bronchitis, asthma), the quantity of secretion produced daily in the lungs increases and it is quite common for chronic bronchitics to produce up to 200 ml of sputum in one day during exacerbations of their illness.

The transportation of secretions by the cilia in the lung is sometimes referred to as the "mucociliary escalator". However, unlike mechanical escalators that travel at a constant speed, the "mucociliary escalator" is one in which the speed progressively increases cephalad. In health the speed of the mucus in the trachea is of the order of 5 mm min^{-1}, in the main bronchi approximately half of that (Foster *et al.*, 1980) and in the terminal bronchioles 1/20 – 1/40 of the speed in the trachea (Yeates and Aspin, 1978). It has been suggested that the increase of the flow of the mucus cephalad, together with the progressive increase in the thickness of the epiphase is essential in order to handle: (a) the secretions that are converging from airways, with a total cumulative circumference at the foot of the "escalator" (i.e. 16th airway generation) of several metres to that at the top of the "escalator" (i.e. the trachea), which is only a few centimetres and (b) the extra secretions encountered *en route* and produced by the submucosal glands. Even though some allowance may be made for the loss of secretions due to evaporation, it has been found necessary to postulate that a certain amount of reabsorption of lung secretions—primarily in the distal ciliated airways where the secretions are more "watery"—must also be taking place (Asmundsson and Kilburn, 1970). This hypothesis evolved in order to explain how the fluid load of the "escalator", from the convergence of thousands of bronchioles leading to the trachea, does not give rise to a "log-jam" effect.

Tracheobronchial mucus, a non-Newtonian fluid, is viscoelastic in nature. There is evidence from studies carried out with synthetic materials of an optimal range of apparent viscosity and elasticity for mucus transport *in vitro*, using the frog palate technique. It is worth noting that *in vivo* lung mucociliary clearance in man has a weak correlation with the *in vitro* transport of sputum. Investigators, in trying to come to terms with the factors that play a role with the transportation of secretions, turned their attention to some other physical properties (Lopez-Vidriero *et al.*, 1986). Spinability —the capacity of the mucus to be drawn into threads under stretching—is a physical property of mucus, which is attracting attention (Puchelle *et al.*, 1983). Spinability is inversely proportional to apparent viscosity, but there appears to be no association between spinability and elasticity. Mucus transport *in vitro* appears to be better correlated with the spinability than with the apparent viscosity or elasticity. Other physical properties of mucus such as surface tension, tackiness and adhesion are under investigation, but their role on the transport of bronchial secretion, if any, has not as yet been elucidated.

Inhaled, insoluble particles, bacteria and viruses that deposit on the conducting ciliated airways, as well as locally produced biological debris will be trapped in the mucus and transported to the epiglottis, where they will either be swallowed into the stomach or expectorated and thus removed from the body. In health, particles deposited in the most distal ciliated airways will be cleared in a matter of hours and certainly within a day (Camner and Philipson, 1978). In lung disease, where this host defence mechanism may be compromised, clearance of particles from the most distal ciliated airways may well take in excess of 24 hours (Agnew *et al.*, 1981a). The efficacy of lung mucociliary clearance depends on the intricate inter-relationship between: (a) the integrity of the ciliated epithelium, (b) the ciliary beat frequency and co-ordination, (c) the ephiphase thickness as well as its biochemical and physical properties and (d) the thickness and consistency of the periciliary layer.

II EFFECT OF PHYSIOLOGICAL FACTORS ON LUNG MUCOCILIARY CLEARANCE

The effects of various physiological factors on lung mucociliary clearance have been investigated in man. There is no evidence of a difference in lung mucociliary clearance between males and females. On the other hand, lung mucociliary clearance has been reported to be reduced with age (Goodman *et al.*, 1978; Puchelle *et al.*, 1979). Although, in patients with hypersecretion, posture appears to play a role in the rate of clearance of their lung secretions and indeed is incorporated in chest physiotherapy in the form of postural drainage, in healthy subjects change of posture (e.g. from supine to upright position) makes no difference to the rate of removal of mucus from the lungs (Wong *et al.*, 1977; Pavia, 1984b).

In a study on healthy subjects (Pavia, 1984b) circadian rhythm (i.e. measuring clearance during the day vs during the night whilst awake) was found to have no effect on mucociliary clearance. Simple exercise, such as performing routine duties within a hospital, compared to relaxing (lying in a bed awake) does not have any effect on the rate of the removal of lung secretions in healthy subjects. However, vigorous exercise such as brisk pedalling on a bicycle ergometer, for say half-an-hour, compared to quiet breathing has been shown to result in a significant enhancement of lung mucociliary clearance in both healthy subjects (Wolff *et al.*, 1977) and chronic bronchitics (Oldenburg *et al.*, 1979). The healthy subjects during controlled eucapnic hyperventiliation increased their mucociliary clearance, though to only 50% of that achieved during exercise. In a carefully carried out study on healthy subjects it was shown that during "natural" night sleep *per se* lung mucociliary clearance was dramatically reduced (Bateman *et al.*, 1978; Pavia, 1984b).

A Smoking and lung mucociliary clearance

The histological changes that have been observed (Auerbach *et al.*, 1962) in the bronchial epithelium of cigarette smokers together with the reported *in vitro* ciliotoxic effects of cigarette smoke (Dalhamn and Rylander, 1965), gave rise to numerous studies seeking to establish the long-term and acute effects of cigarette smoke on lung mucociliary clearance in man.

Studies of the acute effects of cigarette smoke on lung mucociliary clearance have yielded conflicting results and are difficult to interpret because the number of cigarettes smoked and the period of time over which these cigarettes were smoked varies greatly. Our study (Pavia *et al.*, 1971) on 22 subjects who chain-smoked 2–5 cigarettes showed a significant retardation in whole lung clearance. This impairment however was reversible soon after cessation of chain-smoking.

Studies of the long-term effects of tobacco smoking have, on balance, shown an impairment of lung mucociliary clearance (Lourenço *et al.*, 1971). Camner and colleagues (1973b) studied the effect of giving up cigarette smoking in relatively asymptomatic smokers. This study revealed that the observed, depressed lung mucociliary clearance in these smokers returned to normal values within three months of cessation of smoking. In a group of patients with chronic bronchitis, who had given up cigarette smoking for at least one year, we were unable to show any difference in their mucociliary clearance compared to a matched group of chronic bronchitics, who were still smoking (Agnew *et al.*, 1982).

III TECHNIQUES FOR MEASURING LUNG MUCOCILIARY CLEARANCE IN MAN (Pavia *et al.*, 1983)

The measurement of the efficiency of mucus transport in the lungs is achieved primarily in two ways (Pavia *et al.*, 1980). The first entails the actual measurement of the flow of the mucus and the second the rate of removal of the deposited aerosols resulting in an index of mucus flow efficiency.

A Mucus velocity

Measurement of the linear flow of mucus involves the timing of the movement of marker(s), placed on the mucus, over a given distance in an anatomically well-defined airway, usually the trachea. Measurements of the mucus flow have been reported for the main bronchi. However, with the present state of technology, the measurement of flow of mucus from more distal airways is complicated by either the degree of invasiveness of the technique and/or the amount of overlap of the airways when visualized in a two-dimensional display.

There are essentially four techniques for measuring the speed of mucus in the human lung although only three of these, outlined here, are used by investigators at present (Fig. 1). The *cinefibrescopic technique*, developed by Sackner et al. (1973), utilizes Teflon discs (0.68 mm in diameter, 0.13 mm in thickness and weighing 0.13 mg) that are insufflated through the inner channel of the fibreoptic bronchoscope onto the tracheal mucosa in a circumferential distribution. The movement of these discs, which serve as markers of mucus flow, is filmed (Fig. 1a). By measuring the time taken to move a given distance a measure of tracheal mucus velocity (TMV) is obtained; usually the TMV quoted is the mean of measurements made on 10–20 discs. Using such a technique TMVs of 2.15 $\pm$ 0.55 cm min^{-1} have been reported for healthy, non-smokers (Santa Cruz *et al.*, 1974).

A modified version of the cinefibrescopic method is the *roentgenographic technique* (Friedman *et al.*, 1977). In this instance, Teflon discs coated with a radio-opaque substance, bismuth trioxide, are blown through the inner channel of a bronchoscope (located at the vocal cord level) into the trachea. The cephalad motion of the radiopaque particles in the trachea is recorded with a fluoroscopic unit provided with an image intensifier, television monitor and videotape. Several tracheal X-rays are taken at one minute intervals and the average distance travelled by several discs during the procedure is measured resulting in an average measurement of TMV (Fig. 1b). A lower (mean $\pm$ SD) TMV of 1.14 $\pm$ 0.38 cm min^{-1} has been reported using this technique for healthy, non-smokers compared to the more invasive cinebronchofibrescopic method.

The *radioaerosol boli technique* due to Yeates *et al.* (1975) entails the fast inhalation of radioaerosol from near total lung capacity so that the radioaerosol deposits predominantly in local concentrations in the large airways. The boli of radioaerosol transported up the trachea by ciliary action and their position can be recorded by a γ-camera (Fig. 1c). The TMV can then be determined from the measurement of distance moved by boli in a given time. This non-invasive technique gives a (mean ± SD) TMV of 0.44 ± 0.13 cm min^{-1}. The degree of invasiveness of a technique appears to be related to the measure of the rate of mucus flow (Clarke and Pavia, 1981).

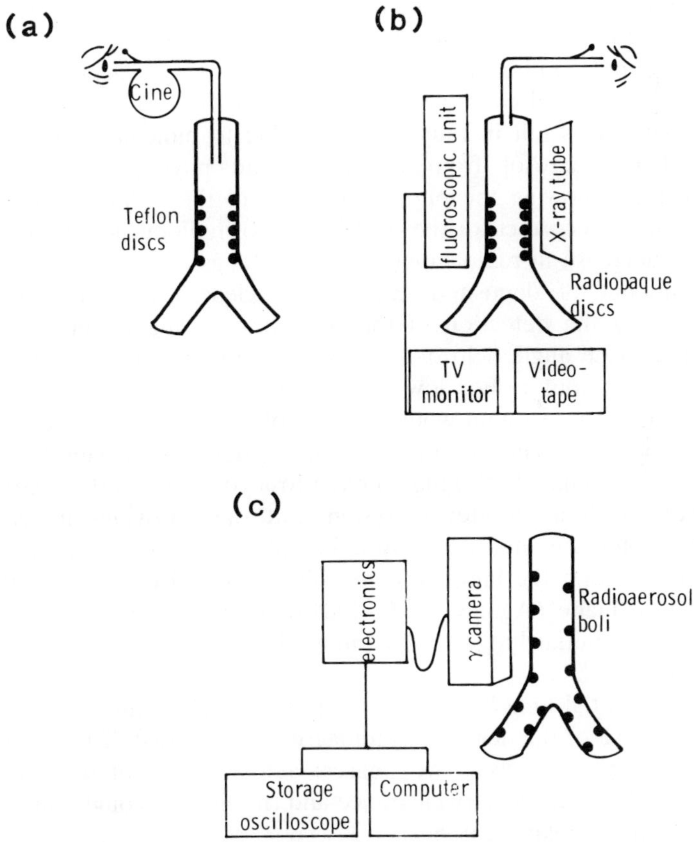

Fig. 1 Schematic diagrams of (a) the cinefibreoptic technique, (b) the roentgenographic technique and (c) the radioaerosol boli technique for measuring tracheal mucus velocity in man.

B Tracheobronchial clearance

The second approach for assessing lung mucociliary clearance efficiency involves the use of inhaled radioaerosol and was first reported by Albert and Arnett (1955). The method involves the inhalation of an aerosol that has been labelled in a fairly unleachable manner with a γ-emitting radionuclide. The aerosol particles must be insoluble in the fluids of the lungs and several types of materials have been used for measuring lung mucociliary clearance: Teflon, polystyrene, albumin microspheres, erythrocytes, iron oxide and resin (Amberlite IRP 67). Technetium – 99m (physical half-life: 6 hours; γ-ray energy: 140 keV) has been widely used to label the above aerosols. Measurement of the radiation emanating from the subject's chest, immediately after inhalation, gives a measure of the amount of radioaerosol which has been initially deposited within the lungs. Sequential counting after inhalation shows a decrease in lung radioactivity. This fall in radioactivity is due to biological clearance of deposited radioaerosol from the lungs and physical decay of the radionuclide. Knowing the physical half-life of the radionuclide, it is a simple matter to correct for the contribution of radionuclide decay to the observed decrease in radioactivity from the lungs.

The amount of deposited radioaerosol cleared from the lungs is monitored by the detection of the γ-radiation using either a suitably collimated (wide angle field of view) scintillation counter or a γ-camera linked to a computer. For low lung burdens (e.g. 1 μCi of 99mTc) a suitable monitoring system would be a whole body scanner, located in a well shielded room (Foord *et al.*, 1977). A large field of view γ-camera (in order to visualize both lungs) linked to a computer is the instrument of choice. Such a monitoring system not only provides information regarding retention of radioaerosol, but also permits a measure of its distribution within the lungs, thus enabling regional clearance measurements to be made (Agnew *et al.*, 1984b). If a γ-camera is to be used then a higher initial lung burden (approximately 100 μCi of 99mTc) is necessary.

A plot of initial lung burden (%) versus time after inhalation yields a clearance curve of the deposited radioaerosol (Fig. 2(a)). The whole lung clearance curve comprises two phases: a fast phase, of several hours duration, due to mucociliary clearance and (in disease) cough, and a slow phase due to alveolar clearance.

Clearance of deposited radioaerosol from the non-ciliated, alveolated regions is slow with a biological half-life of 3–4 months depending to some extent on the size and the type of material that is deposited there. The amount of radioaerosol present in the lungs after 24 hours is taken to represent the proportion of radioaerosol initially deposited beyond the

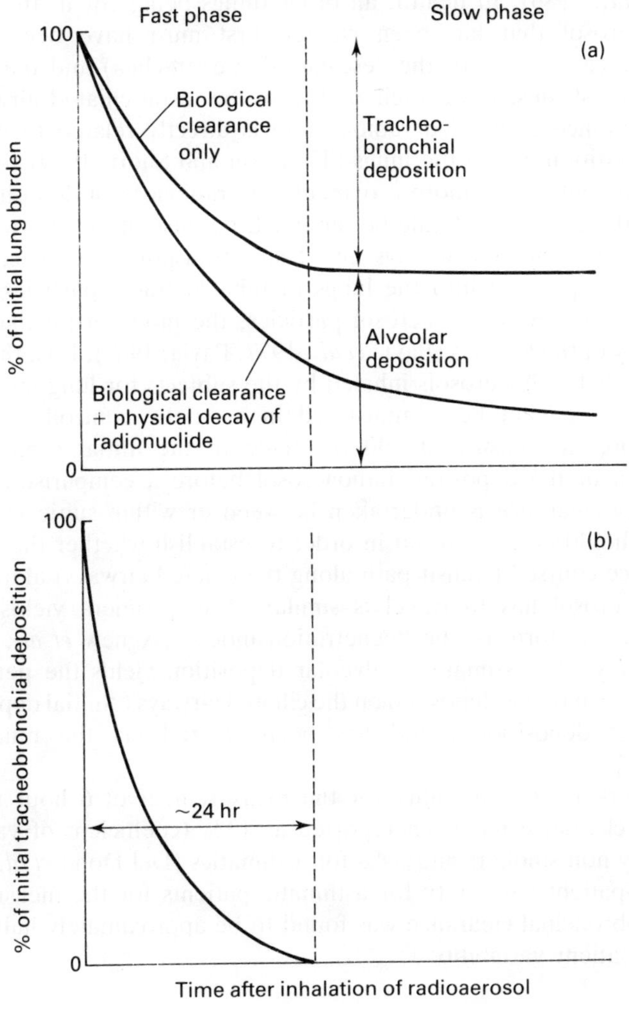

Fig. 2 Schematic diagrams for (a) whole lung and (b) tracheobronchial clearance curves of deposited radioaerosol.

reach of the "mucociliary escalator" (i.e. alveolar deposition) and is not available for mucus clearance (Camner and Philipson, 1978; Agnew *et al.*, 1981a). By subtracting this estimate of alveolar deposition from the whole lung clearance curve a 24 hour tracheobronchial clearance curve (Fig. 2(b)) can be obtained (Sutton *et al.*, 1981; Yeates *et al.*, 1981;

Foster *et al.*, 1980). In health, all other things being equal, the amount of radioaerosol that has been cleared first must have been initially deposited near the top of the "escalator" (i.e. trachea) and the amount coming up last must have originated from the distal ciliated airways.

The clearance of inhaled radioaerosol is directly related to its initial site of deposition within the lungs (Thomson and Short, 1969). All other things being equal, the more proximally the radioaerosol deposits within the lungs the quicker it should be removed, because of the shorter transit path along the ciliated airways and faster transport rate. Factors that govern the deposition into the lungs of inhaled tracer particles are the physical properties of the aerosol particles, the mode of inhalation and the patency of the airways (Pavia *et al.*, 1977; Pavia, 1988). It is, therefore, important that radioaerosols inhaled by the subjects for lung mucociliary clearance assessment be administered in a strictly controlled manner. Furthermore, a measure should be made of the initial topographical distribution of the deposited radioaerosol before a comparison of lung mucociliary clearance is undertaken between or within subjects. Such a measure should be carried out in order to establish whether the distance of the "race course" (transit path along the ciliated airways) along which the radioaerosol has to travel is similar. The γ-camera yields such a measure in the form of the "penetration index" (Agnew *et al.*, 1981b). Alternatively, the estimate of alveolar deposition yields the percentage of radioaerosol that is deposited on the ciliated airways ("initial deposition" – "alveolar deposition") and has been cleared via the mucociliary "escalator".

The inter-subject variability for the measurement of 6 hour tracheobronchial clearance has been reported as 13% (coefficient of variation) for healthy non-smokers and 39% for asthmatics (Del Dono *et al.*, 1988). The intra-patient variability for asthmatic patients for the measurement of tracheobronchial clearance was found to be approximately half that of the inter-patient variability.

IV EFFECT OF CHEMICAL MEDIATORS

A Cilia

Dulfano *et al.* (1982) reported the presence of a cilioinhibitory factor in the sputum of asthmatic patients, when incubated with strips of frog palate mucosa that has ciliated epithelium. The slowing down of the ciliary beat frequency was found, however, to be reversible and there was no evidence to suggest that it was related to structural damage. The same group (Dulfano and Luk, 1982) also showed the presence of this cilioinhibitory factor when they incubated human bronchial explants with the sputa taken from asthmatic (atopic and intrinsic type) patients. This cilioinhibitory factor was found in both types of asthmatic patients and was not related to the degree of eosinophilia. It is worth noting that a major basic protein isolated from the eosinophils of asthmatic patients, in whom it is found in large quantities, has been reported to induce ciliotasis (Frigas *et al.*, 1980, 1981). The cilioinhibitory factor was related to the "slurry" type of sputum produced by patients, it manifested itself more frequently during clinical exacerbations and its effect could be reversed by the removal of the sputum from the ciliated epithelium.

The cilioinhibitory factor was identified as having a molecular weight of 6000–8000.

Wanner *et al.* (1983) investigated the effects of several chemical mediators of anaphylaxis on ciliary beat frequency *in vitro*. The ciliated cells were obtained from the trachea of conscious sheep with a cytology brush. Leukotriene C_4 (LTC_4), prostaglandin E_1 (PGE_1) and prostaglandin E_2 (PGE_2) were found to be ciliostimulators; ciliary beat frequency increased by 7–33%. Histamine gave rise to a modest increase in ciliary beat frequency and then only at a relatively high concentration (in excess of 10^{-5} M). Prostaglandin $F_{2\alpha}$ ($PGF_{2\alpha}$) was without effect. No discoordination of ciliary movement was noted with any of the chemical mediators used.

The neuropeptide substance P (SP) is another agent involved in inflammatory reactions. Capsaicin induces an acute release of SP-like immunoreactivity from central and peripheral sensory nerve endings. Lindberg and Mercke (1986) reported that the administration of capsaicin (3.0–150 μg kg^{-1}) resulted in ciliostimulation in the rabbit maxillary sinus, which has ciliated epithelium, *in vivo*. This effect was attributed to the release of both SP and acetylcholine.

Yeates *et al.* (1988a) using the irritant capsaicin, which was delivered in aerosol form (3×10^{-9} M) to the lungs of anaesthetized dogs, confirmed the results of Lindberg and Mercke (1986). The ciliostimulation attributable to capsaicin appeared to involve multiple neurally initiated pathways, one of which may be peptidergic and two of which may involve the release of prostaglandins.

The ciliary beat frequency *in vitro* of ciliated epithelium, obtained with a cytology brush from the upper trachea of sheep with hypersensitivity to *Ascaris suum*, was measured before and after challenge with this antigen (Maurer *et al.*, 1982). Ciliary beat frequency showed a statistically significant increase of 14% after challenge, compared to baseline with return to normal values at 2 hours post-challenge.

Bradykinin is another mediator that is released in the airway during allergic challenge. Aerosolized bradykinin (10^{-5} M) given to anaesthetized dogs resulted in an enhancement of tracheal beat frequency (Yeates *et al.*, 1988b). The ciliostimulatory effect was completely inhibited by both hexamethonium bromide (2 mg kg^{-1}, i.v.) and indomethacin (2 mg kg^{-1}, i.v.), indicating that the stimulation of ciliary beat frequency by bradykinin requires both neural and cyclogenase pathways.

B Secretions

Alteration of the rate of water flow into the lumen of the airways as a result of the changes in the Na^+/Cl^- "ionic pump", enhancing chloride and water transport across the tracheal mucosa into the lumen, has been demonstrated with histamine (Marin *et al.*, 1977). Such an effect can, in theory, alter (a) the thickness and consistency of the periciliary layer and/or epiphase and (b) the coupling of the cilia with the epiphase thereby altering mucociliary transport.

Marom *et al.* (1982) used cultured human airways as a model for studying control of secretion. LTC_4 and LTD_4 were found to be potent secretagogues. Other mediators of anaphylaxis as a result of allergen interaction with IgE-sensitized mast cells, such as histamine and the prostaglandins $PGF_{2\alpha}$, PGD_2, PGI_2, PGE_1 and PGA_2 have also been reported to be secretagogues, although their potency is far less than those for leukotrienes. PGE_2 has been found to inhibit mucus secretion (Marom *et al.*, 1981).

Such alteration in the production of mucus output, with any accompanying changes in its physicochemical properties, may well give rise to altered mucociliary transport in the lungs.

V ASTHMA AND LUNG MUCOCILIARY CLEARANCE

The effect of various chemical mediators of anaphylaxis on mucus flow has been studied both in animals and man.

Maurer *et al.* (1982) challenged sheep with hyperresponsiveness to inhaled *Ascaris suum* with this antigen and measured their tracheal mucous velocity TMV before and after challenge. TMV was found to be statistically significantly reduced to 57% of baseline value following challenge. The same group (Russi *et al.*, 1983) administered aerosolized LTD_4 to sheep with hypersensitivity to inhaled *Ascaris suum* and examined its effect on tracheal mucus flow. Low doses of LTD_4 that were insufficient to induce bronchoconstriction resulted in a reduction in TMV. However, higher doses of LTD_4 that resulted in bronchoconstriction had no apparent effect on the flow of mucus in the trachea. This apparent discrepancy was attributed to opposing, but dose related, effects of LTD_4 on mucus output and ciliary beat frequency. These findings and those reported by Wanner *et al.* (1983) on the effects of chemical mediators of anaphylaxis on ciliary function would indicate that the reduction in mucociliary clearance during an allergic reaction is not due to a reduction in ciliary beat frequency.

In contrast to the above, histamine and acetylcholine, have been shown in dogs to enhance mucociliary clearance (Wanner *et al.*, 1975). In humans, the role of slow reacting substance of anaphylaxis (SRS-A) in mediating mucociliary dysfunction in allergic asthma was studied by Ahmed *et al.* (1981). Asymptomatic non-smokers with ragweed asthma had their specific airway conductance and TMV measured before and after bronchial challenge with ragweed extract. Doses of ragweed extract, which resulted in a decrease of specific airway conductance in excess of 35% from baseline, gave rise to an immediate decrease in TMV of approximately 26% from baseline with return to baseline values within 2 hours. These results suggested that SRS-A liberated during airway anaphylaxis impairs mucociliary clearance.

A Stable asthma

TMV was measured (Foster *et al.*, 1982) in stable asthmatic patients and healthy subjects and found to be (mean ± SEM) 0.25 ± 0.16 cm min^{-1} and 0.55 ± 0.04 cm min^{-1} respectively. These investigators also measured the main bronchus mucus velocity and found it to be in asthmatics 33% of that in healthy subjects. We have measured the lung mucociliary clearance of 25 stable asthmatics, none of whom were on oral steroid therapy (Bateman *et al.*, 1983b). The data of these patients were compared with those from 25 healthy, non-smoking subjects matched for sex and age. All patients and healthy subjects were non-smokers. Due to the statistically significant reduction in ventilatory function, the asthmatic group had a more central initial tracheobronchial deposition of inhaled radioaerosol compared to the healthy group. Despite this "unfair advantage", i.e. shorter transit path along the ciliated airways for the radioaerosol in the asthmatic group, mucociliary clearance was found to be significantly slower than in the healthy control group (Fig. 3).

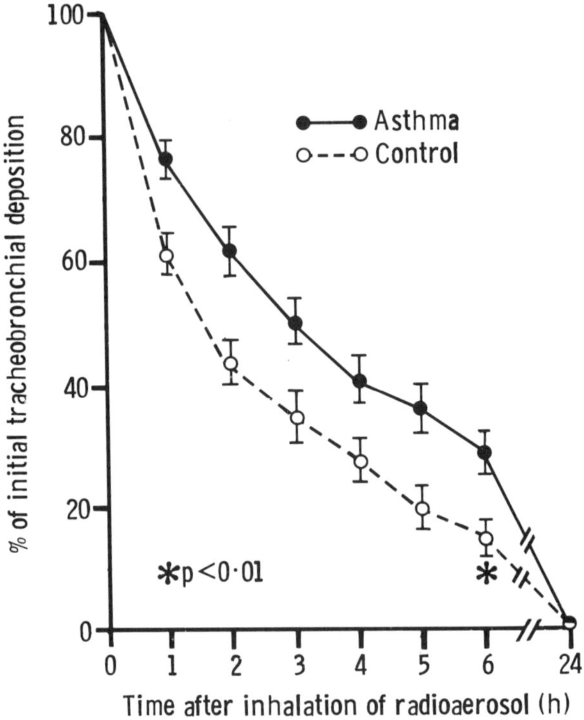

Fig. 3 Mean (±SEM) tracheobronchial retention curves for 25 patients with stable, mild asthma and 25 healthy control subjects. (With permission from Bateman *et al.*, 1983b).

B Asthma in remission

Reduction in mucociliary transport has also been reported in asymptomatic asthmatics. Mezey *et al.* (1978) found the TMV in six asymptomatic asthmatics with hypersensitivity to ragweed to be only 54% of that observed in healthy non-smokers. We have also measured lung mucociliary clearance in eight asthmatics, who were in complete remission at the time (Pavia *et al.*, 1985b), these patients were symptom free and required no medication whatsoever for a period of 1–6 months before entering the study. Their pulmonary function indices (for large and small airways) were within normal limits. The patients' data were compared with those of a control, non-smoking healthy group of subjects with similar physical characteristics and pulmonary function to those of the asthmatics.

Under identical experimental conditions the inhaled radioaerosol was deposited statistically significantly more proximally in the asthmatics than in the control group. This suggested an abnormal lung architecture (e.g. narrowing of the airways) in the asthmatics resulting in enhanced turbulence and premature deposition by impaction of the inhaled aerosol. When the healthy subjects were studied for a second time and inhaled the radioaerosol, on average, twice as fast as in their first assessment (i.e. under turbulent inspiratory flow conditions) they achieved approximately the same radioaerosol topographical deposition in their lungs as the asthmatics. Under such "fair race-course" conditions (i.e. similar transit paths along the ciliated airways) the lung mucociliary clearance for the asthmatics was found to be significantly poorer compared with the healthy group. These findings raised the question whether asthma ever remits completely, and if it does not, whether medication should be maintained during periods of apparent remission. Mucociliary clearance which is depressed after infection with *Influenza* A virus (Camner *et al.*, 1973a) and *Mycoplasma pneumoniae* (Jarstrand *et al.*, 1974) reverts back to normal levels after a period of several months.

In another study (Bateman *et al.*, 1983a), we measured the lung mucociliary clearance in a group of asthmatic patients who were hospitalized because of an acute exacerbation of their asthma. The first measurement was performed within 5 days of their admission to hospital. Their lung mucociliary clearance was also measured 2 weeks and 2–4 months after admission to hospital. The data suggest that the reduced lung mucociliary clearance that was observed in these patients following their hospitalization showed no sign of improvement 2–4 months later.

C Sleep

The observed retardation in lung mucociliary clearance during sleep, *per se* in healthy subjects, raised the question as to whether the same was true in asthmatics. Any such further delay in clearance of secretions in asthmatics during sleep may contribute to airways obstruction and early-morning cough, sputum and wheeze. Ten stable asthmatics with an (mean ± SEM) age of 34 ± 4 years, were studied on two occasions in a randomized, cross-over fashion. The two assessments involved a day-active and a night-asleep run with a mean period of sleep of 5.25 hours. A statistically significant delay in lung mucociliary clearance was observed during sleep (Fig. 4), which was approximately 60% of that achieved during the day-active run (Pavia, 1984b; Pavia *et al.*, 1985a).

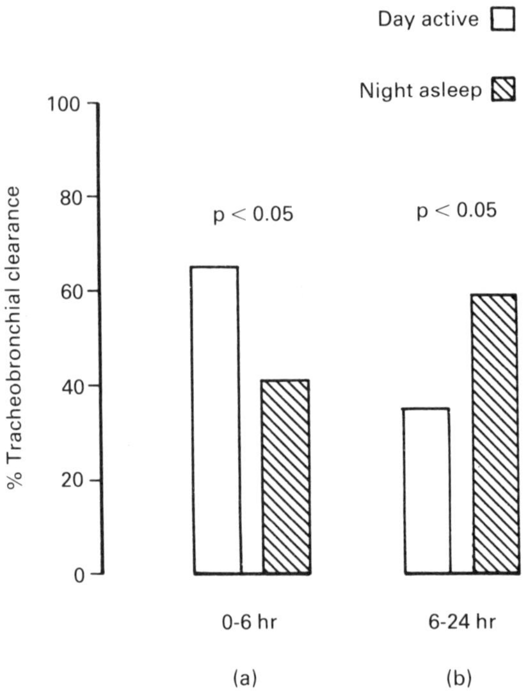

Fig. 4 Mean tracheobronchial clearance for ten asthmatics measured during day-active and night-asleep runs for (a) the initial 6 hours when the patients were asleep during the night as opposed to being awake during the day run and (b) the ensuing 18 hours (i.e. 6–24 hours after inhalation of the test radioaerosol). (With permission from: D. Pavia *et al.*, 1985a).

VI EFFECT OF PHARMACOLOGICAL AGENTS ON LUNG MUCOCILIARY CLEARANCE

A β-Agonists

β_2 adrenoceptor agonists are potent bronchodilators and are widely used in the therapy of obstructive lung disease. Such drugs, however, have an additional role of enhancing depressed clearance of lung secretions. This enhancement of lung mucociliary clearance has been attributed to stimulation of ciliary beat frequency and/or type of mucus secretion. β_2 adrenoceptor agonists have been shown to increase the rate of glycoprotein secretion in human bronchi *in vitro* and this is a strong indication that they must increase the rate of mucus production (Phipps *et al.*, 1982). β_2 agonists apparently have been found not to have an effect on ion flux in human bronchial epithelium (Knowles *et al.*, 1982); this finding is in contrast to the positive effect reported in dogs (Davis *et al.*, 1979). *In vitro* studies have shown that isoproterenol (Verdugo *et al.*, 1980) and terbutaline (Clarke and Lopez-Vidriero, 1982) stimulate the activity of ciliated cells of the respiratory epithelium, obtained from animals or humans, and that this effect is β-adrenoceptor specific as the observed stimulation can be blocked by propanolol.

Studies of oral, subcutaneous or topical administration of β^2 adrenoceptor drugs on lung mucociliary clearance of healthy subjects and patients, although they have yielded some conflicting results, they have, in general, demonstrated an enhancement of mucus clearance (Sackner, 1973; Wanner, 1979). It would appear that one needs to administer at least 2.5 times the normal recommended therapeutic dose (for bronchodilatation) from metered-dose inhalers to achieve enhancement of mucus clearance as well (Pavia *et al.*, 1984; 1987).

B Anticholinergics

The bronchodilator properties of anticholinergic drugs are well known (Kennedy *et al.*, 1964). However, their widespread use has not been advocated, mainly because of the possibility of mucus retention in the lungs. Anticholinergic drugs have been shown to reduce sputum production and ciliary beat frequency. Both of these effects could, in theory, inhibit the removal of lung secretions in asthmatic patients who already have an inefficient clearance of lung secretions and potentially cause plugging. Some studies have shown that the oral or parenteral administration of anticholinergic drugs, such as hyoscine (Pavia and Thomson, 1971) and atropine (Annis *et al.*, 1976) results in a slowing of lung mucociliary clearance. Interestingly the topical administration of the synthetic anticholinergic bronchodilator ipratropium bromide when given to asthmatic patients as a single dose (Foster *et al.*, 1983) or as a high dose (five times the normal recommended dose) for up to four weeks (Taylor *et al.*, 1986) has been shown not to alter mucociliary clearance (Fig. 5). More recently, we have demonstrated that the longer acting synthetic anticholinergic bronchodilator oxitropium bromide has no effect on lung mucociliary clearance in asthmatics after four weeks' treatment (Pavia *et al.*, 1989). It is worth noting that the dose of a bronchodilating drug delivered to the lungs from a metered-dose inhaler is small, since less

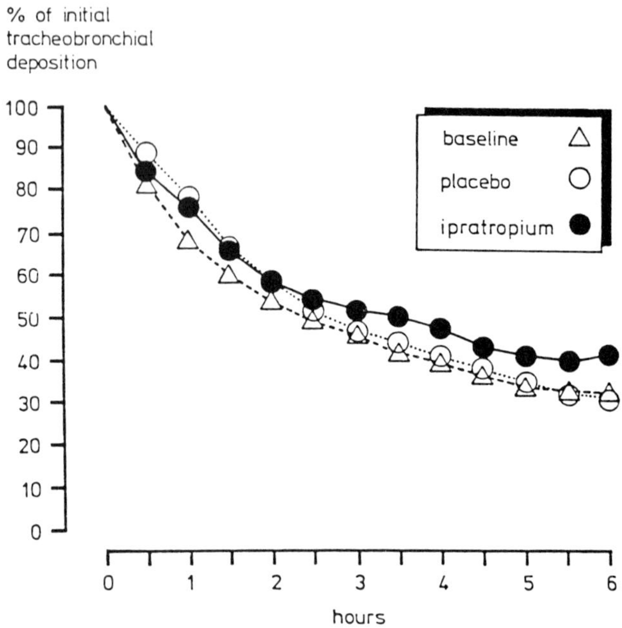

Fig. 5 Mean tracheobronchial retention at half hourly intervals for 15 patients (8 chronic bronchitics and 7 asthmatics) for baseline run and after four weeks' treatment with placebo and ipratropium bromide 200 μg t.d.s. from metered-dose inhaler. (With permission from Taylor *et al.*, 1986).

than 10% of the metered dose is likely to reach the lungs (Newman *et al.*, 1981). It is conceivable that the small doses of these synthetic anticholinergic bronchodilators required to achieve bronchodilatation do not play a role on mucus clearance, unlike the relatively high doses of the atropine-like drugs, which were given orally or parenterally, and have been shown to adversely affect clearance.

C Methylxanthines

Theophylline derivatives may well share other properties, besides bronchodilatation, with β agonist agents including the ability to enhance mucociliary clearance. The addition of aminophylline has been shown (Iravani and Melville, 1975) to increase ciliary beat frequency in an *in vitro* preparation. Furthermore, the addition of theophylline increases discharge in normal and hypertrophied submucosal glands (Whimster and Reid, 1973) – possibly by potentiation of the cyclic AMP system. Either or both of these two alternatives could affect the transport of mucus in the lungs. Serafini *et al.* (1976) showed that intravenous aminophylline increased the TMV in dogs by almost 60% and in the main bronchi by 27%, but no effect on transport was detected in the more distal ciliated airways. The administration of theophylline in healthy subjects, which resulted in low therapeutic serum theophylline levels (mean: 7.8 $\mu g\ ml^{-1}$), has been reported to have increased mucociliary transport rates (Cotromanes *et al.*, 1985). Matthys and Kohler (1980) have also reported that the infusion of aminophylline at a dose of 6 mg kg^{-1} (bodyweight) gave rise to improved mucociliary clearance rates in some normal subjects and infertile males with a reduced tracheobronchial clearance. The administration of the β_2 agonist hexoprenaline (0.4 mg by inhalation) to 14 patients with chronic obstructive lung disease had no effect on mucociliary clearance compared to the run when the patients inhaled 0.9% NaCl as an aerosol. However, the combination of aminophylline (6 mg kg^{-1} bodyweight i.v.) and hexoprenaline resulted in a significant enhancement of mucociliary clearance compared with 0.9% NaCl (Vastag *et al.*, 1982). In our laboratories we have found that the oral administration of 450 mg of aminophylline (b.d.) for seven days in patients with airways obstruction resulted in a significant enhancement of lung mucociliary clearance (Fig. 6) compared to the placebo run (Sutton *et al.*, 1981).

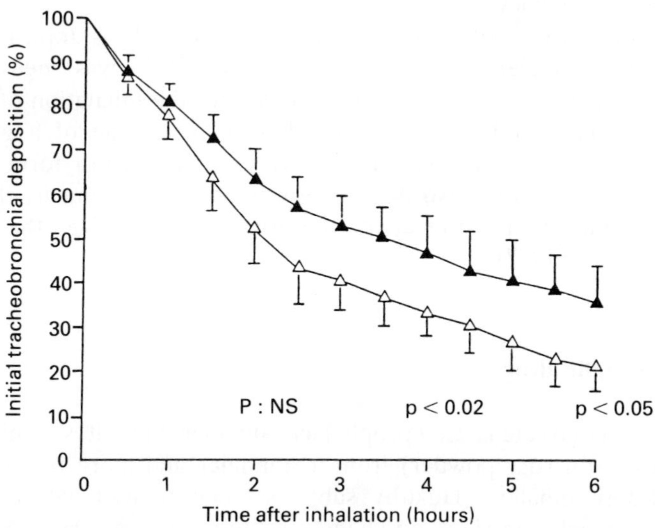

Fig. 6 Mean (±SEM) tracheobronchial clearance curves for 12 patients with obstructive lung disease following therapy with oral aminophylline (450 mg b.d. for 7 days) (open triangles) and placebo (filled triangles). (With permission from Sutton *et al.*, 1981).

D Corticosteroids

Corticosteroids are widely used for the treatment of patients with asthma. Their pharmacological action in asthma is largely unknown and there is little that is quantitatively known about their effect on respiratory secretions and patients' abilities to clear mucus from the conducting airways. Plugs of mucus can be found in the airways of asthmatic patients with severe disease and there is some tendency towards plugging within the peripheral airways when asthma is in remission. In acute asthma, corticosteroids may reduce the serum transudate component of the bronchial secretion and thereby affect mucus–cilia coupling. Glucocorticosteroids have been found to decrease the rate of mucin secretion in some, but not all, human bronchial strips in organ culture.

Agnew *et al.* (1983, 1984a) treated stable asthmatics with medium followed by high dose oral corticosteroids (2 weeks on 15 mg prednisolone each day, plus 2 weeks on 30 mg) and measured the patients' lung mucociliary clearance. A reduction in cough frequency and sputum production was observed following treatment, indicating less reliance of tracheobronchial clearance transport on cough. Mucociliary clearance from the peripheral zone of the lungs showed significant improvement after four weeks of steroid treatment. It is also worth noting that Iravani and Melville (1975) reported that the topical administration of prednisolone to isolated preparations of rat bronchi resulted in a modest increase in ciliary beat frequency.

A common route of administering corticosteroids is topically from metered-dose inhalers or as a dry powder. TMV was measured in conscious sheep before and 30–60 minutes after the inhalation of 4 puffs (50 μg per puff) of beclomethasone dipropionate—one of a group of insoluble corticosteroids that are widely used in aerosol form for the treatment of asthmatics. No difference was observed in mucus clearance between groups of sheep receiving the drug and those given the placebo (Sackner *et al.*, 1977).

E Prophylactic drugs

Sodium cromoglycate is used prophylactically in asthma; it is administered in aerosol form (dry powder) from a spinhaler and more recently from metered-dose inhalers. Healthy subjects when treated with 20 mg of sodium cromoglycate show no change in their baseline TMV. Asymptomatic asthmatics with ragweed hypersensitivity already have reduced mucus velocities that are further depressed to 72% of baseline immediately after challenge with ragweed and to a level of 47% of baseline values one hour after challenge. Pre-treatment with 20 mg sodium cromoglycate, however, gave rise to a 32% increase in TMV compared to baseline with a further 62% increase after bronchial provocation with ragweed (Mezey *et al.*, 1978).

FPL-55712 is a slow reacting substance of anaphylaxis (SRS-A) antagonist and its effect on TMV has been studied in asymptomatic non-smokers with ragweed asthma (Ahmed *et al.*, 1981). Such patients when challenged with doses of ragweed that resulted in a 35% decrease of specific airway conductance (SGaw) and their TMV fell immediately to 74% of baseline value, returning to baseline within two hours. When these patients were pre-treated with 0.5 and 1.0% FPL-55712 and then challenged until SGaw was reduced by at least 35%, this was found to be accompanied by increases in TMVs to 138% and 126% respectively with return to baseline within two hours. If FPL-55712 was given following ragweed challenge then it prevented the slowing down of TMV only. This study indicates that SRS-A liberated during airway anaphylaxis reduces mucus transport and the antigen-induced increase in mucus transport after pre-treatment with an SRS-A antagonist may reflect a stimulatory effect of other chemical mediators of anaphylaxis, e.g. histamine, acetylcholine.

REFERENCES

Agnew, J.E., Bateman, J.R.M., Watts, M., Paramananda, V., Pavia, D. and Clarke, S.W. (1981a). The importance of aerosol penetration for lung mucociliary clearance studies. *Chest* **80** (Suppl.), 843–846.

Agnew, J.E., Pavia, D. and Clarke, S.W. (1981b). Airway penetration of inhaled radioaerosol: An index to small airway function? *Eur. J. Respir. Dis.* **62**, 239–255.

Agnew, J.E., Little, F., Pavia, D. and Clarke, S.W. (1982). Mucus clearance from the airways in chronic bronchitis—smokers and ex-smokers. *Bull. Eur. Physiopathol. Respir.* **18**, 473–484.

Agnew, J.E., Bateman, J.R.M., Sheahan, N.F., Lennard-Jones, A.M., Pavia, D. and Clarke, S.W. (1983). Effect of oral corticosteroids on mucus clearance by cough and mucociliary transport in stable asthma. *Bull. Eur. Physiopathol. Respir.* **19**, 37–41.

Agnew, J.E., Bateman, J.R.M., Pavia, D. and Clarke, S.W. (1984a). Peripheral airways mucus clearance in stable asthmatics improved by oral corticosteroid therapy. *Bull. Eur. Physiopathol. Respir.* **20**, 295–301.

Agnew, J.E., Bateman, J.R.M., Pavia, D. and Clarke, S.W. (1984b). A model for assessing bronchial mucus transport. *J. Nucl. Med.* **24**, 170–176.

Ahmed, T., Greenblatt, D.W., Birch, S., Marchette, B. and Wanner, A. (1981). Abnormal mucociliary transport in allergic patients with antigen-induced bronchospasm: role of slow reacting substance of anaphylaxis. *Am. Rev. Respir. Dis.* **124**, 110–114.

Albert, R.E. and Arnett, L.C. (1955). Clearance of radioactivity dust from the lung. *Arch. Environ. Hlth* **12**, 99–106.

Annis, P., Landa, J. and Lichtiger, M. (1976). Effects of atropine on velocity of tracheal mucus in anesthetized patients. *Anaesthesiology* **44**, 74–77.

Asmundsson, T. and Kilburn, K.H. (1970). Mucociliary clearance rates at various levels in dog lungs. *Am. Rev. Respir. Dis.* **102**, 388–397.

Auerbach, O., Stout, A.P., Hammond, E.C. and Garfinkel, L. (1962). Changes in bronchial epithelium in relation to sex, age, residence, smoking and pneumonia. Bronchial epithelium in former smokers. *New Eng. J. Med.* **267**, 111–125.

Bateman, J.R.M., Pavia, D. and Clarke, S.W. (1978). The retention of lung secretions during the night in normal subjects. *Clin. Sci. Mol. Med.* **55**, 523–527.

Bateman, J.R.M., Newman, S.P., Sheahan, N.F., Pavia, D. and Clarke, S.W. (1983a). Tracheobronchial clearance during recovery from acute severe asthma. *Thorax* **38**, 220.

Bateman, J.R.M., Pavia, D. Sheahan, N.F., Agnew, J.E. and Clarke, S.W. (1983b). Impaired tracheobronchial clearance in patients with mild stable asthma. *Thorax* **38**. 463–467.

Camner, P. and Philipson, K. (1978). Human alveolar deposition of 4 μm Teflon particles. *Arch. Environ. Hlth* **36**, 181–185.

Camner, P., Jarstrand, C. and Philipson, K. (1973a). Tracheobronchial clearance in patients with influenza. *Am. Rev. Respir. Dis.* **108**, 131–135.

Camner, P., Philipson, K. and Arvidsson, T. (1973b). Withdrawal of cigarette smoking. A study of tracheobronchial clearance. *Arch. Environ. Hlth* **26**, 90–92.

Clarke, S.W. and Lopez-Vidriero, M.T. (1982). The effect of β_2-agonist on the activity of human bronchial cilia *in vitro*. *J. Physiol.* **336**, 40P–41P.

Clarke, S.W. and Pavia, D. (1981). Comparison of techniques for measuring tracheal mucus velocities *in vitro* in man. In *Bronchology: Research, Diagnostic, and Therapeutic Aspects* (eds J.A. Nakhosteen and W. Massen), pp. 469–471. Martinus Nijhoff, The Hague.

Cotromanes, E., Gerrity, T.R., Garrard, C.S., Harshbarger, R.D., Yeates, D.B., Kendzierski, D.L. and Lourenço, R.V. (1985). Aerosol penetration and mucociliary transport in the healthy human lung. Effect of low serum theophylline levels. *Chest* **88**. 194–200.

Dalhamn, T. and Rylander, R. (1965). Ciliastatic action of cigarette smoke. *Arch. Otolaryng.* **81**, 379–382.

Davis, B., Marin, M.G., Yee, J.W. and Nadel, J.A. (1979). Effect of terbutaline on movement of Cl^- and Na^+ across the trachea of the dog *in vitro*. *Am. Rev. Respir. Dis.* **120**, 547–552.

Del Donno, M., Pavia, D., Agnew, J.E., Lopez-Vidriero, M.T. and Clarke, S.W. (1988). Variability and reproducibility in the measurement of tracheobronchial clearance in healthy subjects and patients with different obstructive lung diseases. *Eur. Respir. J.* **1**, 613–620.

Dulfano, M.J. and Luk, C.K. (1982). Sputum and ciliary inhibition in asthma. *Thorax* **37**, 646–651.

Dulfano, M.J., Luck, C.K., Beckage, M. and Wooten, O. (1982). Ciliary inhibitory effect of asthma patients' sputum. *Clin. Sci.* **63**, 393–396.

Foster, W.M., Langeback, E. and Bergofsky, E.H. (1980). Measurement of tracheal and bronchial mucus velocities in man: relation to lung clearance. *J. Appl. Physiol.: Respirat. Environ. Exercise Physiol.* **48**, 965–971.

Foster, W.M., Langenback, E.G. and Bergofsky, E.H. (1982). Lung mucociliary function in man: interdependence of bronchial and tracheal mucus transport velocities with lung clearance in bronchial asthma and healthy subjects. *Ann. Occup. Hyg.* **26**, 227–244.

Foster, W.M., Langenback, E.G., Glaser, M.L. and Bergofsky, E.H. (1983). Acute effect of ipratropium bromide at therapeutic dose on mucus transport of adult asthmatics. *Eur. J. Respir. Dis.* **64** (Suppl. 128), 554–557.

Foord, N., Black, A. and Walsh, M. (1977). Pulmonary deposition of inhaled particles with diameters in the range of 2.5 to 7.5 μm. In *Inhaled Particles IV* (ed. W.H. Walton), pp. 137–148. Pergamon Press, Oxford.

Friedman, M., Stott, E.D., Poole, D., Dougherty, R., Chapman, G., Watson, H. and Sackner, M.A. (1977). A new roentgenographic method for estimating mucus velocity in airways. *Am. Rev. Respir. Dis.* **115**, 67–72.

Frigas, E., Loegering, D.A. and Gliech, G.J. (1980). Cytotoxic effects of the guinea-pig eosinophil major basic protein on tracheal epithelium. *Lab. Invest.* **42**, 35–43.

Frigas, E., Loegering, D.A., Solley, G.O., Farrow, G.M. and Gliech, G.J. (1981). Elevated levels of the eosinophil granule major basic protein in the sputum of patients with bronchial asthma. *Mayo Clin. Proc.* **56**, 345–353.

Goodman, R.M., Yergin, B.M., Landa, J.F., Golinvaux, M.H. and Sackner, M.A. (1978). Relationship of smoking history and pulmonary function tests to tracheal mucus velocity in non-smokers, ex-smokers, and patients with chronic bronchitis. *Am. Rev. Respir. Dis.* **117**, 205–214.

Iravani, J. and Melville, G.N. (1975). Effects of drugs and environmental factors on ciliary movement. *Respiration* **32**, 157–164.

Jarstrand, C., Camner, P. and Philipson, K. (1974). Mycoplasma pneumoniae and tracheobronchial clearance. *Am. Rev. Respir. Dis.* **110**, 415–419.

Jeffery, P.K. (1987). The origins of secretions in the lower respiratory tract. *Eur. J. Respir. Dis.* **71** (suppl. 153), 34–42.

Kennedy, M.C. and Thursby Pelham, D.C. (1964). Some adrenergic drugs and atropine methonitrate given by inhalation for asthma: a comparative study. *Br. Med. J.* **1**, 1018–1021.

Knowles, M.R., Murray, G.F., Shallal, J.A, Gatzy, J.T. and Boucher, R.C. (1982). Ion transport in excised human bronchi and in neurohumoral control. *Chest* **81** (Suppl. 5), 11S–13S.

Lindberg, S. and Mercke, V. (1986). Capsaicin stimulates mucociliary activity by releasing substance P and acetylcholine. *Eur. J. Respir. Dis.* **68**, 96–106.

Lopez-Vidriero, M.T. (1984). Lung secretions. In *Aerosols and the Lung: Clinical and Experimental Aspects* (eds S.W. Clarke and D. Pavia), pp. 19–48. Butterworths, London.

Lopez-Vidriero, M.T., Allegra, L., Sackner, M.A. and Puchelle, E. (1986). The physical properties of mucus and their clinical significance. *Bull. Eur. Physiopathol. Respir.* **22**, 207–212.

Lourenço, R.V., Klimeck, M.F. and Borowski, C.J. (1971). Deposition and clearance of 2 micron particles in the tracheobronchial tree of normal subjects—smokers and non-smokers. *J. Clin. Invest.* **50**, 1411–1420.

Marin, M.G., Davis, B. and Nadel, J.A. (1977). Effect of histamine on electrical and ion transport properties of tracheal epithelium. *J. Appl. Physiol.: Respirat. Environ. Exercise Physiol.* **42**, 735–738.

Marom, Z., Shelhamer, J.H. and Kaliner, M. (1981). The effect of arachidonic acid, monohydroxyeiosatetraenoic acid and prostaglandins on the release of mucous glycoproteins from human airways *in vitro*. *J. Clin. Invest.* **67**, 1695–1702.

Marom, Z., Shelhamer, J.H., Bach, M.K., Morton, D.R. and Kaliner, M. (1982). Slow-reacting substances, leukotrienes C_4 and D_4, increase the release of mucus from human airways *in vitro*. *Am. Rev. Respir. Dis.* **126**, 449–451.

Matthys, H. and Kohler, D. (1980). Effect of theophylline on mucociliary clearance in man. *Eur. J. Respir. Dis.* **61** (Suppl. 109), 98–102.

Maurer, D.R., Sielezak, M., Oliver, Jr, W., Abraham, W.M. and Wanner, A. (1982). Role of ciliary motility in acute allergic mucociliary dysfunction. *J. Appl. Physiol.: Respirat. Environ. Exercise Physiol.* **52**, 1018–1023.

Melville, G.N. and Iravani, J. (1974). Factors affecting ciliary beat frequency in the intrapulmonary airways of rats. *Can. J. Physiol. Pharmacol.* **53**, 1122–1128.

Mezey, R.J., Cohn, M.A., Fernandez, R.J., Janszkiewicz, A.J. and Wanner, A. (1978). Mucociliary transport in allergic patients with antigen-induced bronchospasm. *Am. Rev. Respir. Dis.* **118**, 677–684.

Newman, S.P., Pavia, D., Móren, F., Sheahan, N.F. and Clarke, S.W. (1981). Deposition of pressurised aerosols in the human respiratory tract. *Thorax* **36**, 52–55.

Oldenburg, F.A., Dolovich, M.B., Montgomery, J.H. and Newhouse, M.T. (1979). Effects of postural drainage, exercise and cough on mucus clearance in chronic bronchitis. *Am. Rev. Respir. Dis.* **120**, 739–745.

Pavia, D. (1984a). Lung mucociliary clearance. In *Aerosols and the Lung: Clinical and Experimental Aspects* (eds S.W. Clarke and D. Pavia), pp. 127–155. Butterworths, London.

Pavia, D. (1984b). Mucociliary clearance at night—effect of physical activity, posture, and circadian rhythm. In *Nocturnal Asthma* (eds P.J. Barnes and J. Levy), pp. 29–38. Royal Society of Medicine International Congress and Symposium Series no. 73, London.

Pavia, D. (1988). Radioaerosols for the study of lung function. In *Methods in Bronchial Mucology* (eds P.C. Braga and L. Allegra), pp. 367–375. Raven Press, New York.

Pavia, D. and Thomson, M.L. (1971). Inhibition of mucociliary clearance from the human lung by hyoscine. *Lancet* **1**, 449–450.

Pavia, D., Thomson, M.L. and Pocock, S.J. (1971). Evidence for temporary slowing of mucociliary clearance in the lung caused by tobacco smoking. *Nature* **231**, 325–326.

Pavia, D., Thomson, M.L., Clarke, S.W. and Shannon, H.S. (1977). Effect of lung function and mode of inhalation on penetration of aerosol into the human lung. *Thorax* **32**, 194–197.

Pavia, D., Bateman, J.R.M., Sheahan, N.F., Agnew, J.E., Newman, S.P. and Clarke S.W. (1980). Techniques for measuring lung mucociliary clearance. *Eur. J. Respir. Dis.* **61** (suppl. 110), 157–177.

Pavia, D., Sutton, P.P., Agnew, J.E., Lopez-Vidriero, M.T., Newman, S.P. and Clarke, S.W. (1983). Measurement of bronchial mucociliary clearance. *Eur. J. Respir. Dis.* **64** (suppl. 127), 41–56.

Pavia, D., Agnew, J.E., Lopez-Vidriero, M.T., Newman, S.P. and Clarke, S.W. (1984). The effect of metered dose aerosols on the viscoelastic properties and clearance of bronchial secretions. In *Metered Dose Inhalers* (ed. S.W. Epstein), pp. 38–48. Astra, Mississauga (Canada).

Pavia, D., Agnew, J.E. and Clarke, S.W. (1985a). Physiological, pathological and drug-induced alterations in the tracheobronchial mucociliary clearance. In *Sustained Release Theophylline and Nocturnal Asthma* (eds A.F. Isles and P. Von Wichert), pp. 44–59. Excerpta Medica, Amsterdam.

Pavia, D., Bateman, J.R.M., Sheahan, N.F., Agnew, J.E. and Clarke, S.W. (1985b). Tracheobronchial mucociliary clearance in asthma: impairment during remission. *Thorax* **40**, 171–175.

Pavia, D., Agnew, J.E., Sutton, P.P., Lopez-Vidriero, M.T., Clay, M.M., Killip, M. and Clarke, S.W. (1987). Effect of terbutaline administered from metered dose inhaler (2 mg) and subcutaneously (0.25 mg) on tracheobronchial clearance in asthma. *Br. J. Dis. Chest* **81**, 361–370.

Pavia, D., Lopez-Vidriero, M.T., Agnew, J.E., Taylor, R.G., Eyre-Brook, A., Lawton, W.A., Pellow, P.G.D. and Clarke, S.W. (1989). Effect of four-week treatment with oxitropium bromide on lung mucociliary clearance in patients with chronic bronchitis or asthma. *Respiration* **55**, 33–43.

Phipps, R.J., Williams, I.P., Richardson, P.S., Pell, J., Pack, R.J. and Wright, N. (1982).

Sympathomimetic drugs stimulate the output of secretory glycoproteins from human bronchi *in vitro*. *Clin. Sci.* **63**, 23–28.

Puchelle, E., Zahm, J-M. and Bertrand, A. (1979). Influence of age on bronchial mucociliary transport. *Scand. J. Respir. Dis.* **60**, 307–313.

Puchelle, E., Zahm, J-M. and Duvivier, C. (1983). Spinability of bronchial mucus. Relationships with viscoelasticity and mucous transport properties. *Biorheology* **20**, 239–249.

Russi, E., Chapman, G.A., Marchette, B., Abraham, W.M. and Wanner, A. (1983). Effect of leukotriene D_4 on mucociliary function and airway mechanics in allergic sheep. *Am. Rev. Respir. Dis.* **127** (No. 4, part 2 of 2 parts), 70.

Sackner, M.A. (1978). Effect of respiratory drugs on mucociliary clearance. *Chest* **73** (Suppl.), 958–964.

Sackner, M.A., Rosen, M.J. and Wanner, A. (1973). Estimation of tracheal mucus velocity by bronchofiberscopy. *J. Appl. Physiol.* **34**, 495–499.

Sackner, M.A., Reinhart, M. and Arkin, B. (1977). Effects of beclomethasone diproprionate on tracheal mucus velocity. *Am. Rev. Respir. Dis.* **115**, 1009–1070.

Santa Cruz, R., Landa, J., Hirsch, J. and Sackner, M.A. (1974). Tracheal mucus velocity in normal man and in patients with obstructive lung disease; effects of terbutaline. *Am. Rev. Respir. Dis.* **109**, 458–463.

Serafini, S.M. and Michaelson, E.D. (1977). Length and distribution of cilia in human and canine airways. *Bull. Eur. Physiolpathol. Respir.* **13**, 551–559.

Serafini, S.M., Wanner, A. and Michaelson, E.D. (1976). Effects of aminophylline. *Bull. Eur. Physiopathol. Respir.* **12**, 415–422.

Sleigh, M.A. (1981). Ciliary function in mucus transport. *Chest* **80** (Suppl.), 791–795.

Sutton, P.P., Pavia, D., Bateman, J.R.M. and Clarke, S.W. (1981). The effect of oral aminophylline on lung clearance in man. *Chest* **80** (Suppl.), 889–891.

Taylor, R.G., Pavia, D., Agnew, J.E., Lopez-Vidriero, M.T., Newman, S.P., Lennard-Jones, T. and Clarke, S.W. (1986). Effect of four weeks' high dose ipratropium bromide treatment on lung mucociliary clearance. *Thorax* **41**, 295–300.

Thomson, M.L. and Short, M.D. (1969). Mucociliary function in health, chronic obstructive airway disease and asbestosis. *J. Appl. Physiol.* **26**, 535–539.

Torelmalm, N.G. (1960). The daily amount of tracheobronchial secretions in man. *Acta Otolaryng.* **158** (Suppl.), 43.

Vastag, E., Kohler, D., Fischer, J., Daikeler, G. and Matthys, H. (1982). The influence of hexoprenaline and aminophylline on mucociliary clearance of the bronchial system in patients with chronic obstructive airway diseases. *Atemw.- Lungenkrkh. Jahrgang* **8**, 205–208.

Verdugo, P., Johnson, N.T. and Tam, P.Y. (1980). Beta-adrenergic stimulation of respiratory ciliary activity. *J. Appl. Physiol.: Respirat. Environ. Exercise Physiol.* **48**, 868–871.

Wanner, A. (1979). The role of mucociliary dysfunction in bronchial asthma. *Am. J. Med.* **67**, 477–485.

Wanner, A., Zarzecki, S., Hirsch, J. and Epstein, S. (1975). Tracheal mucus transport in experimental canine asthma. *J. Appl. Physiol.* **39**, 950–957.

Wanner, A., Maurer, D., Abraham, W.M., Szepfalusi, Z. and Sielczak, M. (1983). Effects of chemical mediators of anaphylaxis on ciliary function. *J. Allergy Clin. Immunol.* **72**, 663–667.

Whimster, W.F. and Reid, L. (1973). The influence of dibutysyl cyclic adenosine monophosphate and other substances on human bronchial mucus gland discharge. *Exp. Mol. Pathol.* **18**, 234–240.

Wiebel, E.R. (1963). *Morphotometry of the Human Lung*. Springer-Verlag, Berlin.
Wolff, R.K., Dolovich, M.B., Obminski, G. and Newhouse, M.T. (1977). Effects of exercise and eucapnic hyperventilation on bronchial clearance. *J. Appl. Physiol.* **43**, 46–50.
Wong, J.W., Keens, T.G., Wammamaker, E.M., Douglas, P.T., Crozier, N., Levison, H. and Aspin, N. (1977). Effects of gravity on tracheral mucus transport rates in normal subjects and in patients with cystic fibrosis. *Paediatrics* **60**, 146–152.
Yeates, D.B. and Aspin, N. (1978). A mathematical description of the airways of the human lung. *Respir. Physiol.* **39**, 91–104.
Yeates, D.B., Aspin, N., Levison, H., Jones, M.T. and Bryan, A.C. (1975). Mucociliary tracheal transport rates in man. *J. Appl. Physiol.* **39**, 487–495.
Yeates, D.B., Pitt, B.R., Spektor, D.M., Karron, G.A. and Albert, R.E. (1981). Coordination of mucociliary transport in the human trachea and intrapulmonary airways. *J. Appl. Physiol.: Respir. Environ. Exercise Physiol.* **51**, 1057–1064.
Yeates, D.B., Wong, L.B. and Miller, I.F. (1988a). Capsaicin stimulation of ciliary beat is mediated by both neural and humoral mechanisms. *Eur. Respir. J.* **1** (Suppl.1), 114s.
Yeates, D.B., Wong, L.B. and Miller, I.F. (1988b). Stimulation of tracheal ciliary beat frequency of bradykinin. *Eur. Respir. J.* **1** (Suppl.1), 114s.

5

Mast cell heterogeneity

[1]R. Christopher Benyon, Mark A. Lowman, Paul H. Rees, Stephen T. Holgate and Martin K. Church

Immunopharmacology Group, Clinical Pharmacology, University of Southampton, Centre Block, Southampton General Hospital, Southampton, Hampshire SO9 4XY, UK
[1] Present address: Department of Microbiology and Infectious Diseases, Faculty of Medicine, The University of Calgary Health Sciences Centre, 3330 Hospital Drive N.W., Calgary, Alberta T2N 4N1, Canada

I MAST CELL HETEROGENEITY IN RODENTS

In a series of studies published in 1966, Enerback (1966a,b) described two types of mast cells within the tissues of rat. As well as differing in gross morphology, these types could clearly be distinguished by their ability to be stained by basic dyes following treatment with fixatives containing formalin. Granules of mast cells of rat skin had a high affinity for toluidine blue or Alcian blue following fixation in aldehyde fixatives, such as neutral buffered formalin, whereas staining of mast cells of the intestinal mucosa was blocked by this treatment. The granules of these cells could, however, be stained following treatment with fixatives such as Carnoy's solution, containing isotonic chloroform and acetic acid, or Mota's lead acetate. Mast cells from the mucosa further differed from those of skin by having a higher affinity for copper phthalocyanin dyes, such that when Carnoy's-fixed cells were subjected to a staining sequence of Alcian blue followed by safranin O, mucosal mast cells stained a deep blue whilst those of skin stained mainly red. Staining with the basic dye berberine sulphate also differentiated between the two sub-types, the granules of skin mast cells showing a bright yellow fluorescence whilst

ASTHMA REVIEWS VOLUME 2
ISBN 0-12-040922-4

those of mucosal mast cells remained unstained. These staining differences are considered to reflect differences in the density of negatively-charged groups of granule glycosaminoglycans and their intragranular environment which differs in the two types of mast cells due to the presence of different granule proteoglycans and neutral proteases.

These observations of histochemical differences gave rise to the hypothesis that there are at least two distinct types of mast cells in rodents, formalin-insensitive connective-tissue mast cells (CTMC), which predominate in skin, small intestine submucosa and peritoneum, and formalin-sensitive mucosal mast cells (MMC) types predominating in intestinal mucosa and bronchial epithelium. The concept of mast cell heterogeneity in rodents, particularly the rat, is supported by a wide variety of studies done since the pioneering work of Enerback. It is now known that rat CTMC and MMC differ in several respects including morphology, mediator content, sensitivity to secretagogues and modulation of histamine release by drugs (Table 1). In the following sections, we will highlight some of the differences between rat CTMC and MMC focusing particularly on rat peritoneal mast cells (RPMC) and intestinal mucosal mast cells (IMMC), which to date are the most well-characterized studied examples of CTMC and MMC.

Apart from the more obvious phenotypic differences between RPMC and IMMC such as size and granule structure, these cells have both qualitative and quantitative differences in the content of their mediators. Considering first their amine content, the former contain approximately ten times more histamine than the latter (15–20 pg per cell compared to 1–2 pg per cell) and also more 5-hydroxytryptamine (Befus *et al.*, 1982). Neutral proteases represent a large proportion of the macromolecular constituents of the granule matrix, with mast cells of both sites containing large quantities of serine endoproteinases that, because of their chymotrypsin-like substrate specificity, have been termed chymases. The chymase of RPMC, designated rat mast cell protease I (RMCP I), has a molecular weight of 29,000 Da and constitutes a major cell product (30 $\mu g/10^6$ mast cells). Unlike α-chymotrypsin, RMCP I is not inhibited by basic pancreatic trypsin inhibitor (Seppa and Jarvinen, 1978). The chymase of IMMC, known as RMCP II, has a molecular weight of 25,000 Da and is less tightly bound to granule proteoglycan than is RMCP I. Although both chymases have a high degree of amino acid sequence homology (Woodbury *et al.*, 1978), they differ in their substrate specificity and antigenic determinants (Yurt and Austen, 1977; Woodbury *et al.*, 1978; Gibson and Miller, 1986). RMCP II may have a role in the expulsion of intestinal parasites as *in vivo* studies have shown that this protease is released into the intestinal lumen of rats infected with *Nippostrongylus*

Table 1 A comparison of rat intestinal and peritoneal mast cells.

	Intestinal mucosal	Peritoneal
Staining characteristics	Stain poorly with Alcian blue dye following formalin fixation. Stain mainly blue following Alcian blue/safranin staining sequence.	Insensitive to formalin fixation. Stain mainly brown in this sequence.
Morphology	~10 μm in diameter with few granules and smooth surface.	~20 μm in diameter with many granules and microvilli.
Ontogeny	Dependent on T-lymphocyte factors for maturation. Short half-life of <40 days.	Independent of T-cell factors for maturation. Half life of >6 months.
Mediator content	<2 pg histamine per cell. Contain chondroitin sulphate as major proteoglycan. Contain chymotryptic RMCP II IgE-dependent production of mainly LTC_4 with smaller amounts of LTB_4 and PGD_2.	~15 pg histamine per cell. Contain heparin as major proteglycan. Contain chymotryptic RMCP I IgE-dependent production of mainly PGD_2.
Secretory stimuli	Respond to antigen (~40 000 IgE receptors/cell) and concanavalin A but unresponsive to compound 48/80 and neuropeptides. Poor response to substance P. IgE-dependent secretion unaffected by phosphatidylserine.	Respond to antigen (~300 000 IgE receptors/cell), concanavalin A and many non-immunological stimuli including compound 48/80 and neuropeptides. IgE-dependent secretion potentiated by phosphatidylserine.
Drug modulation of histamine release	Secretion unaffected by cromoglycate, theophylline. Inhibition by doxantrazole and quercetin.	Secretion inhibited by cromoglycate, theophylline, doxantrazole and quercetin.

brasiliensis, this release being associated with a dramatic increase in mucosal permeability which may reflect the ability of RMCP II to degrade connective tissue (Woodbury and Miller, 1982).

Other proteolytic enzymes are known to be present within the granules of RPMC, but have been less well studied in IMMC. Carboxypeptidase A, which cleaves C-terminal aromatic amino acids from polypeptides (Everitt and Neurath, 1980), is a major RPMC granule constituent (~25 μg/10^6 cells) which, together with RMCP I, can constitute more than 20% of the total cell protein of RPMC (Schwartz *et al.*, 1981c).

These cells also contain a variety of acid hydrolases including β-hexosaminidase, β-glucuronidase and β-galactosidase (Schwartz *et al.*, 1979). Following mast cell activation, these enzymes are released in parallel with histamine and assay of their extracellular concentrations using synthetic substrates has been used to monitor mast cell degranulation (Schwartz *et al.*, 1979; Holgate *et al.*, 1980). Although RPMC contain arylsulphates types A and B, only the former is released with histamine following IgE-dependent challenge (Lynch *et al.*, 1978) suggesting that arylsulphatase B is not associated with the granule.

The secretory granules of both RPMC and IMMC contain proteoglycans; the avid binding of basic dyes to these macromolecules allows easy identification of mast cells by microscopy and led to their initial discovery by Paul Ehrlich (1876). Mast cell proteoglycans have a complex structure consisting of a polypeptide core, largely composed of glycine, and serine to which are linked side-chain branches of modified carbohydrate polymers. The side chains contain repeating heterodimers of iduronic acid and N-sulphated glucosamine in heparin/heparan proteoglycans and glucuronic acid and N-acetyl-galactosamine in the chondroitin sulphate proteoglycans. Both types of proteoglycan are highly acidic due to the presence of O-sulphate groups at various positions of the uronic acids and hexosamines (Silbert, 1967; Hook *et al.*, 1975). These heteropolymers are attached by a carbohydrate linkage of xylose–galactose–galactose to serine hydroxyl groups of the polypeptide core. The high density of negative charges on mast cell proteoglycans allows the tight binding of histamine and neutral proteases to the molecules, thereby facilitating the packaging and inactivation of these mediators within the granule. Rat peritoneal mast cells contain 10–20 pg per cell of heparin with a molecular weight of ~750 000 Da, each molecule containing ~10 glycan side chains of 60–80 000 Da. There are approximately 2000 carboxyl groups and 4000 sulphate groups per molecule (Yurt *et al.*, 1977; Robinson *et al.*, 1978).

IMMC contain little, if any, heparin (Tas and Berndsen, 1977) but instead contain chondroitin sulphate di-B as their major granule proteoglycan (Stevens *et al.*, 1986). These cells, therefore, belong to the group of non-heparin containing mast cells, which include rat and mouse cultured mast cells and mouse mucosal mast cells, the latter containing chondroitin sulphate E (Metcalfe *et al.*, 1984). The difference in sulphation between RPMC heparin and IMMC chondroitin sulphate is presumed to account for the binding of safranin O to the former, but not to the latter, in the Alcian blue/safranin staining sequence.

Following stimulation with either calcium ionophore or anti-IgE, rat mast cells oxidatively metabolize membrane-derived arachidonic acid via lipoxygenase and/or cyclooxygenase pathways to form leukotrienes (LTs) and prostaglandins (PGs) respectively. RPMC preferentially generate PGD_2, the amounts generated being related to the concentration and nature of the secretory stimulus and closely correlated with histamine release (Lewis *et al.*, 1982). The latter observation suggests that the release of both pre-formed and newly-generated mediators are interrelated events. With anti-IgE as stimulus, RPMC release approximately 37 pmol of PGD_2 per 10^6 mast cells (Lewis *et al.*, 1982) with the 5-lipoxygenase products LTB_4 and LTC_4 being undetectable. In contrast, rat IMMC release all three eicosanoids following IgE-dependent stimulation. In a recent study, Heavey *et al.* (1988) compared the anti-IgE dependent release of PGD_2, histamine, LTC_4 and LTD_4 from IMMC and PMC of the same *Nippostrongylus brasiliensis* infected rats. Following activation of each cell type with the same concentration of anti-IgE, IMMC released 13, 1486, 46 and 36 pmol/10^6 mast cells of these mediators respectively, compared with the release of 21 pmol of PGD_2 and 51 nmol of histamine per 10^6 RPMC. The ability of IMMC to release leukotrienes may account for the presence of increased levels of LTC_4 and LTD_4 in enteral and plasma samples taken from parasitized rats at the time of appearance within the intestinal lumen of RMCP II (Moqbel *et al.*, 1986a).

One major difference between RPMC and IMMC lies in their responsiveness to different secretagogues. RPMC release histamine following activation not only with IgE-dependent stimuli such as antigen, anti-IgE and concanavalin A but also with a wide range of agents including polybasic compounds (compound 48/80, poly-L-lysine and poly-L-arginine), opioids (morphine, codeine, dynorphin and β-endorphin), neuropeptides (substance P, vasoactive intestinal polypeptide, somatostatin, bradykinin and neurotensin), the complement fragments C5a and C3a, and calcium ionophores A23187 and ionomycin (Ellis *et al.*, 1970; Johnson and Erdos, 1973; Foreman and Lichtenstein, 1980; Grosman, 1981; Lagunoff *et al.*, 1983; Shanahan *et al.*, 1984, 1985; Piotrowski and Foreman, 1985). In contrast, rat IMMC respond to far fewer stimuli. Although these cells respond to IgE-dependent stimuli and calcium ionophores, they are unresponsive to compound 48/80 (Enerback, 1966c) and to a variety of neuropeptides and endorphins (Shanahan *et al.*, 1984, 1985) with the exception of substance P to which they have a reduced response compared to RPMC. The biological significance of the insensitivity of rat IMMC to peptides is uncertain, but it has been suggested that this property may prevent them from being activated by peptides derived from the breakdown of dietary proteins (Shanahan *et al.*, 1984).

Various drugs differ in their effects on histamine release from RPMC and IMMC. Sodium cromoglycate (SCG) is an effective inhibitor of secretion from RPMC activated with IgE-dependent stimuli (Orr *et al.*, 1971; Garland, 1973), calcium ionophore A23187 (Johnson and Bach, 1975), compound 48/80 (Orr *et al.*, 1971), phospholipase A (Orr and Cox, 1969) and substance P (Shanahan *et al.*, 1986). In contrast, IgE-dependent and substance P-induced histamine release from rat IMMC are unaffected by this drug (Pearce *et al.*, 1982; Shanahan *et al.*, 1985). Secretion from these cells initiated by IgE-dependent stimuli is also unaffected by theophylline which inhibits secretion from RPMC (Pearce *et al.*, 1982). However, some drugs have similar effects on both cell types. For example, the anti-allergic compound doxantrazole and the flavonoid quercetin, inhibit histamine release from both RPMC and rat IMMC to a similar degree (Pearce *et al.*, 1982).

II ONTOGENY OF MAST CELL SUB-TYPES IN RODENTS

There has been much interest recently in both why and how mast cell heterogeneity has arisen in rodents. It is believed that *in vivo*, mature mast cells are derived from multipotential haematopoietic cells that migrate in the blood-stream to their final site of deposition where, under the influence of the surrounding tissue environment, they develop into recognizable mature mast cells (Hatanaka *et al.*, 1979; Kitamura *et al.*, 1981; Zucker-Franklin *et al.*, 1981; Galli *et al.*, 1984). The type of mast cell that develops at a particular site presumably adopts characteristics appropriate to its particular function at that site. It has been proposed that one function of the mast cells of intestinal mucosa is the expulsion of parasites. Evidence for this derives from the observations that infection of the rat intestine with helminths is associated with a massive proliferation of mast cells within the mucosa and their migration into the epidermis at 12–14 days following infection only in those areas of tissue in contact with helminths (Jarrett *et al.*, 1982). Mast cell proliferation is accompanied by increases in the content of histamine, 5-hydroxytryptamine and mast cell chymase in the mucosa (Befus *et al.*, 1979; Woodbury *et al.*, 1982) during the time when parasites are being expelled. The proliferative response of IMMC requires the integrity of the host immune system of which T-lymphocytes, in particular, are considered to have an obligatory role (Ruitenberg and Elgersma, 1976; Mayrhofer, 1979; Befus and Bienenstock, 1979; Haig *et al.*, 1982). In being T-lymphocyte dependent, IMMC are similar to rodent mast cells cultured *in vitro* from precursor cells of lymphoid organs and bone marrow (Nabel *et al.*, 1981; Razin *et al.*, 1981). Metachromatic cells from both sources have granules that are Alcian blue-positive and safranin-negative, contain chondroitin sulphate E proteoglycans (Razin *et al.*, 1982) and RMCP II. In the case of cultured mast cells, the T-lymphocyte factor responsible for their growth and differentiation has been identified as a lymphokine, the 29 000 Da glycoprotein interleukin 3 (IL-3) (Ihle *et al.*, 1983; Razin *et al.*, 1984). IL-3 is probably required for IMMC proliferation *in vivo* as T-lymphocyte deficient rats have a reduced mast cell response to intestinal parasites (Miller, 1980).

The development of CTMC may require different lymphokines such as IL-4 (Hamaguchi *et al.*, 1987). However, there is some evidence that their development is T-lymphocyte independent, as Ginsburg *et al.* (1982) showed that these CTMC developed from progenitors added to cultures of embryonic fibroblasts in the absence of T-lymphocytes, and congenitally athymic rats have numerous CTMC in their skin (Keller *et al.*, 1976). Fibroblasts may have an important role in the development and maintenance of CTMC phenotype. Provided that fibroblasts are present in the culture (Levi-Schaffer *et al.*, 1986), mouse bone marrow-derived mast cells incubated with IL-3 and initially having MMC phenotype will take on several of the properties of CTMC such as increased histamine content, initiation of heparin synthesis and release of substantial quantities of PGD_2 following activation. Also, rodent mature peritoneal mast cells maintain their phenotype and viability for up to 30 days, although do not proliferate, when co-cultured with fibroblasts (Levi-Schaffer *et al.*, 1985).

Whilst studies using cultured cells have been useful for dissecting the individual processes of mast cell differentiation, it is unlikely that such systems can duplicate the complex cell–cell interactions which occur *in vivo*. However, the experimental model of Kitamura and co-workers has addressed this problem. These workers have gained valuable information about mast cell development by studying the reconstitution of mast cells from progenitors injected into various sites of mast cell-deficient mice of strain $WBB6F_1$-W/W^v. These animals are profoundly deficient in mast cells, having less than 1% of the mast cell number of the $WBB6F_1$−+/+ strain at various anatomic sites (Kitamura *et al.*, 1978). The defect in W/W^v strain rats is uncertain; they apparently produce circulating mast cell progenitors, but these do not take up residence and mature at tissue sites (Suda *et al.*, 1985), suggesting that the precursors are not interacting normally with their environment. Injection of bone-marrow cells from +/+ congenic mice into W/W^v strain leads to appearance after several weeks of virtually normal levels of mature mast cells in the animals. The effect of bone-marrow cells is mimicked by intraperitoneal injection of culture +/+ strain bone-marrow derived mast cells (Nakano *et al.*, 1985). Although, as stated above, these cells have the phenotype of MMC, the phenotypes of the cells that arise from them, in the tissues of the W/W^v mice, depends upon the tissue site in which they are deposited. Mast cells which appear in the peritoneal cavity, spleen, skin and muscularis propria of the stomach resemble CTMC in staining and phenotype whilst those found in mucosa of stomach resemble MMC. These results indicate that CTMC and MMC can arise from cultured, MMC-like cells provided that appropriate conditions for maturation are available. The studies of Sonoda *et al.* (1986) also demonstrated that both types of mast cells may arise from CTMC. These workers showed that single peritoneal mast cells of $WBB6F_1-+/+$ mice, which are known to have low proliferative potential *in vivo* (Padawer, 1974), when injected into W/W^v mice developed into either CTMC or MMC depending on the injection site. In about 5% of the W/W^v mice in which peritoneal mast cells were injected into the skin, there was a loss of peritoneal mast cell morphology, which was followed by an abrupt appearance at 15–20 days of clusters of 400–8000 CTMC at injection sites (Sonoda *et al.*, 1984). This was considered to show that the peritoneal mast cells had de-differentiated, i.e. lost recognizable mast cell phenotype in the skin sites and, had then proliferated and re-differentiated into recognizable CTMC. Taken overall, the important findings of Kitamura and co-workers suggest that CTMC and MMC are interconvertible by a sequence of de-differentiation (possibly followed by proliferation) and redifferentiation, a process that has been termed "transdifferentiation" (Kitamura *et al.*, 1986).

III HETEROGENEITY WITHIN THE HUMAN MAST CELL POPULATION

A Morphological differences

Mast cells of those human sites so far investigated appear to have a similar appearance, having a single spherical nucleus which is generally displaced to one side of the cell. They contain varying numbers of approximately spherical electron-dense, membrane-bound secretory granules of 0.2–0.5 μm diameter, which contain the mast cell pre-formed mediators (Orr, 1977; Fujita *et al.*, 1969). These granules, which originate in the Golgi apparatus, are considered to be modified phagolysosomes on account of their high content of acid hydrolases (Schwartz *et al.*, 1981a). Human mast cell granules differ from those of rodents in having a readily discernible crystalline ultrastructure observable by electron microscopy. Whorl, scroll, lattice and grating patterns with distinct periodicity have been variously described in mast cells of human skin (Bowyer, 1968; Fujita *et al.*, 1969; Lagunoff, 1972; Orr, 1977), intestine

(Dobbins *et al.*, 1969; Fox *et al.*, 1985), nasal mucosa (Friedman and Kaliner, 1985) and rheumatoid synovium (Gruber *et al.*, 1986). The different granule sub-structures observed in different lung mast cells appears to relate to their content of the neutral proteases tryptase and chymase (Craig *et al.*, 1988).

B Differences in mediator content

In the following sections, the pre-formed and newly-generated mediator content of mast cells of various human anatomic sites will be compared to examine the evidence for heterogeneity amongst these cells.

1 *Proteoglycans*

Mast cells of different human anatomical sites differ in their proteoglycan content. Studies with mastocytosis skin tissue suggest that human skin mast cells contain mainly heparin (Metcalfe *et al.*, 1980). Our preliminary studies with dispersed human skin mast cells, conducted in collaboration with Drs H. Thompson and D. Metcalfe of the National Institutes of Health, USA, confirm that they contain mainly heparin (~60% of total proteoglycan) with the remainder being chondroitin sulphates. In this respect, they resemble mast cells dispersed from human lung, which contain mainly heparin (62% of total proteoglycan), and chondroitin sulphates A and E (Metcalfe *et al.*, 1979; Thompson *et al.*, 1988). Human lung mast cell heparin has an average molecular weight of 60 000 Da distinguishing it from the larger rat mast cell heparin of >750 000 Da (Yurt *et al.*, 1977). Studies with colon biopsies suggest that human intestinal mast cells have chondroitin sulphate E as their major proteoglycan (Eliakim *et al.*, 1986; Gilead *et al.* 1987). The release of this mediator into the medium correlates closely with that of histamine suggesting that a close stoichiometric relationship exists between these mediators in the mast cell granule. Human basophils differ from mast cells so far investigated in containing only chondroitin sulphate A (Metcalfe *et al.*, 1984).

Mast cell proteoglycans may have several biological functions. Within the mast cell granule, these highly negative molecules might assist in the packing and inactivation of mediators by binding tightly to histamine and proteases. Once released, proteoglycans may have several effects relevant to inflammation and allergy. Firstly, heparin stabilizes tryptase tetramers allowing expression of their catalytic activity (Schwartz and Bradford, 1986). Secondly, heparin is a potent anti-coagulant, although chondroitin sulphate E is less active in this respect (Scully *et al.*, 1986). Thirdly, heparin amplifies the alternative complement pathway (Schwartz and Austen, 1984). Mast cell hyperplasia is commonly observed in tissues surrounding healing wounds (Pessinger *et al.*, 1983; Atkins and Clark, 1987) and increased release of heparin at these sites may assist tissue growth and re-structuring by enhancing neutrophil elastase activity (Lonky *et al.*, 1978), activating fibroblasts in the presence of tryptase (Pillarisetti *et al.*, 1983) and stimulating capillary endothelial cell migration (Marks *et al.*, 1986).

2 *Histamine*

Although both histamine and 5-hydroxytryptamine (5-HT) are present in the granules of rat mast cells (Benditt *et al.*, 1955), the latter has not been detected in human mast cells although it may be released from platelets activated by mast cell-derived platelet-activating factor. Histamine is tightly bound within the secretory granule by ionic interaction with negatively-charged carboxyl and sulphate groups of proteoglycans (Uvnas *et al.*, 1970). During mast cell secretion, histamine slowly dissociates from the granule mediator complex by ionic exchange with sodium ions (Uvnas, 1967) and then exerts its effects on cells and tissues by binding to either H_1- or H_2-receptors (Black *et al.*, 1972). Activities mediated via H_1-receptors include vasodilation, increased vascular permeability, contraction of visceral and bronchial smooth muscle whilst those mediated through H_2-receptors include inhibition of histamine release from basophils and increased gastric acid production by parietal cells.

Our studies have shown that mast cells dispersed from foreskin of children in the range 1–12 years contain 3–5 pg per cell of histamine (Benyon *et al.*, 1987a) whilst other workers (Schwartz *et al.*, 1987a) have calculated values of 1.6 pg per cell for mast cells of neonate foreskin and 1.9 pg per cell for mast cells of adult foreskin. Mast cells dispersed from human lung have a content of histamine that depends on cell size. Using countercurrent elutriation centrifugation to obtain lung mast cells of different size ranges, Schulman *et al.* (1982) reported histamine contents of 2.5 pg per cell for mast cells of the smallest size (9.9 μm mean diameter) increasing to 10.1 pg per cell for the largest cells (18.4 μm mean diameter). Unseparated dispersates of mast cells of human intestine (Fox *et al.*, 1985; Befus *et al.*, 1987; Benyon *et al.*, 1987b; Rees *et al.*, 1988) contain 1–3 pg per cell of histamine whilst those dispersed from rheumatoid synovium (Gruber *et al.*, 1986) and mastocytosis spleen (Robinson *et al.*, 1988) contain 1–2 pg and 7.7 pg per cell respectively. Mast cells recovered by human bronchoalveolar lavage (BAL) contain 2–10 pg of histamine per cell (Flint *et al.*, 1985b). These findings suggest that, although mast cells of these various anatomical sites differ in their content of histamine, there are no observations of marked differences as seen in rat mast cells where IMMC contain ~10-fold less histamine than RPMC (Befus *et al.*, 1982).

3 Tryptase and chymase

Proteases of human mast cells fall into two groups, those with tryptic activity (tryptases) and those with chymotryptic activity (chymases). There is currently a great deal of interest in these proteases, due to the realization that these enzymes may provide a useful means of discriminating between different mast cell sub-types and also serve as specific markers of mast cell activation.

Tryptase of human lung mast cells is the most extensively characterized human mast cell-derived protease (Schwartz *et al.*, 1981a,b; Smith *et al.*, 1984). This serine protease has a tetrameric structure of two pairs of non-identical subunits of molecular weight 31 500 and 33 000 Da with each subunit having a single active site. Heparin stabilizes the tetrameric structure that is required for optimal enzymatic activity, and dissociation of tryptase from this proteoglycan may be the major mechanism of inactivation of the enzyme (Schwartz and Bradford, 1986). Due to the long half-life of immunoreactive tryptase in serum compared to histamine (>2 hours versus <2 minutes) and the findings of negligible quantities of tryptase in basophils (Castells *et al.*, 1986), this enzyme should prove to be useful in evaluating the specific *in vivo* involvement of mast cells in various biological processes. Towards this end, increased concentrations of tryptase have been detected in plasma of patients with active systemic mastocytosis and during anaphylaxis (Schwartz *et al.*, 1987b).

Tryptase has several biological activities pertinent to its function as a pro-inflammatory mediator. It generates the anaphylatoxin and vasoactive agent C3a from C3 (Schwartz *et al.*., 1983), protects fibrinogen from the activity of thrombin (Schwartz *et al.*, 1985a) and inactivates high molecular weight kininogen (Maier *et al.*, 1983). Tryptase apparently neither has collagenolytic activity (Gruber *et al.*, 1988) nor activates procollagenase (Johnson and Cawston, 1985).

Immunocytochemical techniques have demonstrated the association of tryptase with mast cells of human lung cell dispersates (Schwartz, 1985; Schwartz *et al.*, 1985b; Irani *et al.*, 1986). Specific immunoassay shows that these cells contain ~10 pg of tryptase (Wenzel *et al.*, 1986; Schwartz *et al.*, 1987a), this protease being released in parallel with histamine following activation of these cells with anti-IgE (Schwartz *et al.*, 1981b).

Both tryptase and chymase are present in high salt extracts of human skin (Glenner and Cohen, 1960; Fraki and Hopsu-Havu, 1972a, b, c, 1975; Schechter *et al.*, 1983). Immunohistochemical techniques using monoclonal antibodies raised against human lung tryptase have localized tryptase to human skin mast cells (Schwartz *et al.*, 1985b; Irani *et al.*, 1986). Tryptase appears to be ubiquitously distributed in the human mast cell population with this enzyme, or a structurally related protein, having been detected in mast cells of a variety of human anatomical sites in addition to lung and skin, including both the mucosa and submucosa of large and small intestine and the conjunctiva (Irani *et al.*, 1986; Schwartz *et al.*, 1987a; Irani *et al.*, 1988). The tryptase content of mast cells may vary with age as mast cells of adult foreskin contain 2- to 3-fold higher levels of tryptase than those of infant foreskin, although histamine content is similar in each case (Schwartz *et al.*, 1987a). This suggests that production and storage of tryptase is delayed relative to histamine during maturation of these cells.

Several studies suggest that human skin mast cells contain chymase in addition to tryptase (Schechter *et al.*, 1983, 1986; Irani *et al.*, 1986; Schwartz *et al.*, 1987a). Human skin chymase is a monomeric serine protease with a molecular weight of 30 000 Da (Schechter *et al.*, 1983) which is antigenically distinct from bovine chymotrypsin, human neutrophil cathepsin G and RMCP I (Schechter *et al.*, 1983; Starkey and Barrett, 1985; Wintroub *et al.*, 1986). The biological properties of human chymase have not been as extensively investigated as those of tryptase, but this enzyme may degrade connective tissue at the junction between epidermis and dermis (Briggaman *et al.*, 1984) and, therefore, may play a key role in the formation of the blisters that are characteristic of the bullous form of mastocytosis and bullous pemphigoid.

Although mast cells of all human tissues examined so far contain tryptase, chymase-containing mast cells exist in higher concentrations in some regions than in others. Irani *et al.* (1986), using a polyclonal antibody raised against skin chymase, demonstrated that chymase was present in <10% of mast cells of dispersed lung and intestinal mucosa, whereas mast cells of intestinal submucosa and skin were approximately 90% chymase-containing cells (Fig. 1). On the basis of these observations, these workers suggested that human mast cells fall into one of two groups, those containing only tryptase (designated MC_T) and those containing both tryptase and chymase (designated MC_{TC}). These observations provide some evidence for human mast cell heterogeneity on the basis of protease content. The detailed morphology of human mast cells may depend on their content of these proteins as Craig *et al.* (1988) have observed that MC_{TC} granules are more uniformly shaped, are larger and are present in greater numbers per cell than MC_T granules. The former

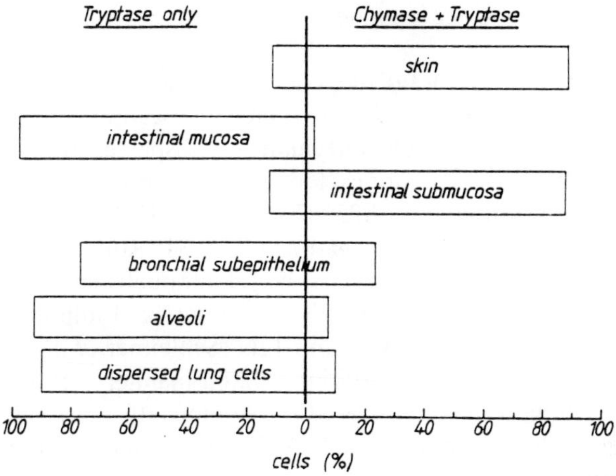

Fig. 1 Comparison of the neutral protease content of human mast cells. (Data derived from Irani *et al.*, 1986)

also contain lattice and grating structures, which were not seen in the latter.

The chymase, tryptase and histamine content of mast cells of lung and skin have been compared by Schwartz *et al.* (1987a). Both adult dispersed lung and skin mast cells contain tryptase amounting to 10.8 and 35 pg per mast cell respectively, whereas the latter contain 25-fold greater quantities of chymase (0.04 and 1 pg per mast cell respectively). As was seen with tryptase, adult foreskin mast cells contain larger quantities of chymase than those of newborn (0.09 pg per mast cell).

The heterogeneity of human mast cell protease content may be compared with the situation in rat mast cells, in which mucosal and connective tissue populations contain different neutral proteases, although in this case both enzymes have chymotryptic activity. In this species, the development of MMC depends on the presence of T-lymphocyte factors, particularly interleukin 3 (Razin *et al.*, 1984; Ihle, 1983). In humans, similar factors may be required for the development of MC_T mast cells; Irani *et al.* (1987) have shown that in individuals with severe combined immunodeficiency disease, acquired immune deficiency syndrome and Omenn's syndrome, all diseases in which there are T-lymphocyte deficiencies, there were greatly decreased numbers of MC_T mast cells in the mucosa of different regions of the intestine whilst the numbers of MC_{TC} were relatively unaffected, suggesting their development to be independent of T-lymphocyte factors.

4 Prostaglandins and leukotrienes

Following activation with IgE-dependent or calcium ionophore stimuli, human mast cells synthesize *de novo* and release products derived from arachidonic acid. In mast cells enzymatically dispersed from human lung parenchyma, PGD_2 is the major cyclooxygenase product released following stimulation with ionophore A23187 or anti-IgE (Lewis *et al.*, 1982; Schleimer *et al.*, 1983, 1986; Holgate *et al.*, 1984; Robinson and Holgate, 1986; Campbell and Robinson, 1988), although small amounts of thromboxane B_2 and $PGF_{2\alpha}$ have also been detected following activation of highly-purified mast cells with anti-IgE (Schleimer *et al.*, 1983). Anti-IgE releases PGD_2 in a concentration-related manner with release of this mediator reaching a maximum of 100–280 pmol/10^6 mast cells in a ratio to histamine of 9–33 pmol per nmol. Although calcium ionophore A23187 is an effective liberator of PGD_2 from lung mast cells, in comparison with anti-IgE, it releases only approximately half the amount of eicosanoid per unit amount of histamine, Holgate *et al.* (1984) reporting releases of 24 and 10 pmol of PGD_2 per nmol of histamine with anti-IgE and A23187 respectively.

Human lung parenchymal fragments (Dahlén *et al.*, 1983; Sautebin *et al.*, 1985) and unfractionated lung dispersates (Harvey *et al.*, 1985; Robinson *et al.*, 1986; Campbell and Robinson, 1988) release sulpidopeptide leukotrienes following challenge with IgE-dependent stimuli or A23187. Although several studies suggest that lung mast cells synthesize and release LTC_4 (MacGlashan *et al.*, 1982; Peters *et al.*, 1984a; Harvey *et al.*, 1985; Robinson and Holgate, 1986; Levi-Schaffer *et al.*, 1985), the quantities reported to be released vary widely between laboratories, varying from undetectable levels to >80 pmol/10^6 mast cells. The reason for this disparity is uncertain, but may result from different groups using different methods for cell dispersion and challenge and the specificity of antibodies used for radioimmunoassay. In addition, LTC_4 released from mast cells may be metabolized rapidly by other cells present in dispersates to LTD_4 and LTE_4 that are less easily detected with available antibodies against LTC_4. In this laboratory, we have found that the quantitative relationship between immunoreactive LTC_4, LTD_4 and LTE_4 released from dispersates of human lung activated with anti-IgE varies with the concentration of the stimulus, with LTE_4 being the major product at high concentrations (75 $\mu g\ ml^{-1}$) of anti-IgE (Campbell and Robinson, 1988).

Eicosanoid release by mast cells of other human anatomical sites has also been studied. When activated with ionophore A23187 or anti-IgE, cells enzymatically dispersed from the spleen of a patient with mastocytosis release both PGD_2 and histamine (Robinson *et al.*, 1988). Separation of these cells into populations that were enriched or depleted in mast cell content allowed the study of the association of mediators with these cells. There was a clear correlation between the release of histamine and PGD_2 following activation of gradient fractions with anti-IgE or A23187. Although, relative to histamine PGD_2 release from these cells was only one-fifth to one-sixth that seen in lung parenchymal mast cells (Holgate *et al.*, 1984), these preparations were similar in one respect, namely that anti-IgE released ~2-fold more PGD_2 per unit amount of histamine than did A23187 (4.1 pmol per nmol and 1.9 pmol per nmol histamine respectively).

IgE-dependent activation of mast cells recovered by human bronchoalveolar lavage (BAL) releases negligible quantities of LTC_4 (Flint *et al.*, 1985a). Prostaglandin D_2 is released from these cells by anti-IgE or A23187 but, in contrast to human lung parenchymal mast cells, the ratio of PGD_2 to histamine is higher with A23187 (27 pmol $nmol^{-1}$) than with anti-IgE (13.5 pmol $nmol^{-1}$) (Agius *et al.*, 1988). Maximum release of PGD_2 was 162 pmol/10^6 mast cells in these studies. Although mast cells normally constitute a small percentage (<1%) of the BAL cells, the findings of close correlations between anti-IgE-induced net release of PGD_2, LTC_4 and histamine suggest that these eicosanoids originate from the mast cell population. Density-gradient centrifugation of BAL cells followed by IgE-dependent challenge of individual fractions supports the view that PGD_2 originated from the mast cell population.

Unpurified dispersates of intestinal mucosa containing 3–5% mast cells respond to anti-IgE with the release of PGD_2 and variable amounts of sulphidopeptide leukotrienes (Fox *et al.*, 1985). Release of 60 pmol/10^6 mast cells of PGD_2 was measured at the maximum concentration of anti-IgE used; we have calculated from the data presented by these workers that this corresponds to release of ~11 pmol PGD_2 per nmol of histamine. High-performance liquid chromatographic separation of leukotrienes showed that LTE_4 was the major 5-lipoxygenase product, with only small amounts of LTC_4 and LTD_4 being detected. Taking into account the assay sensitivity for LTE_4, Fox and co-workers (1985) calculated that intestinal mast cells produce ~50 pmol of LTC_4/10^6 cells, corresponding to 8.8 pmol per nmol of histamine. Work done at this laboratory confirms that dispersates of human intestinal mucosa/submucosa and muscle layers, containing 3–5% mast cells release PGD_2 following anti-IgE stimulation (Rees, Hillier and Church, unpublished observations). At the highest concentration of anti-IgE used, 121 and 177 pmol/10^6 mast cells of PGD_2 were released from these preparations respectively, in ratios of 20.8 and 26.3 pmol per nmol of histamine. The close correlation of PGD_2 release to that of histamine observed over a wide range of anti-IgE concentrations is highly suggestive that mast cells were the major source of PGD_2, although further studies with preparations of purified mast cells will be required to show this definitively.

Various studies indicate that human skin mast cells produce PGD_2. Firstly, patients with heat-induced urticaria (Koro *et al.*, 1986), cold-induced urticaria (Heavey *et al.*, 1986; Kobza-Black *et al.*, 1988) and cholinergic urticaria (Kaplan *et al.*, 1975), all of which are inflammatory conditions considered to involve mast cell activation, have increased levels of PGD_2 in association with histamine their circulation. Secondly, Barr *et al.* (1988) showed that epicutaneous challenge of exposed dermal surfaces with allergens causes exudation of PGD_2 and histamine into skin chambers covering the site. In the same studies, these workers also showed release of these mediators from passively-sensitized, allergen-challenged skin slices. Fewer studies have examined the possible lipoxygenase products of human skin mast cells. Talbot *et al.* (1985) examined the appearance of LTB_4, C_4, D_4 and E_4 in fluid of skin chambers placed over allergen-challenged human skin and found that LTC_4 comprised >85% of the sulphidopeptide leukotrienes released with minimal changes in the other leukotrienes.

More recently, products of arachidonic acid metabolism have been examined in mast cells dispersed from human skin by treatment with collagenase and hyaluronidase (Benyon *et al.*, 1986; Benyon *et al.*, 1987a). Human dispersed skin mast cells are present at a cell purity of 4–8% in dispersates, but may be prepared in a range of purities from <1% to >85% by Percoll density-gradient centrifugation (Benyon *et al.*, 1987a). High-performance liquid chromatographic analysis of the radiolabelled cyclooxygenase and lipoxygenase products released following ionophore A23187 stimulation of [$^3H_8$]-arachidonic acid-labelled, density-gradient-separated, skin cells suggested that PGD_2 and LTC_4 were the major products of the mast cell population. Challenge of gradient-separated human dispersed skin cells with calcium ionophore A23187 induced release of histamine and immunoreactive PGD_2 (Benyon *et al.*, 1987c), the net quantities of i-PGD_2 released in each gradient fraction being significantly correlated with both mast cell numbers and net release of histamine. This provides strong evidence that PGD_2 originates from the mast cell population. In unseparated dispersates, maximum release of PGD_2 occurred with a 1 μM concentration of A23187 and was 163 pmol/10^6 mast cells with a released PGD_2/histamine ratio of 18.6 pmol $nmol^{-1}$. Similar correlations between PGD_2 and histamine release were noted when anti-IgE was used to stimulate gradient fractions. As in lung parenchymal and spleen mast cells, this stimulus was more effective than A23187 in generating PGD_2 relative to histamine. In unseparated dispersates, anti-IgE elicited maximum releases of 106 pmol PGD_2 per 10^6 mast cells in a ratio to histamine of 30 pmol $nmol^{-1}$ (Benyon, Robinson, Church and Holgate, unpublished observations). Immunoreactive LTC_4 was also detected and, as with PGD_2, the release of this mediator significantly correlated with that of histamine. In unseparated dispersates, the maximum anti-IgE-dependent release of immunoreactive LTC_4 was 7.4 pmol/10^6 mast cells with a ratio to histamine of 1.7 pmol $nmol^{-1}$. In highly-purified preparations (75–85%) of human dispersed skin mast cells, anti-IgE stimulated concentration-dependent release of histamine and immunoreactive PGD_2 and LTC_4, maximum release being 4267, 115 and 9 pmol/10^6 mast cells respectively (Fig. 2).

These *in vitro* studies provide strong evidence that human skin mast cells release PGD_2 and LTC_4 as their major, if not only, eicosanoid products. However, the role of these eicosanoids in the development of allergic reactions and inflammation in skin is uncertain. Intradermal injection of sub-nanomolar quantities of PGD_2 and LTC_4 causes rapidly-developing weal and flare reactions (Bisgaard *et al.*, 1982; Camp *et al.*, 1983; Soter *et al.*, 1983; Maurice *et al.*, 1987). However, PGD_2 released by the skin mast cells may also act at non-vascular sites to promote inflammation. This eicosanoid potentiates histamine release from allergen-activated human basophils (Peters *et al.*, 1984b), is chemokinetic for leucocytes (Goetzl *et al.*, 1976), chemotactic for neutrophils (Soter *et al.*, 1983) and inhibits platelet aggregation (Smith *et al.*, 1974).

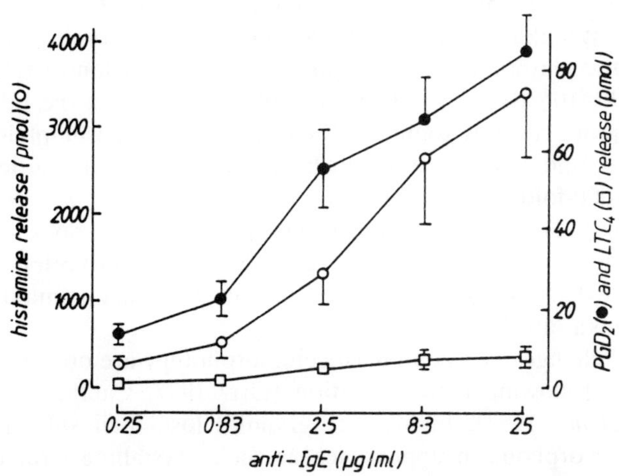

Fig. 2 Release of histamine, PGD_2 and LTC_4 from human dispersed skin mast cells activated with anti-IgE. Results are mean (±SEM) of 4 experiments. Net release is expressed as pmol/10^6 nucleated cells. Mast cell purity was 76.2 ± 4.4% of total nucleated cells.

In summary, mast cells from various human tissues have the capacity to release PGD_2 following activation with IgE- or calcium-dependent stimuli. Release of smaller and more variable amounts of LTC_4 and other sulphidopeptide leukotrienes has also been reported. These different studies have used preparations of human mast cells, dispersed using various enzymatic methods, which vary in mast cell purity and contain a variety of cells other than mast cells that may release eicosanoids. The techniques used for cell isolation and subsequent challenge may critically affect release of eicosanoids. Interaction of mast cells with other cells in the dispersate may also influence mast cell eicosanoid production. For example, co-culture of human dispersed lung mast cells with fibroblasts has been reported to augment their IgE-dependent release of PGD_2 and LTC_4 (Levi-Schaffer *et al.*, 1985). Bearing this in mind caution should be exercised in interpreting apparent quantitative differences in eicosanoid generation between mast cells of different human anatomical sites as being evidence of mast cell heterogeneity as suggested by Lawrence *et al.* (1987).

IV ACTIVATION OF MAST CELL MEDIATOR SECRETION BY IgE-DEPENDENT STIMULI

Mast cells bear cell-surface receptors for immunoglobulin E (IgE). These receptors ($Fc_{\epsilon}R_I$), of which there are approximately 10^4 to 10^5 per cell (Conrad *et al.*, 1975; Coleman and Godfrey, 1981), have been shown in rat basophil leukaemia cells to be tetrameric glycoprotein structures that traverse the plasma membrane and bind the Fc portion of IgE with high affinity ($K=10^9$–10^{12} M^{-1}). These receptors differ from the IgE-receptors ($Fc_{\epsilon}R_{II}$) more recently found on the cell-surface of eosinophils, platelets, monocytes and lymphocytes which are probably monomeric and have 100- to 1000-fold lower affinity for IgE (Lawrence *et al.*, 1975; Capron *et al.*, 1986). The binding of IgE to mast cell receptors does not, in itself, activate mediator secretion, rather, cross-linkage of mast cell IgE-receptors by multi-valent antigen or anti-IgE is the necessary stimulus (Ishizaka and Ishizaka, 1984).

Several changes in human mast cell morphology are observed in human mast cells following their activation (Orr, 1977; Caulfield *et al.*, 1980; Dvorak *et al.*, 1983). Firstly, the granules lose their sub-structure and become amorphous in appearance as their crystalline structure is lost. Granules swell as anions move across the granule membrane and finally granules, which were formerly separate, fuse with each other to form extensive lacunae. These eventually form channels with the cell exterior through which mediators are released at various rates according to their solubility and affinity for the intragranular membrane.

Following IgE-dependent activation, several changes in mast cell biochemistry occur. These have been most easily and extensively studied in rat basophil leukaemia cells, RPMC and human lung mast cells and include alterations in phospho- and polyphospho-inositide metabolism, increased calcium flux into the cytoplasm, stimulation of adenylate cyclase, increased activity of protein kinase C, increased protein phosphorylation and changes in microfilament and microtubule disposition. Several of these biochemical events are thought to be involved in the coupling of IgE-receptor activation to mediator secretion as discussed in detail elsewhere (Ishizaka and Ishizaka, 1984; Metzger *et al.*, 1986; Benyon, 1988).

A Characteristics of histamine secretion by IgE-dependent stimuli

Mast cells of human skin (Greaves *et al.*, 1972; Tharp *et al.*, 1983; Clegg *et al.*, 1985; Benyon *et al.*, 1986, 1987a), lung (Church *et al.*, 1982; Ennis, 1982; Lowman *et al.*, 1988a), tonsil (Church *et al.*, 1983; Lowman *et al.*, 1988a), adenoid (Lowman *et al.*, 1988a), heart (Vurek *et al.*, 1967; Assem and Ghanem, 1988), rheumatoid synovium (Gruber *et al.*, 1986), broncho-alveolar lumen (Flint *et al.*, 1985) and intestinal mucosa and submucosa (Fox *et al.*, 1985; Befus *et al.*, 1987; Rees *et al.*, 1988; Lowman *et al.*, 1988a) release histamine following activation with IgE-dependent stimuli and calcium ionophores. The time course of histamine release by anti-IgE is similar in each case in which it has been studied, with 2–6 minutes being required for secretion to reach completion. In contrast, secretion from mast cells of intestinal mucosa reaches a plateau within 45 seconds (Rees *et al.*, 1988). In a recent study in which similar enzymatic techniques were used to disperse mast cells from various human tissues, it was shown that maximum net IgE-dependent histamine release from mast cells of tonsil, adult breast skin and lung was 25–30% of cell total whilst that from mast cells of foreskin was 14–18% (Lowman *et al.*, 1988a). Calcium ionophore A23187 elicited release of larger amounts of histamine from these cells, there being maximum net release from adenoids, lung and tonsils of 60–75%, colon and breast skin of ~50% and foreskin of 25–30% of total histamine. Anti-IgE and calcium ionophore-induced histamine release from human foreskin (Benyon *et al.*, 1987a; Lowman *et al.*, 1988a), lung (Church *et al.*, 1982), tonsil (Church *et al.*, 1983) and intestinal mucosa and muscle (Rees *et al.*, 1988) is presumed to be non-cytotoxic, being greatly reduced by inhibitors of cellular ATP generation.

V DIFFERENCES IN RESPONSIVENESS TO NON-IMMUNOLOGICAL STIMULI. EVIDENCE FOR FUNCTIONAL HETEROGENEITY OF HUMAN MAST CELLS

Mast cells of human skin differ from those of other human anatomical sites so far investigated, with the possible exception of mast cells of rheumatoid synovium, in releasing histamine in response to a variety of non-immunological stimuli including compound 48/80, poly-L-lysine, morphine, dynorphin, substance P, vasoactive intestinal polypeptide (VIP) and somatostatin (Casale *et al.*, 1984; Hermens *et al.*, 1985; Clegg *et al.*, 1985; Ebertz, 1986; 1987; Tharp *et al.*, 1987; Benyon *et al.*, 1987a; Lowman *et al.*, 1988a). Agents that induce histamine release from human dispersed skin mast cells are shown in Table 2. A variety of other peptides tested including pentagastrin, bradykinin, lysyl-bradykinin and neurokinin B release negligible amounts of histamine, whilst neurokinin A and calcitonin gene-related peptide release small, but significant, amounts at 30 μM concentrations (Benyon *et al.*, 1987a; Lowman *et al.*, 1988b).

As described above, immunocytochemical studies of mast cells from a limited number of tissues suggest that the human mast cell population may be divided into a tryptase-only containing or tryptase and chymase containing mast cells (MC_T and MC_{TC} cells respectively) (Irani *et al.*, 1986) (Fig. 1). Although the majority of mast cells of both skin and intestinal muscle both fall into the latter group, the observation that mast

Table 2 Histamine release from human dispersed skin mast cells activated by various secretagogues.

Compound	Concentration range[1]	Maximum release (% of cell total)
Anti-IgE	0.25–25 μg ml^{-1}	15–20
Ionophore A23187	0.03–10μM	25–30
Compound 48/80	0.1–10 μg ml^{-1}	10–15
Poly-L-lysine	0.1–10 μM	10–15
Morphine	30–1000 μM	10–15
Dynorphin	10–300 μM	10–15
Substance P	1–30 μM	10–15
Somatostatin	1–30 μM	15–20
VIP	1–30 μM	15–20
Neurokinin A	10–30 μM	<5
CGRP	30 μM	<5

[1]Range over which histamine release was significantly ($p<0.05$) greater than spontaneous secretion. (Data derived from Benyon *et al.*, 1987a and Lowman *et al*, 1988b).

cells of skin respond to non-immunological stimuli whereas those of intestinal muscle do not, demonstrates that mast cell sensitivity to these two groups of stimuli does not correlate with mast cell chymase and tryptase content.

The observations that skin mast cells are activated *in vitro* by the above non-immunological stimuli are, perhaps, not surprising considering the ability of these compounds to induce weal and flare reactions *in vivo* in human skin (Lewis, 1927; Anand *et al.*, 1983; Foreman *et al.*, 1983; Casale *et al.*, 1984; Fuller *et al.*, 1987). However, *in vitro* systems have allowed the mechanism of mediator release by these agents to be studied in detail. The studies so far performed (Benyon *et al.*, 1987a; Lowman *et al.*, 1988b) indicate that histamine release by non-immunological stimuli differs in several respects from that activated by IgE-dependent stimuli in being more rapid (complete in <20 seconds) and being only partially-dependent on the presence of extracellular calcium ions. Histamine release by nonimmunological stimuli does not appear to be cytotoxic as it resembles that by anti-IgE and A23187 in being blocked by inhibitors of ATP production. The characteristics of histamine secretion by anti-IgE and substance P are compared in Fig. 3.

Another difference between the two types of stimuli lies in their ability to activate release of eicosanoids from skin mast cells. Skin mast cells purified to 76% purity by density-gradient centrifugation release similar amounts of histamine following stimulation with either anti-IgE or substance P. However, the IgE-dependent stimulus is a more effective stimulus of eicosanoid release, releasing of 22-fold more PGD_2 and 13-fold more LTC_4 than the peptide (Benyon, Robinson and Church, unpublished observations). Compound 48/80, morphine, poly-L-lysine, VIP and somatostatin all gave similar results to substance P. The biochemical mechanism explaining these differences has not yet been investigated, but one possibility is that non-immunological stimuli are less effective than anti-IgE in mobilizing precursor arachidonic acid from membrane lipids.

The physiological role of the nonimmunological pathway of secretion from skin mast cells has yet to be fully evaluated. It is likely that neuropeptides, particularly substance P, VIP and somatostatin released from dermal nerve endings represent the major nonimmunological stimuli of human skin mast cells *in vivo*. Lewis (1927) first described the triple response to histamine in skin and suggested that the flare component was mediated by a neurogenic mechanism involving antidromic impulses conducted along primary afferent neurones. The flare component requires an intact sensory nervous system being blocked by section of the sensory fibres innervating the relevant area of skin, by topical application of local

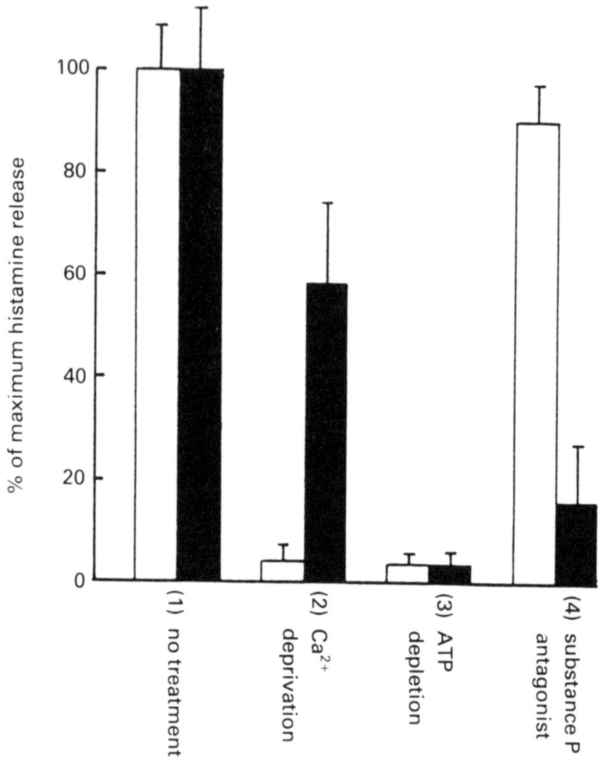

Fig. 3 Comparison of histamine release from human skin mast cells activated by anti-IgE and substance P. Treatments were as follows: (1) Challenge in HEPES-buffered salts solution (HBSS) containing 1.8 mM Ca^{2+} and 5 mM D-glucose; (2) Challenge in HBSS lacking Ca^{2+} and containing 2 mM EDTA; (3) Cells preincubated for 20 minutes in HBSS lacking glucose and containing 5 mM 2-deoxy-D-glucose and 1 μM antimycin A before challenge; (4) cells preincubated for 5 minutes with the substance P antagonist [D-Pro^{4}, D-$Trp^{7,9,10}$] substance P_{4-11} fragment before challenge.

anaesthetics (Lewis, 1927; Foreman *et al.*, 1983) or by topical application of capsaicin (*trans*-8-methyl-*N*-vanillyl-6-noneamide), which depletes sensory neurones of their peptides (Theriault *et al.*, 1979; Anand *et al.*, 1983). The relevant primary afferent neurones are now considered to be unmyelinated C-fibres (Hinsey and Gasser, 1930) that branch within the dermis. One branch generally terminates at a polymodal nociceptor responsive to deep pressure, heat and various chemicals including histamine and 5-HT (Celander and Folkow, 1953; Torebjork and Hallin, 1974; Kenins, 1981; Orwin and Fozard, 1986). Stimulation of these nociceptors activates the release of neuropeptides from the terminals of further branches of the same nerve. Such nerve endings have been observed in close anatomical association with mast cells (Wiesner-Menzel *et al.*, 1981; Newson *et al.*, 1983; Foreman and Piotrowski, 1984; Skotfisch *et al.*, 1985).

A variety of mast cell-stimulating neuropeptides have been localized in mammalian sensory nerves including substance P (Hokfelt *et al.*, 1975), somatostatin (Hokfelt *et al.*, 1976) and VIP (Hartschuh *et al.*, 1983; Johansson, 1986). These neuropeptides may be involved in the homeostatis of the dermal vasculature as they induce weal and flare reactions when injected intradermally into humans (Anand *et al.*, 1983; Jorizzo *et al.*, 1983; Foreman and Piotrowski, 1984). The flare which follows substance P injection is probably mediated by released histamine, as it is blocked by H_1-histamine antagonists (Hagermark *et al.*, 1978; Foreman *et al.*, 1983) or by prior addition to the test site of compound 48/80, which depletes skin mast cells of their histamine stores (Lambeck and Holzer, 1979).

Thus, there is a bi-directional communication between skin mast cells and sensory nerves. The ability of peptides to activate the rapid release of histamine, presumably in conjunction with other pre-formed mediators provides a mechanism by which neuropeptides may control a variety of functions such as cutaneous blood flow (Schayer, 1962), angiogenesis (Marks *et al.*, 1986) and fibroblast proliferation (Pillarisetti *et al.*, 1983). There is increasing evidence that neuropeptides modulate the activity of a variety of immuno-competent leucocytes including macrophages, monocytes and lymphocytes (Hartung and Toyka, 1983; Stanisz *et al.*, 1986; McGillis *et al.*, 1987; O'Dorisio, 1987). The findings that skin mast cells are activated by neuropeptides suggest that these cells may also be included amongst those involved in neuro-immune interactions.

The characteristics of mast cell activation by nonimmunological stimuli have been studied in some detail (Benyon *et al.*, 1987a; Lowman *et al.*, 1988b). Histamine release induced by compound 48/80, poly-L-lysine, morphine, substance P, somatostatin and VIP is blocked by a substance P octapeptide fragment, [D-Pro^4, D-Trp^{7,9,10}] substance P fragment 4–11 (SPA), which antagonizes the binding of tachykinins to smooth muscle receptors. This suggests that each of these stimuli activates secretion following binding either to the same receptor population or to populations of receptors with structural similarities. However, the relative potency of a variety of tachykinins in stimulating human skin mast cells secretion suggests that the receptor is not one of the NK-1, NK-2 or NK-3 subtypes of tachykinin receptor previously characterized on smooth muscle (Lee *et al.*, 1986).

Studies with substance P fragments indicate that both the basic amino-terminal tetrapeptide (Arg^{2+}-Pro-Lys^{+}-Pro) and hydrophobic carboxyl-terminal sequence (Gln-Gln-Phe-Phe-Gly-Leu-MetNH_2) contribute to the ability of substance P to release histamine. Available evidence indicates that the human skin mast cell receptor for substance P resembles that of rat peritoneal mast cells. These receptors are considered to have two domains, one of which is highly lipophilic and binds and constrains the carboxyl-terminal sequence of substance P, which allows the amino-terminal positively-charged region of substance P to interact with the second receptor domain to trigger histamine release (Repke *et al.*, 1987).

VI COMPARISONS OF HUMAN MAST CELL RESPONSIVENESS TO PHARMACOLOGICAL AGENTS

The purported pivotal role of mast cells in allergic disorders has made them obvious targets for drug development and many pharmaceutical companies synthesize compounds to modulate the release of mast cell mediators.

Perhaps the most important group of drugs introduced recently for the treatment of allergic diseases are the anti-allergic drugs, initially called "mast cell stabilizers", including sodium cromoglycate (SCG) and nedocromil sodium. The mechanism of action of SCG, initially discovered by its ability to suppress allergen-induced bronchoconstriction in a human volunteer, was suggested by its ability to prevent IgE-dependent mediator release from rat mast cells (Cox, 1967; Cox and Altounyan, 1970). Whilst it is clear that some of the beneficial actions of SCG derive from other effects such as inhibition of neuronal reflexes in the lung (Dixon *et al.*, 1980) and leucocyte activation (Moqbel *et al.*, 1986b, c) only the aspects of drug activity relating to mast cell heterogeneity will be discussed here.

Studies with SCG have revealed large inter-species and intra-species differences in the sensitivity of mast cells to its inhibitory actions. For example, it is a potent inhibitor of histamine release from peritoneal mast cells of the rat, is less effective on those from the hamster and is inactive against those of the mouse (Pearce *et al.*, 1985). Similarly, SCG is an effective inhibitor of histamine release from mast cells dispersed from lung of rat but not those from lung of cow, dog or guinea-pig (Sheard and Blair, 1970; Burka and Eyre, 1975; Krell and Chakrin, 1976; Pearce *et al.*, 1985) and rat, but not guinea-pig skin (Tay *et al.*, 1972). Against this background, we and others have studied the heterogeneous effects of SCG on human mast cells. IgE-dependent histamine release from human lung fragments (Church and Young, 1983) and mast cells dispersed from lung parenchymal tissue (Church and Hiroi, 1987; Pearce, 1986) are poorly responsive to SCG, concentrations of 100–1000 μM being required to cause inhibition of approximately 30%. Furthermore, these cell show rapid tachyphylaxis to this drug (Church and Hiroi, 1987; Pearce *et al.*, 1986) similar to that seen in rat peritoneal mast cells (Sung *et al.*, 1977a, b). A different profile of activity is observed in mast cells obtained by bronchoalveolar lavage (Flint *et al.*, 1985b; Leung *et al.*, 1988) and dispersed from the intestine (Rees and Church, unpublished observations) where SCG is not only effective, but also shows no evidence of tachyphylaxis. This may be particularly important in asthma as the mast cells lining the bronchial tree and found within the bronchial lumen are likely to be the first stimulated by inhaled allergens. In contrast, mast cells dispersed from human skin are insensitive to the inhibitory effects of SCG (Lowman *et al.*, 1988c) or nedocromil sodium (Benyon, Lowman and Church, unpublished observations) at concentrations up to 1 mM, thus, confirming the results of previous studies with skin slices (Pearce *et al.*, 1974; Clegg *et al.*, 1985) and *in vivo* (Ting *et al.*, 1983).

Agents which elevate intracellular levels of cyclic AMP, such as β-adrenoceptor agonists, are inhibitors of histamine secretion from human mast cells. This has been demonstrated repeatedly in human lung fragments and cells dispersed from lung parenchyma where nanomolar concentrations of β-adrenoceptor agonists are effective inhibitors of IgE-dependent release of histamine and eicosanoids (Church and Young, 1983; Church and Hiroi, 1987; Butchers *et al.*, 1979; Assem and Schild, 1969; Schulman *et al.*, 1982). More recently, the β-agonist salbutamol has been shown to inhibit histamine release from human dispersed skin mast cells activated by substance P and anti-IgE (Lowman *et al.*, 1988c) and histamine and PGD_2 release from human intestinal mast cells (Rees and Church, unpublished results).

VII CONCLUSION

The origins and functions of mast cell heterogeneity have been investigated using a wide variety of strategies. Perhaps no one has become more associated with the subject of mast cell heterogeneity than Lennart Enerback, whose pioneering studies of differences in fixation, dye binding and reactivity to stimuli between rodent mucosal and connective tissue mast cells laid the foundations of this subject. Now it is known that mast cell heterogeneity, both between species and within the mast cell population of single species, is a widespread phenomenon. The studies of Kitamura and co-workers of the ontogeny of mast cell sub-types have made elegant use of mast cell-deficient strains of mice. These studies, combined with those of the factors required by mast cells for development in cell culture, have drawn our attention to the importance of cellular interactions in the development of mast cell sub-types in rodents.

These studies have helped address the question of how mast cell heterogeneity has evolved, but there remains the question of the consequences of mast cell heterogeneity. An understanding of the functional differences between mast cells requires knowledge of the mediators released by these cells under different circumstances. Since their discovery by Paul Ehrlich in 1876, it has become clearly established that mast cells play an important part in the development of allergic responses. Their activation by allergens which cross-link their cell-surface receptors for IgE initiates the release of pre-formed and newly generated mediators that exert their pro-inflammatory actions by interacting with a variety of target cells. In accord with an important defensive role, mast cells are present in abundance in intestine, lung, skin and other tissues that form barriers between animals and their external environment. Although mast cells and their associated complement of pro-inflammatory mediators have traditionally been associated with allergy, the recent observations of the ability of human rheumatoid synovial and skin mast cells to be activated by a wide variety of IgE-independent stimuli suggest that they may have evolved to perform other functions. Probably, the most relevant agents that activate skin mast cells by the non-immunological pathway *in vivo* are neuropeptides localized to the dermis. There is an increasing awareness that there are extensive interactions between the peptidergic nervous system and immunocompetent leucocytes such as macrophages, monocytes and lymphocytes (Hartung and Toyka, 1983; McGillis *et al.*, 1987; O'Dorisio, 1987). The ability of mast cells to respond to peptides suggests that these cells may now be included amongst those involved in the neuro-immune axis. These two possible pathways of skin mast cell activation effectively allows these cells to be bi-functional. Whilst they have retained the capacity to release a wide spectrum of mediators presumably required for the mounting of an effective allergic response, skin mast cells may also play a role in the neurogenic control of homeostatic activities such as microvascular blood flow, angiogenesis and fibroblast proliferation. It is therefore apparent that, at least in skin mast cells, the presence of an IgE-independent pathway for mast cell activation may have great physiological relevance.

REFERENCES

Agius, R.M., Robinson, C., Church, M.K. and Holgate, S.T. (1988). Prostaglandin (PG) D_2 synthesis by human bronchoalveolar mast cells. *Br. J. Pharmacol.* **93**, 51P.

Anand, P., Bloom, S.R. and McGregor, G.P. (1983). Topical capsaicin pretreatment inhibits axon reflex vasodilation caused by somatostatin and vasoactive polypeptide in human skin. *Br. J. Pharmacol.* **78**, 665–669.

Assem, E.S.K. and Ghanem, N.S. (1988). Demonstration of IgE-sensitised mast cells in human heart and kidney. *Int. Arch. Allergy Appl. Immunol.* **87**, 101–104.

Assem, E.S.K. and Schild, H.O. (1969). Inhibition by sympathomimetic amines of histamine release induced by antigen in passively sensitized human lung. *Nature* **224**, 1028–1029.

Atkins, F.M. and Clark, R.A.F. (1987). Mast cells and fibrosis. *Arch. Dermatol.* **123**, 191–193.

Barr, R.M., Koro, O., Francis, D.M., Kobza-Black, A., Numata, T. and Greaves, M.W. (1988). The release of prostaglandin D_2 from human skin *in vivo* and *in vitro* during immediate allergic reactions. *Br. J. Pharmacol.* **94**, 773–780.

Befus, A.D. and Bienenstock, J. (1979). Immunologically-mediated intestinal mastocytosis in *Nippostrongylus brasiliensis* infected rats. *Immunology* **38**, 95–101.

Befus, A.D., Johnston, N. and Bienenstock, J. (1979). *Nippostrongylus brasiliensis*: Mast cells and histamine levels in tissues of infected and normal rats. *Exp. Parasitol.* **48**, 1–8.

Befus, A.D., Pearce, F.L., Gauldie, J., Horsewood, P. and Bienenstock, J. (1982). Mucosal mast cells. I. Isolation and functional characteristics of rat intestinal mast cells. *J. Immunol.* **128**, 2475–2480.

Befus, A.D., Dyck, N., Goodacre, R. and Bienenstock, J. (1987). Mast cells from the human intestinal lamina propria: isolation, histochemical subtypes, and functional characterization. *J. Immunol.* **138**, 2604–2610.

Benditt, E.P., Wong, R.L. and Arase, M. (1955). 5-Hydroxytryptamine in mast cells. *Proc. Soc. Exp. Biol. Med.* **90**, 303–304.

Benyon, R.C. (1988). Stimulus-secretion coupling in mast cells and basophils. In *Mast cells, Mediators and Disease* (ed. S.T. Holgate), pp. 195–226. MTP Press, Lancaster.

Benyon, R.C., Church, M.K., Clegg, L.S. and Holgate, S.T. (1986). Dispersion and characterization of mast cells from human skin. *Int. Arch. Allergy Appl. Immunol.* **79**, 332–334.

Benyon, R.C., Lowman, M.A. and Church, M.K. (1987a). Human skin mast cells: their dispersion, purification and secretory characterization. *J. Immunol.* **138**, 861–867.

Benyon, R.C., Church, M.K., Hillier, K. and Rees, P.H. (1987b). Human colon dispersed mast cells: isolation and characterization *Br. J. Pharmacol.* **90** (Proceedings Suppl), 158P.

Benyon, R.C., Robinson, C., Holgate, S.T. and Church, M.K. (1987c). Prostaglandin D_2 release from human skin mast cells in response to ionophore A23187. *Br. J. Pharmacol.* **92**, 635–638.

Bisgaard, H., Kristensen, J. and Sondergaard, J. (1982). The effect of leukotriene C_4 and D_4 on cutaneous blood flow in humans. *Prostaglandins* **23**, 797–801.

Black, J.W., Duncan, W.A.M., Durant, C.J., Ganellin, C.R. and Parsons, E.M. (1972). Definition and antagonism of histamine H_2-receptors. *Nature* **236**, 385–390.

Bowyer, A. (1968). Observations on the granularity of mast cells in human skin. *Acta Derm. Venereol.* **48**, 574–577.

Briggaman, R.A., Schechter, N.M., Fraki, J.E. and Lazarus, G.S. (1984). Degradation of the epidermal-dermal junction by a proteolytic enzyme from human skin and human polymorphonuclear leukocytes. *J. Exp. Med.* **160**, 1027–1042.

Burka, J.F. and Eyre, P. (1975). Modulation of the formation and release of bovine SRS-A *in vitro* by several anti-anaphylactic drugs. *Int. Arch. Allergy Appl. Immunol.* **49**, 774–781.

Butchers, P.R., Fullerton, J.R., Skidmore, I.F., Thomson, L.E., Vardey, C.J. and Wheeldon, A. (1979). A comparison of the anti-anaphylactic activities of salbutamol and disodium cromoglycate in the rat, the rat mast cell and in human lung tissue. *Br. J. Pharmacol.* **67**, 23–32.

Camp, R.D.R., Coutts, A.A., Greaves, M.W., Kay, A.B. and Walport, M.J. (1983). Responses of human skin to intradermal injection of leukotrienes C_4, D_4 and B_4. *Br. J. Pharmacol.* **80**, 497–502.

Campbell, A.M. and Robinson, C. (1988). Further studies on IgE-mediated eicosanoid release from human dispersed lung cells. *Br. J. Pharmacol.* **95** (Proceedings Suppl), 674P.

Capron, A., Dessaint, J.P., Capron, M., Joseph, M., Ameisen, J.C. and Tonnel, A.B. (1986). From parasites to allergy: the second receptor for IgE. *Immunology Today* **7**, 15–18.

Casale, T.B., Bowman, S. and Kaliner, M. (1984). Induction of human cutaneous mast cell degranulation by opiates and endogenous opioid peptides: evidence for opiate and nonopiate receptor participation. *J. Allergy Clin. Immunol.* **73**, 775–781.

Castells, M., Irani, A.A. and Schwartz, L.B. (1986). Evaluation of human peripheral blood leukocytes for mast cell protease. *J. Allergy Clin. Immunol.* **77** (Suppl), 246.

Caulfield, J.P., Lewis, R.A., Hein, A. and Austen, K.F. (1980). Secretion of dissociated human pulmonary mast cells: evidence for solubilization of granule contents before discharge. *J. Cell Biol.* **85**, 299–311.

Celander, O. and Folkow, B. (1953). The nature and distribution of afferent fibres provided with the axon reflex arrangement. *Acta Physiol. Scand.* **29**, 359–370.

Church, M.K. and Young, K.D. (1983). The characteristics of inhibition of histamine release from human lung fragments by sodium cromoglycate, salbutamol and chlorpromazine. *Br. J. Pharmacol.* **78**, 671–679.

Church, M.K. and Hiroi, J. (1987). Inhibition of IgE-dependent histamine release from human dispersed lung mast cells by anti-allergic drugs and salbutamol. *Br. J. Pharmacol.* **90**, 421–429.

Church, M.K., Pao, GJ-K and Holgate, S.T. (1982). Characterization of histamine secretion from dispersed human lung mast cells: effects of anti-IgE, calcium ionophore A23187, compound 48/80 and basic polypeptides. *J. Immunol.* **129**, 2116–2121.

Church, M.K., Mageed, R.A.K. and Holgate, S.T. (1983). Human tonsillar mast cells: characterization of histamine secretion and methods of dispersion. *Int. Arch. Allergy Appl. Immunol.* **72**, 188–190.

Clegg, L.S., Church, M.K. and Holgate, S.T. (1985). Histamine secretion from human skin slices induced by anti-IgE and artificial secretagogues and the effects of sodium cromoglycate and salbutamol. *Clin. Allergy* **15**, 321–328.

Coleman, J.W. and Godfrey, R.C. (1981). The number and affinity of IgE receptors on dispersed human lung mast cells. *Immunology* **44**, 859–863.

Conrad, D.H., Bazin, H., Sehon, A.H. and Froese, A. (1975). Binding parameters of the interaction between rat IgE and rat mast cell receptors. *J. Immunol.* **114**, 1688–1691.

Cox, J.S.G. (1967). Disodium cromoglycate (FPL 670, Intal): a specific inhibitor of reaginic antibody-antigen mechanisms. *Nature* **216**, 1328–1329.

Cox, J.S.G. and Altounyan, R.E.C. (1970). Nature and modes of action of disodium cromoglycate (Lomudal). *Respiration* **27** (Suppl), 292–309.

Craig, S.S., Schechter, N.M. and Schwartz, L.B. (1988). Ultrastructural analysis of human

T and TC mast cells identified by immunoelectron microscopy. *Lab. Invest.* **58**, 682–691.

Dahlén, S.E., Hansson, G., Hedqvist, P., Bjorck, T., Granstrom, E. and Dahlen, B. (1983). Allergen challenge of lung tissue from asthmatics elicits bronchial contraction that correlates with the release of leukotrienes C_4, D_4, and E_4. *Proc. Natl. Acad. Sci. USA.* **80**, 1712–1716.

Dixon, M., Jackson, D.M. and Richards, I.M. (1980). The action of sodium cromoglycate on "C" fibre endings in the dog lung. *Br. J. Pharmacol.* **70**, 11–13.

Dobbins, W.O., Tomasini, J.T. and Rollins, E.L. (1969). Electron and light microscopic identification of the mast cell of the gastrointestinal tract. *Gastroenterology* **56**, 268–279.

Dvorak, A.M., Galli, S.J., Schulman, E.S., Lichtenstein, L.M. and Dvorak, H.F. (1983). Basophil and mast cell degranulation: ultrastructural analysis of mechanisms of mediator release. *Fed. Proc.* **42**, 2510–2515.

Ebertz, J.M., Hermens, J.M., McMillan, J.C., Uno, H., Hirshman, C.A. and Hanafin, J.M. (1986). Functional differences between human cutaneous mast cells and basophils: a comparison of morphine-induced histamine release. *Agents and Actions* **18**, 455–462.

Ebertz, J.M., Hirshman, C.A., Kettelkamp, N.S., Uno, H. and Hanifin, J.M. (1987). Substance P-induced histamine release in human cutaneous mast cells. *J. Invest. Dermatol.* **88**, 682–685.

Ehrlich, P. (1876). Beitrage zur Kenntnis der Anilinfarbungen und ihrer Verwendung in der Mikroskopischen Technik. *Arch. Mikr. Anat.* **13**, 263–277.

Eliakim, R., Gilead, L., Ligumsky, M., Okon, E., Rachmilewitz, D. and Razin, E. (1986). Histamine and chondroitin sulfate E proteoglycan released by cultured human colonic mucosa: indication for possible presence of E mast cells. *Proc. Natl. Acad. Sci. USA.* **83**, 461–464.

Ellis, H.V., Johnson, A.R. and Moran, N.C. (1970). Selective release of histamine from rat mast cells by several drugs. *J. Pharmacol. Exp. Ther.* **175**, 627–631.

Enerback, L. (1966a). Mast cells in the gastrointestinal mucosa. I. Effects of fixation. *Acta Path. Microbiol. Scand.* **66**, 289–302.

Enerback, L. (1966b). Mast cells in the gastrointestinal mucosa. II. Dye binding and metachromatic properties. *Acta Path. Microbiol. Scand.* **66**, 303–312.

Enerback, L. (1966c). Mast cells in the gastrointestinal mucosa. III. Reactivity towards compound 48/80. *Acta Path. Microbiol. Scand.* **66**, 313–322.

Ennis, M. (1982). Histamine release from pulmonary mast cells. *Agents and Actions* **12**, 60–63.

Everitt, M. and Neurath, H. (1980). Rat peritoneal mast cell carboxypeptidase: localization, purification and enzymatic properties. *FEBS Lett.* **110**, 292–296.

Flint, K.C., Hudspith, B.N., Leung, K.B.P., Pearce, F.L., Seiger, K., Hammond, M.D.H., Brostoff, J. and Johnson, N.Mc.I. (1985a). IgE-dependent release of leukotriene C_4 and prostaglandin D_2 from human bronchoalveolar cells. *Thorax* **40**, Abstract 716.

Flint, K.C., Leung, K.B.P., Pearce, F.L., Hudspith, B.N., Brostoff, J. and Johnson, N.Mc.I. (1985b). Human mast cells recovered from bronchoalveolar lavage: their morphology, histamine release and effects of sodium cromoglycate. *Clin. Sci.* **68**, 427–432.

Foreman, J.C. and Lichtenstein, L.M. (1980). Induction of histamine secretion by polycations. *Biochim. Biophys. Acta* **629**, 587–603.

Foreman, J.C. and Piotrowski, W. (1984). Peptides and histamine release. *J. Allergy Clin. Immunol.* **74**, 127–131.

Foreman, J.C., Jordan, C.C., Oehme, P. and Renner, H. (1983). Structure–activity relationships for some substance P-related peptides that cause wheal and flare reactions in human skin. *J. Physiol.* **335**, 449–465.

Fox, C.C., Dvorak, A.M., Peters, S.P., Kagey-Sobotka, A. and Lichtenstein, L.M. (1985). Isolation and characterization of human intestinal mucosal mast cells. *J. Immunol.* **135**, 483–491.

Fraki, J.E. and Hopsu-Havu, V.K. (1972a). Human skin proteases. Differential extraction of proteases and of endogenous protease inhibitors. *Arch. Derm. Forsch.* **242**, 329–342.

Fraki, J.E. and Hopsu-Havu, V.K. (1972b). Human skin proteases. Partial purification and chracterisation of a protease inhibitor. *Arch. Derm. Forsch.* **243**, 153–163.

Fraki, J.E. and Hopsu-Havu, V.K. (1972c). Human skin proteases. Fractionation and characterisation. *Arch. Derm. Forsch.* **243**. 52–66.

Fraki, J.E. and Hopsu-Havu, V.K. (1975). Human skin proteases. Separation and characterization of two alkaline proteases, one splitting trypsin and the other chymotrypsin substrates. *Arch. Dermatol. Res.* **253**, 261–276.

Friedman, M.M. and Kaliner, M. (1985). In situ degranulation of human nasal mucosal mast cells: ultrastructural features and cell–cell associations. *J. Allergy Clin. Immunol.* **76**, 70–82.

Fujita, H., Asagami, C., Murozumi, S., Yamamoto, K. and Kinoshita, K. (1969). Electron microscopic studies of mast cells of human fetal skins. *J. Ultrastruct. Res.* **28**, 353–370.

Fuller, R.W., Conradson, T.B., Dixon, C.M.S., Crossman, D.C. and Barnes, P.J. (1987). Sensory neuropeptide effects in human skin. *Br. J. Pharmacol.* **92**, 781–788.

Galli, S.J., Dvorak, A.M. and Dvorak, H.F. (1984). Basophils and mast cells: morphologic insights into their biology, secretory patterns, and function. *Prog. Allergy* **34**, 1–141.

Garland, L.G. (1973). Effect of cromoglycate on anaphylactic histamine release from rat peritoneal mast cells. *Br. J. Pharmacol.* **49**, 128–130.

Gibson, S. and Miller, H.R.P. (1986). Mast cell subsets in the rat distinguished immunohistochemically by their content of serine proteinases. *Immunology* **58**, 101–104.

Gilead, L., Livni, N., Eliakim, R., Ligumski, M., Fich, A., Okon, E., Rachmilewitz, D. and Raxin, E. (1987). Human gastric mucosal mast cells are chondroitin sulfate E-containing mast cells. *Immunology* **62**, 23–28.

Ginsburg, H., Ben-Shahar, D. and Ben-David, E. (1982). Mast cell growth on fibroblast monolayers: two cell entities. *Immunology* **45**, 371–380.

Glenner, C.G. and Cohen, L.A. (1960). Histochemical demonstration of a species-specific trypsin-like enzyme in mast cells. *Nature* **185**, 846–847.

Goetzl, E.J., Weller, P.F. and Valone, F.H. (1976). Biochemical and functional bases of the regulatory and protective roles of the human eosinophil. *Adv. Inflamm. Res.* **1**, 157–167.

Greaves, M.W., Yamamoto, S. and Fairley M. (1972). IgE-mediated hypersensitivity in human skin studied using a new *in vitro* method. *Immunology* **23**, 239–248.

Grosman, N. (1981). Histamine release from isolated rat mast cells: effect of morphine and related drugs and their interaction with compound 48/80. *Agents and Action* **11**, 196–203.

Gruber, B., Poznansky, M., Boss, E., Partin, J., Gorevic, P. and Kaplan, A.P. (1986). Characterization and functional studies of rheumatoid synovial mast cells-activation by secretagogues, anti-IgE and a histamine-releasing lymphokine. *Arthritis Rheum.* **29**, 944–955.

Gruber, B.L., Marchese, M.J., Kiely, J., Schwartz, L.B. and Schechter, N.M. (1988). Human mast cell products degrade connective tissue matrix. *Int. Arch. Allergy Appl. Immunol.* **81**, 133–137.

Hagermark, O., Hokfelt, T. and Pernow, B. (1978). Flare and itch induced by substance P in human skin. *J. Invest. Dermatol.* **71**, 233–235.

Haig, D.M., McKee, T.A., Jarrett, E.E.E., Woodbury, R. and Miller, H.R.P. (1982).

Generation of mucosal mast cells is stimulated in *in vitro* by factors derived from T cells of helminth infected rats. *Nature* **300**, 188–190.

Hamaguchi, Y., Kanakura, Y., Fujita, J., Tajeda, S., Nakano, T., Tasui, S., Honjo, T. and Kitamura, Y. (1987). Interleukin 4 as an essential factor for *in vitro* growth of murine connective tissue type mast cells. *J. Exp. Med.* **165**, 268–273.

Hartschuh, W., Weihe, E. and Reinecke, M. (1983). Peptidergic (neurotensin, VIP, substance P) nerve fibres in the skin. Immunohistochemical evidence of an involvement of neuropeptides in nociception, pruritis and inflammation. *Br. J. Dermatol.* **109** (Suppl. 25), 14–17.

Hartung, H.P. and Toyka, K.V. (1983). Activation of macrophages by substance P: induction of oxidative burst and thromboxane release. *Eur. J. Pharmacol.* **89**, 301–305.

Harvey, J., Holgate, S.T., Peters, B.J., Robinson, C. and Walker, J.R. (1985). Oxidative transformations of arachidonic acid in human dispersed lung cells: disparity between utilization of endogenous and exogenous substrate. *Br. J. Pharmacol.* **86**, 417–426.

Hatanaka, K., Kitamura, Y. and Nishimune, Y. (1979). Local development of bone marrow-derived precursors in the skin of mice. *Blood* **53**, 142–147.

Heavey, D.J., Ernst, P.B., Stevens, R.L., Befus, A.D., Bienenstock, J. and Austen, K.F. (1988). Generation of leukotrienes C_4, leukotriene B_4, and prostaglandin D_2 by immunologically activated rat intestinal mucosa mast cells. *J. Immunol.* **140**, 1953–1957.

Hermens, J.M., Ebertz, J.M., Hanafin, J.M. and Hirshman, C.A. (1985). Comparison of histamine release in human skin mast cells induced by morphine, fentanyl and oxomorphine. *Anesthesiology* **62**, 124–129.

Hinsey, J.C. and Gasser, H.S. (1930). The component of the dorsal root mediating vasodilation and the Sherrington contracture. *Am. J. Physiol.* **92**, 679–689.

Hokfelt, T., Kellerth, J.O., Nillson, G. and Pernow, B. (1975). Experimental immunohistochemical studies on the localization and distribution of substance P in cat primary sensory neurones. *Brain Res.* **100**, 235–252.

Hokfelt, T., Elde, R., Johansson, O., Luft, R., Nillson, G. and Arimura, A. (1976). Immunohistochemical evidence for separate populations of somatostatin-containing and substance P-containing primary afferent neurones in the rat. *Neuroscience* **1**, 131–136.

Holgate, S.T., Lewis, R.A., Maguire, J.F., Roberts, L.J., Oates, J.A. and Austen, K.F. (1980). Effects of prostaglandin D2 on rat serosal mast cells: Discordance between immunologic mediator release and cyclic AMP levels. *J. Immunol.* **125**, 1367–1373.

Holgate, S.T., Burns, G.B., Robinson, C. and Church, M.K. (1984). Anaphylactic and calcium dependent generation of prostaglandin D_2 (PGD_2), thromboxane B_2 and other cyclooxygenase products of arachidonic acid by dispersed human lung cells and relationship to histamine release. *J. Immunol.* **133**, 2138–2144.

Hook, M., Lindahl, U., Hallen, A. and Backstrom, G. (1975). Biosynthesis of heparin: studies on the microsomal sulfation process. *J. Biol. Chem.* **250**, 6065–6071.

Ihle, J.N., Keller, J., Oroszlan, S., Henderson, L.E., Copeland, T.D., Fitch, F., Prytsowsky, M.B., Goldwasser, E., Schrader, J.W., Palaszynski, E., Dy, M. and Lebel, B. (1983). Biological properties of homogenous interleukin 3: Demonstration of WEHI-3 growth factor activity, mast cell growth factor activity, P-cell stimulating factor activity, colony-stimulating activity and histamine producing cell stimulating factor activity. *J. Immunol.* **131**, 282–287.

Irani, A.A., Butrus, S. and Schwartz, L.B. (1988). Distribution of T and TC mast cell subsets in vernal conjunctivitis (VC) and giant papillary conjunctivitis. *NER Allergy Proc.* **9**, Abstract 451.

Irani, A.A., Craig, S.S., DeBlois, G., Elson, C.O., Schechter, N.M. and Schwartz, L.B. (1987). Deficiency of the tryptase-positive chymase-negative mast cell type in gastrointestinal mucosa of patients with defective T-lymphocyte function. *J. Immunol.* **138**, 4381–4386.

Irani, A.A., Schechter, N.M., Craig, S., DeBlois, G. and Schwartz, L.B. (1986). Two types of human mast cells that have distinct neutral protease compositions. *Proc. Natl. Acad. Sci. USA*. **83**, 4464–4468.

Ishizaka, T. and Ishizaka, K. (1984). Activation of mast cells for mediator release through IgE receptors. *Prog. Allergy* **34**, 188–235.

Jarrett, E.E.E. and Miller, H.R.P. (1982). Production and activities of IgE in helminth infection. *Prog. Allergy* **31**, 178–233.

Johansson, O. (1986). A detailed account of the NPY immunoreactive nerves and cells of the human skin. Comparison with VIP-, substance P- and PHI-containing structures. *Acta Physiol. Scand.* **128**, 147–153.

Johnson, A.R. and Erdos, E.G. (1973). Release of histamine from mast cells by vasoactive peptides. *Proc. Soc. Exp. Biol. Med.* **142**, 1252–1256.

Johnson, D.A. and Cawston, T.E. (1985). Human lung mast cell tryptase fails to activate procollagenase or degrade proteoglycan. *Biochem. Biophys. Res. Commun.* **132**, 453–459.

Johnson, H.G. and Bach, M.K. (1975). Prevention of calcium ionophore-induced release of histamine in rat mast cells by disodium cromoglycate. *J. Immunol.* **114**, 514–516.

Jorizzo, J.L., Coutts, A.A., Eady, R.A.J. and Greaves, M.W. (1983). Vascular responses of human skin to injection of substance P and mechanism of action. *Eur. J. Pharmacol.* **87**, 67–76.

Kaplan, A.P., Gray, L., Shaff, R.E., Horakova, Z. and Beaven, M.A. (1975). *In vivo* studies of mediator release in cold urticaria and cholinergic urticaria. *J. Allergy Clin. Immunol.* **55**, 394–402.

Keller, R., Hess, M.W. and Riley, J.F. (1976). Mast cells in the skin of normal, hairless and athymic mice. *Experientia* **32**, 171–172.

Kenins, P. (1981). Identification of the unmyelinated sensory nerves which evoke plasma extravasation in response to antidromic stimulation. *Neurosci. Lett.* **25**, 137–141.

Kitamura, Y., Go, S. and Hatanaka, K. (1978). Decrease of mast cells in W/W^v mice and their increase by bone marrow transplantation. *Blood* **52**, 447–452.

Kitamura, Y., Yokoyama, M., Matsuda, H., Ohno T. and Mori, K.J. (1981). Spleen colony-forming cell as a common precursor for tissue mast cells and granulocytes. *Nature* **291**, 159–160.

Kitamura, Y., Nakano, T., Sonoda, T., Kanayama, Y., Yamamura, T. and Asai, H. (1986). Probable transdifferation between connective tissue and mucosal mast cells. In *Mast Cell Differentiation and Heterogeneity* (eds A.D. Befus, J. Bienenstock and J.A. Denburg), pp. 135–140. Raven Press, New York.

Kobza-Black, A., Ormerod, A.D., Dawes, J., Murdoch, R.D., Koro, O., Barr, R.M. and Greaves, M.W. (1988). Release of histamine and prostaglandin D_2 in cold urticaria without evidence of platelet activation. *Skin Pharmacol.* **1**, 69.

Koro, O., Dover, J.S., Francis, D.M., Kobza-Black, A., Kelly, R.W., Barr R.M. and Greaves, M.W. (1986). Release of prostaglandin D_2 and histamine in a case of localized heat urticaria and effects of treatments. *Br. J. Dermatol.* **115**, 721–728.

Krell, R.D. and Chakrin, L.W. (1976). An *in vitro* model of canine hypersensitivity reactions. *Int. Arch. Allergy Appl. Immunol.* **51**, 641–655.

Lagunoff, D. (1972). Contributions of electron microscopy to the study of mast cells. *J. Invest. Dermatol.* **58**, 296–311.

Lagunoff, D., Martin, T.W. and Read, G. (1983). Agents that release histamine from mast cells. *Ann. Rev. Pharmacol. Toxicol.* **23**, 331–351.

Lawrence, I.D., Warner, J.A., Cohen, V.L., Hubbard, W.C., Kagey-Sobotka, A. and

Lichtenstein, L.M. (1987). Purification and characterization of human skin mast cells. Evidence for human mast cell heterogeneity. *J. Immunol.* **139**, 3062–3069.

Lee, C.H., Campbell, N.J., Williams, B.J. and Iverson, L.L. (1986). Multiple tachykinin binding sites in peripheral tissues and in brain. *Eur. J. Pharmacol.* **130**, 209–217.

Lembeck, F. and Holzer, P. (1979). Substance P as a neurogenic mediator of antidromic vasodilatation and neurogenic plasma extravasation. *Naunyn Schmiederberg Arch. Pharmacol.* **310**, 175–183.

Leung, K.B.P., Flint, K.C., Brostoff, J., Hudspith, B.N., Johnson, N.Mc.I., Lau, H.Y.A., Liu, W.L. and Pearce, F.L. (1988). Effects of sodium cromoglycate and nedocromil sodium on histamine secretion from human lung mast cells *Thorax*, **43**, 756–761.

Levi-Schaffer, F., Austen, K.F., Caulfield, J.P., Hein, A., Bloes, W.F. and Stevens, R.L. (1985). Fibroblasts maintain the phenotype and viability of the rat heparin-containing mast cell *in vitro*. *J. Immunol.* **135**, 3454–3462.

Levi-Schaffer, F., Austen, K.F., Gravallese, P.M. and Stevens, R.L. (1986). Co-culture of interleukin 3-dependent mouse mast cells with fibroblasts results in a phenotypic change of mast cells. *Proc. Natl. Acad. Sci. USA*. **83**, 6485–6488.

Lewis, R.A., Soter, N.A., Diamond, P.T., Austen, K.F., Oates, J.A. and Roberts, L.J. (1982). Prostaglandin D_2 generation after activation of rat and human mast cells with anti-IgE. *J. Immunol.* **129**, 1627–1631.

Lewis, T. (1927). *The Blood Vessels of the Human Skin and their Responses*. Shaw, London.

Lonky, S.A., Marsh, J. and Wohl, H. (1978). Stimulation of human granulocyte elastase by platelet factor 4 and heparin. *Biochem. Biophys. Res. Commun.* **85**, 1113–1118.

Lowman, M.A., Rees, P.H., Benyon, R.C. and Church, M.K. (1988a). Human mast cell heterogeneity: Histamine release from mast cells dispersed from skin, lung, adenoids, tonsils and intestinal mucosa in response to IgE-dependent and non-immunological stimuli. *J. Allergy Clin. Immunol.* **81**, 590–597.

Lowman, M.A., Benyon, R.C. and Church, M.K. (1988b). Chracterization of neuropeptide-induced histamine released from human dispersed skin mast cells. *Br. J. Pharmacol.* **95**, 121–130.

Lowman, M.A., Benyon, R.C. and Church, M.K. (1988c). Human skin mast cells: Effects of salbutamol and sodium cromoglycate on histamine release induced by anti-IgE and substance P. *Skin Pharmacol.* **1**, 63–64.

Lynch, S.M., Austen, K.F. and Wasserman, S.I. (1978). Release of arylsulphatase A but not B from rat mast cells by non-cytolytic secretory stimuli. *J. Immunol.* **121**, 1394–1399.

MacGlashan, D.W., Schleimer, R.P., Peters, S.P., Schulman, E.S., Adams, G.K., Newball, H.H. and Lichtenstein, L.M. (1982). Generation of leukotrienes by purified human lung mast cells. *J. Clin. Invest.* **70**, 747–751.

Maier, M., Spragg, J. and Schwartz, L.B. (1983). Inactivation of human high molecular weight kininogen by human mast cell tryptase. *J. Immunol.* **130**, 2352–2356.

Marks, R.M., Roche, W.R., Czerniecki, M., Penny, R. and Nelson, D.S. (1986). Mast cell granules cause proliferation of human microvascular endothelial cells. *Lab. Invest.* **55**, 289–294.

Maurice, P.D.L., Barr, R.M., Koro, O. and Greaves, M.W. (1987). The effect of prostaglandin D_2 on the response of human skin to histamine. *J. Invest. Dermatol.* **89**, 245–248.

Mayrhofer, G. (1979). The nature of the thymus dependency of mucosal mast cells. II. The effect of thymectomy and of depleting circulating lymphocytes on the response to Nippostrongylus brasiliensis. *Cell Immunol.* **47**, 312–322.

McGillis, J.P, Organist, M.L. and Payan, D.G. (1987). Substance P and immunoregulation. *Fed. Proc.* **46**, 196–199.

Metcalfe, D.D., Bland, C.E. and Wasserman, S.I. (1984). Biochemical and functional characterisation of proteoglycans isolated from basophils of patients with chronic myelogenous leukemia. *J. Immunol.* **132**, 1943–1950.

Metcalfe, D.D., Lewis, R.A., Silbert, J.E., Rosenberg, R.D., Wasserman, S.I. and Austen, K.F. (1979). Isolation and characterisation of heparin from human lung. *J. Clin. Invest.* **4**, 1537–1543.

Metcalfe, D.D., Soter, N.A., Wasserman, S.I. and Austen, K.F. (1980). Identification of sulfated mucopolysaccharides including heparin in the lesional skin of a patient with mastocytosis. *J. Invest. Dermatol.* **74**, 210–215.

Metzger, H., Alcarez, G., Hohman, R., Kinet, J.-P., Pribluda, V. and Quarto, R. (1986). The receptor with high affinity for immunoglobulin E. *Ann. Rev. Immunol.* **4**, 419–470.

Mikhail, G.R. and Miller-Milinska, A. (1964). Mast cell population in human skin. *J. Invest. Dermatol.* **43**, 249–254.

Miller, H.R.P. (1980). The structure, origin and function of mucosal mast cells: a brief review. *Biol. Cellulaire* **39**, 249–254.

Moqbel, R., King, S.J., MacDonald, A.J., Miller, H.R.P., Cromwell, O., Shaw, R.J. and Kay, A.B. (1986a). Enteral and sytemic release of leukotrienes during anaphylaxis of *Nippostrongylus brasiliensis* primed rats. *J. Immunol.* **137**, 296–301.

Moqbel, R., Walsh, G.M. and Kay, A.B. (1986b). Inhibition of human granulocyte activation by nedocromil sodium. *Eur. J. Respir. Dis.* **69** (Suppl 147), 227–229.

Moqbel, R., Walsh, G.M., MacDonald, A.J. and Kay, A.B. (1986c). Effect of disodium cromoglycate on activation of human eosinophils and neutrophils following reversed (anti-IgE) anaphylaxis. *Clin. Allergy* **16**, 73–83.

Nabel, G., Galli, S.J., Dvorak, A.M., Dvorak, H.F. and Cantor, H. (1981). Inducer T-lymphocytes synthesise a factor that stimulates proliferation of cloned mast cells. *Nature* **291**, 332–334,.

Nakano, T., Sonoda, T., Hayashi, C., Yamatodani, A., Kanayama, Y., Yamamura, T., Asai, H., Yonezawa, T., Kitamura, Y. and Galli, S.J. (1985). Fate of bone marrow-derived cultured mast cells after intracutaneous, intraperitoneal and intravenous transfer into genetically mast cell deficient W/Wv mice: evidence that cultured mast cells can give rise to both connective tissue type and mucosal mast cells. *J. Exp. Med.* **162**, 1025–1043.

Newson, B., Dahlstrom, A., Enerback, L. and Ahlman, H. (1983). Suggestive evidence for a direct innervation of mucosal mast cells. *Neuroscience* **10**, 565–570.

O'Dorisio, M.S. (1987). Biochemical characteristics of receptors for vasoactive intestinal polypeptide in nervous, endocrine and immune systems. *Fed. Proc.* **42**, 192–195.

Orr, T.S.C. (1977). Fine structure of the mast cell with special reference to human cells. *Scand. J. Respir. Dis.* **98** (Suppl), 1–7.

Orr, T.S.C. and Cox, J.S.G. (1969). Disodium cromoglycate, an inhibition of mast cell degranulation and histamine release induced by phospholipase A. *Nature* **233**, 197–198.

Orr, T.S.C., Hall, D.E., Gwilliam, J.M. and Cox, J.S.G. (1971). Effect of disodium cromoglycate on the release of histamine and degranulation of mast cells induced by compound 48/80. *Life Sci.* **10**, 805–812.

Orwin, J.M. and Fozard, J.R. (1986). Blockade of the flare response to intradermal 5-hydroxytryptamine in man by MDL 72,222, a selective antagonist at neuronal 5-hydroxytryptamine receptors. *Eur. J. Clin. Pharmacol.* **30**, 209–212.

Padawer, J. (1974). Mast cells: extended life span and lack of granule turnover under normal *in vivo* conditions. *Exp. Mol. Pathol.* **20**, 269–280.

Pearce, C.A., Greaves, M.W., Plummer, V.M. and Yamamoto, S. (1974). Effect of disodium cromoglycate on antigen evoked histamine release in human skin. *Clin. Exp. Immunol.* **17**, 437–440.

Pearce, F.L. (1986). Functional differences between mast cells from different locations. In *Mast Cell Differentiation and Heterogeneity* (eds A.D. Befus, J. Bienenstock and J.A. Denburg), pp. 215–222. Raven Press, New York.

Pearce, F.L., Ali, H., Barrett, K.E., Befus, A.D., Bienenstock, J., Brostoff, J., Ennis, M., Flint, K.C., Hudspith, B., Johnson, N.M., Leung, K.B.P. and Peachell, P.T. (1985). Functional characteristics of mucosal and connective tissue mast cells of man, the rat and other animals. *Int. Arch. Allergy Appl. Immunol.* **77**, 274–279.

Pearce, F.L., Befus, A.D., Gauldie, J. and Bienenstock, J. (1982). Mucosal mast cells. II. Effects of anti-allergic compounds on histamine secretion by isolated intestinal mast cells. *J. Immunol.* **128**, 2481–2486.

Pessinger, M.A., Lepage, P., Simard, J.P. and Parker, G.H. (1983). Mast cell numbers in incisional wounds in rat skin as a function of distance, time and treatment. *Br. J. Dermatol.* **108**, 179–187.

Peters, S.P., MacGlashan, D.W., Schulman, E.S., Schleimer, R.P., Hayes, E.C., Rokach, J., Adkinson, N.F. and Lichtenstein, L.M. (1984a). Arachidonic acid metabolism in purified human lung mast cells. *J. Immunol.* **132**, 1972–1979.

Peters, S.P., Kagey-Sobotka, A., MacGlashan, D.W. and Lichtenstein, L.M. (1984b). Effect of prostaglandin D_2 in modulating histamine release from human basophils. *J. Pharmacol. Exp. Ther.* **228**, 400–406.

Pillarisetti, V., Rao, S., Friedman, M.M., Atkins, F.M. and Metcalfe, D.D. (1983). Phagacytosis of mast cell granules by cultured fibroblasts. *J. Immunol.* **130**, 341–349.

Piotrowski, W. and Foreman J.C. (1985). On the actions of substance P, somatostatin and vasoactive intestinal polypeptide on rat peritoneal mast cells and in human skin. *Naunyn Schmiederberg Arch. Pharmacol.* **331**, 364–368.

Razin, E., Cordon Cardo, C. and Good R.A. (1981). Growth of a pure population of mouse mast cells *in vitro* with conditioned medium derived from concanavalin A-stimulated splenocytes. *Proc. Natl. Acad. Sci. USA.* **78**, 2559–2561.

Razin, E., Stevens, R.L., Akiyama, F., Schmid, K. and Austen, K.F. (1982). Culture from mouse bone marrow of a subclass of mast cells possessing a distinct chondroitin sulfate proteoglycan with glycosaminoglycans rich in N-acetylgalactosamine-4,6-disulphate. *J. Biol. Chem.* **257**, 7229–7236.

Razin, E.; Ihle, J.N., Seldin, D., Mencia-Huerta, J.M., Katz, H.R., Le Blanc, P.A., Hein, A., Caulfield, J.P., Austen, K.F. and Stevens, R.L. (1984). Interleukin 3: a differentiation and growth factor for the mouse mast cell that contains chondroitin sulfate E proteoglycan. *J. Immunol.* **132**, 1479–1486.

Rees, P.H., Hillier, K. and Church, M.K. (1988). The secretory characteristics of mast cells isolated from human large intestinal mucosa and muscle. *Immunology* **65**, 437–442.

Repke, H., Piotrowski, W., Bienert, M. and Foreman, J.C. (1987). Histamine release induced by Arg-Pro-Lys-Pro(CH2)11CH3 from rat peritoneal mast cells. *J. Pharmacol. Exp. Ther.* **243**, 317–321.

Robinson, C. and Holgate, S.T. (1986). The synthesis, release and effects of prostaglandins in the lung. In *Asthma: Clinical Pharmacology and Therapeutic Progress* (ed. A.B. Kay), pp. 213–225. Blackwell, Oxford.

Robinson, C., Benyon, C., Agius, R.M., Jones, D.B., Wright, D.H. and Holgate, S.T. (1988). The immunological- and calcium-dependent release of histamine and eicosanoids from human dispersed mastocytosis spleen cells. *J. Invest. Dermatol.* **90**, 359–365.

Robinson, H.C., Horner, A.A., Hook, M., Ogren, S. and Lindahl, U. (1978). A proteoglycan form of heparin and its degradation to single chain molecules. *J. Biol. Chem.* **253**, 6687–6693.

Ruitenberg, E.J. and Elgerman, A. (1976). Absence of intestinal mast cell responses in congenitally athymic mice. *Nature* **264**, 258–260.

Sautebin, L., Vigano, T., Grassi, E., Crivellari, M.T., Galli, G., Berti, F., Mezzetti, M. and Folco, G. (1985). Release of leukotrienes, induced by the Ca^{++} ionophore A23187, from human lung parenchyma *in vitro*. *J. Pharmacol. Exp. Ther.* **234**, 217–221.

Schayer, R.W. (1962). Evidence that induced histamine is an intrinsic regulator of the microcirculatory system. *Am. J. Physiol.* **202**, 66–72.

Schechter, N.M., Fraki, J.E., Geesin, J.C. and Lazarus, G.S. (1983). Human skin chymotryptic proteinase: Isolation and relation to cathepsin G and rat mast cell protease. *J. Biol. Chem.* **258**, 2973–2978.

Schechter, N.M., Choi, J.K., Slavin, D.A., Deresienski, D.T., Sayama, S., Dong, G., Lavaker, R.M., Proud, D. and Lazarus, G.S. (1986). Identification of a chymotrypsin-like proteinase from human mast cells. *J. Immunol.* **137**, 962–970.

Schleimer, R.P., Schulman, E.S., MacGlashan, D.W., Peters, S.P., Hayes, E.C., Adams, G.K., Lichtenstein, L.M. and Adkinson, N.F. (1983). Effects of dexamethasone on mediator release from human lung fragments and purified human lung mast cells. *J. Clin. Invest.* **71**, 1830–1835.

Schleimer, R.P., Davidson, D.A., Lichtenstein, L.M. and Adkinson, N.F. (1986). Selective inhibition of arachidonic acid metabolite release from human lung tissue by anti-inflammatory steroids. *J. Immunol.* **136**, 3006–3011.

Schulman, E.S., MacGlashan, D.W., Peters, S.P., Schleimer, R.P., Newball, H.H. and Lichtenstein, L.M. (1982). Human lung mast cells: purification and characterization. *J. Immunol.* **129**, 2662–2667.

Schwartz, L.B. (1985). Monoclonal antibodies against human mast cell tryptase demonstrate shared antigenic sites on subunits of tryptase and selective localization of the enzyme to mast cells. *J. Immunol.* **134**, 526–531.

Schwartz, L.B. and Austen, K.F. (1984). Structure and function of the chemical mediators of mast cells. *Prog. Allergy* **34**, 271–321.

Schwartz, L.B. and Bradford, T.M. (1986). Regulation of tryptase from human lung mast cells by heparin: stabilization of the active tetramer. *J. Biol. Chem.* **261**, 7372–7379.

Schwartz, L.B., Austen, K.F. and Wasserman, S.I. (1979). Immunologic release of beta-hexosaminidase and beta-glucuronidase from purified rat serosal mast cells. *J. Immunol.* **123**, 1445–1450.

Schwartz, L.B., Riedel, C., Caulfield, J.P, Wasserman, S.I. and Austen, K.F. (1981). Cell association of complexes of chymase, heparin proteoglycan and protein after degranulation by rat mast cells. *J. Immunol.* **126**, 2071–2078.

Schwartz, L.B., Lewis, R.A. and Austen, K.F. (1981a). Tryptase from human pulmonary mast cells: purification and characterization. *J. Biol. Chem.* **256**, 11939–11943.

Schwartz, L.B., Lewis, R.A., Seldin, D. and Austen, K.F. (1981b). Acid hydrolases and tryptase from secretory granules of dispersed lung mast cells. *J. Immunol.* **126**, 1290–1294.

Schwartz, L.B., Kawahara, M.S., Hugli, T.E., Vik, D., Fearon, D.T. and Austen, K.F. (1983). Generation of C_{3a} anaphylatoxin from human C_3 by human mast cell tryptase. *J. Immunol.* **130**, 1891–1895.

Schwartz, L.B., Bradford, T.M., Littman, B.L. and Wintroub, B.U. (1985a). The fibrinogenolytic activity of purified tryptase from human lung mast cells. *J. Immunol.* **135**, 2762–2767.

Schwartz, L.B., Foley, J.V., Austen, K.F., Soter, N.A., Shephard, R. and Murphy, G.F. (1985b). Localization of tryptase to human cutaneous mast cells and keratinocytes by immunofluorescence and immunoperoxidase cytochemistry with monoclonal antitryptase antibody. *J. Allergy Clin. Immunol.* **76**, 182–188.

Schwartz, L.B., Irani, A.M., Roller, K., Castells, M. and Schechter, N.M. (1987a). Quantitation of histamine, tryptase, and chymase in dispersed human T and CT mast cells. *J. Immunol.* **138**, 2611–2615.

Schwartz, L.B., Metcalfe, D.D., Miller, J.S., Earl, H. and Sullivan, T. (1987b). Tryptase levels as an indicator of mast cell activation in systemic anaphylaxis and mastocytosis. *N. Eng. J. Med.* **316**, 1622–1626.

Scully, M.F., Ellis, V., Seno, N. and Kakkar, V.V. (1986). The anti-coagulant properties of mast cell product, chondroitin sulphate E. *Biochem. Biophys. Res. Commun.* **137**, 15–22.

Seppa, H.E.J. and Jarvinen, M. (1978). Rat skin main neutral protease: purification and properties. *J. Invest. Dermatol.* **70**, 84–89.

Shanahan, F., Lee, T.D.G., Bienenstock, J. and Befus, A.D. (1984). The influence of endorphins on peritoneal and mucosal mast cell secretion. *J. Allergy Clin. Immunol.* **74**, 499–504.

Shanahan, F., Denburg, J.A., Fox, J., Bienenstock, J. and Befus, D. (1985). Mast cell heterogeneity: effects of neuroenteric peptides on histamine release. *J. Immunol.* **135**, 1331–1337.

Shanahan, F., Lee, T.D.G., Bienenstock, J. and Befus, D. (1986). Mast cell heterogeneity: effect of anti-allergic compounds on neuropeptide-induced histamine release. *Int. Arch. Allergy Appl. Immunol.* **80**, 424–426.

Sheard, P. and Blair, A.M.J.N. (1970). Disodium cromoglycate: activity in three *in vitro* models of the immediate hypersensitivity reaction in lung. *Int. Arch. Allergy Appl. Immunol.* **38**, 217–224.

Silbert, J.E. (1967). Biosynthesis of heparin. *J. Biol. Chem.* **242**, 5146–5152.

Skotfisch, G., Savitt, J.M. and Jacobowitz, D.M. (1985). Suggestive evidence for a functional unit between mast cells and substance P fibres in the rat diaphragm and mesentery. *Histochemistry* **2**, 5–8.

Smith, J.B., Silver, M.J., Ingerman, C.M. and Kocsis, J.J. (1974). Prostaglandin D_2 inhibits the aggregation of human platelets. *Thromb. Res.* **5**, 291–299.

Smith, T.J., Hougland, M.W. and Johnson, D.A. (1984). Human lung tryptase, purification and characterization. *J. Biol. Chem.* **259**, 11046–11051.

Sonoda, T., Kitamura, Y., Haku, Y., Hara, H. and Mori, K.J. (1984). Proliferation of peritoneal mast cells in the skin of W/Wv mice that genetically lack mast cells. *J. Exp. Med.* **160**, 138–151.

Sonoda, S., Sonoda, T., Nakano, T., Kanayama, Y., Kanakura, Y., Asai, H., Yonezawa, T. and Kitamura, Y. (1986). Development of mucosal mast cells after injection of a single connective tissue type mast cell in the stomach mucosa of genetically mast cell-deficient W/W^v mice. *J. Immunol.* **137**, 1319–1322.

Soter, N.A., Lewis, R.A., Corey, E.J. and Austen, K.F. (1983). Local effects of synthetic leukotrienes (LTC_4, LTD_4, LTE_4 and LTB_4) in human skin. *J. Invest. Dermatol.* **80**, 115–119.

Stanisz, A.M., Befus, D. and Bienenstock, J. (1986). Differential effects of vasoactive intestinal peptide, substance P and somatostatin on immunoglobulin synthesis and proliferation by lumphocytes from Peyer's patches, mesenteric lymph nodes, and spleen. *J. Immunol.* **136**, 152–156.

Starkey, P.M. and Barrett, A.J. (1985). Human cathepsin G: catalytic and immunologic properties. *Biochem. J.* **155**, 273–278.

Stevens, R.L., Lee, T.G., Seldin, D.C., Austen, K.F., Befus, A.D. and Bienenstock, J. (1986). Intestinal mast cells of rats infected with *Nippostrongylus brasiliensis* contain protease resistant chondroitin di-B proteoglycan. *J. Immunol.* **137**, 291–295.

Suda, T., Suda, S., Spicer, S.S. and Ogawa, M. (1985). Proliferation and differentiation in culture of mast cell progenitors derived from mast cell deficient mice of genotype

W/W^v. *J. Cell. Physiol.* **122**, 187–192.

Sung, C.P., Saunders, H.L., Krell, R.D. and Chakrin, L.W. (1977a). Studies on the mechanism of tachyphylaxis to disodium cromoglycate. *Int. Arch. Allergy Appl. Immunol.* **55**, 374–384.

Sung, C.P., Saunders, H.L., Lenhardt, E. and Chakrin, L.W. (1977b). Further studies on the tachyphylaxis to disodium cromoglycate: the effects of concentration and temperature. *Int. Arch. Allergy Appl. Immunol.* **55**, 385–394.

Talbot, S.F., Atkins, P.C., Goetzl, E.J. and Zweiman, B. (1985). Accumulation of leukotriene C_4 and histamine on human allergic skin reactions. *J. Clin. Invest.* **76**, 650–656.

Tas, J. and Berndsen, R.G. (1977). Does heparin occur in mucosal mast cells of the rat small intestine? *J. Histochem. Cytochem.* **25**, 1058–1062.

Tay, C.H., Yeoh, T.S. and Greaves, M.W. (1972). Spontaneous and evoked histamine release from guinea-pig skin *in vitro* in presence of disodium cromoglycate. *Int. Arch. Allergy Appl. Immunol.* **43**, 390–394.

Tharp, M.D., Suvunrungsi, R.T. and Sullivan, T.J. (1983). IgE-mediated release of histamine from human cutaneous mast cells. *J. Immunol.* **130**, 1896–1901.

Tharp, M.D., Kagey-Sobotka, A., Fox, C.C., Marone, G., Lichtenstein, L.M. and Sullivan, T.J. (1987). Functional heterogeneity of human mast cells from different anatomic sites: *in vitro* responses to morphine sulfate. *J. Allergy Clin. Immunol.* **79**, 646–653.

Theriault, E., Otsuka, M. and Jessel, T. (1979). Capsaicin-evoked release of substance P from primary sensory neurones. *Brain Res.* **170**, 209–213.

Thompson, H.L., Schulman, E.S. and Metcalfe, D.D. (1988). Identification of chondroitin sulfate E in human lung mast cells. *J. Immunol.* **140**, 2708–2713.

Ting, S., Zweiman, B. and Lavker, R.M. (1983). Cromolyn does not modulate human allergic skin reactions *in vivo*. *J. Allergy Clin. Immunol.* **71**, 12–17.

Torebjork, H.E. and Hallin, R.G. (1974). Identification of afferent C units in intact human skin. *Brain Res.* **67**, 387–403.

Uvnas, B. (1967). Mode of binding and release of histamine in mast cell granules of the rat. *Fed. Proc.* **26**, 219–221.

Uvnas, B., Aborg, C.-H. and Bergendorff, A. (1970). Storage of histamine in mast cells. Evidence for ionic binding of histamine to protein carboxyls in the granule heparin protein complex. *Acta. Physiol. Scand.* **336** (Suppl), 1–26.

Vurek, G.G., Prager, D.J. and Feigen, G.A. (1967). Antibody concentration and temperature as determinants in the *in vitro* sensitisation and histamine release in isolated cardiac tissues. *J. Immunol.* **99**, 1243–1253.

Wenzel, S., Irani, A.M., Sanders, J.M., Bradford, T.R. and Schwartz, L.B. (1986). Immunoassay of tryptase from human mast cells. *J. Immunol. Methods* **86**, 139–142.

Wiesner-Menzel, L., Schulz, B., Vakilzadeh, F. and Czarnetzki, B.M. (1981). Electron microscopical evidence for a direct contact between nerve fibres and mast cells. *Acta Derm. Venereol.* **61**, 465–469.

Wintroub, B.U., Kaempfer, C.E., Schechter, N.M. and Proud, D. (1986). Human lung mast cell chymotrypsin-like enzyme: identification and partial characterization. *J. Clin. Invest.* **77**, 196–201.

Woodbury, R.G. and Miller, H.R.P. (1982). Quantitative analysis of mucosal mast cell protease in the intestine of *Nippostrongylus*-infected rats. *Immunology*, **46**, 487–495.

Woodbury, R.G., Katunuma, N., Kobayashi, K., Titani, K. and Neurath, H. (1978). Covalent structure of a group specific protease from rat small intestine. *Biochemistry* **17**, 811–819.

Yurt, R.W. and Austen, K.F. (1977). Preparative purification of rat mast cell chymase.

Characterization and interaction with granule components. *J. Exp. Med.* **146**, 1405–1419.
Yurt, R.W., Leid, R.W., Austen, K.F. and Silbert, J.E. (1977). Native heparin from rat peritoneal mast cells. *J. Biol. Chem.* **252**, 518–521.
Zucker-Franklin, D., Gusky, G., Hirayama, N. and Schnipper, E. (1981). The presence of mast cell precursors in rat peripheral blood. *Blood* **58**, 544–551.

6

Eosinophil heterogeneity

Takeshi Fukuda, Toshio Numao, Ikuo Akutsu and Sohei Makino

Department of Allergy and Clinical Immunology, Dokkyo University School of Medicine, Tochigi 321–02, Japan

I INTRODUCTION

Eosinophils are primarily tissue-dwelling granulocytes and normally constitute only a small proportion of the circulating leucocytes. Eosinophilia (increased numbers of eosinophils) in circulating blood and/or tissues is common in atopy and is associated with a diversity of diseases, especially parasitic infections. Eosinophilia may also accompany neoplastic, immune, skin and idiopathic disease processes (Weller, 1984). Eosinophils and neutrophils have many properties in common, but eosinophils also possess a number of distinct properties, which include the greatest buoyant density of all peripheral blood leucocytes and a cytoplasmic content of specialized granules containing a number of basic proteins, which are helminthotoxic. Eosinophils generate lipid mediators, preferentially synthesizing leukotriene C_4 and, functionally, eosinophils are distinguished by their ability to kill helminthic parasites (Gleich and Adolphson, 1986).

Early studies focused on comparison between eosinophils from normal subjects and eosinophilic patients. Measurements of a variety of biological parameters demonstrated morphological, metabolic and functional differences (Connell, 1968; Spry and Tai, 1976; Bass *et al.*, 1980; Pincus *et al.*, 1981). More recently, studies using techniques devised to separate leucocytes according to their density (Vadas *et al.*, 1979; Gartner, 1980) have demonstrated that all eosinophil populations are heterogeneous in

ASTHMA REVIEWS VOLUME 2
ISBN 0-12-040922-4

terms of their density. A population of eosinophils of lower than normal density has been discovered and is referred to as light-density or hypodense eosinophils (Winqvist *et al.*, 1982; Prin *et al.*, 1983) as distinct from the normal-density or normodense eosinophils. Density heterogeneity is linked to morphological, biochemical and functional heterogeneity, which has been observed in earlier studies. In this review, current knowledge of heterogeneity of eosinophils has been summarized, giving emphasis to the characteristics and pathogenesis of hypodense eosinophils.

II DENSITY DISTRIBUTION OF EOSINOPHILS

A Normal subjects

The density of eosinophils can be determined using gradients of metrizamide or polyvinylpyrrolidone-coated silica gel (Percoll). Studies using other gradient media or performed under different experimental conditions demonstrated different density ranges for normal eosinophils. When leucocyte preparations isolated from normal subjects were applied to hypertonic (approximately 540 mOsm l^{-1}) metrizamide gradients most of the eosinophils were found in solutions with densities greater than 1.135 g ml^{-1}, hence eosinophils with a density of 1.130 g ml^{-1} or less have been referred to as hypodense (Prin *et al.*, 1984). When isotonic Percoll (pH 7.4) was used as a gradient medium, most eosinophils were found to have densities heavier than 1.082 or 1.081 g ml^{-1} (Fukuda *et al.*, 1985; Shult *et al.*, 1988) and peak eosinophil densities were between 1.085 and 1.094 g ml^{-1}. Only a few eosinophils, with a density lower than 1.081 (Shult *et al.*, 1988) or 1.082 (Fukuda *et al.*, 1985) g ml^{-1}, were designated as hypodense. Additional manipulation of the leucocytes prior to separation on isotonic Percoll gradients caused the eosinophils to localize in solutions with different densities. For example, when leucocyte-rich suspensions were pretreated by centrifugation on a Hypaque–Ficoll cushion to remove mononuclear cells, followed by ammonium chloride (NH_4Cl) lysis of the contaminating erythrocytes before application onto the Percoll gradients, the eosinophils fractionated at higher densities than when the leucocyte suspensions were applied directly on to Percoll gradients (DeSimone *et al.*, 1982). Furthermore, it has been shown that a small shift in pH of the Percoll gradient also influenced the localization of granulocytes (Leonard *et al.*, 1984). These findings raise the question as to whether the eosinophil populations separated according to the different methods are comparable. The populations are probably the same because the percentage of hypodense eosinophils in normal subjects was estimated to be approximately 10% by each method (Fukuda *et al.*, 1985; Shult *et al.*, 1988; Prin *et al.*, 1984). It is evident that the methods are adequately reproducible, since repeat determinations of density distribution for the same normal individuals have shown consistent patterns in each instance (Prin *et al.*, 1983; Fukuda *et al.*, 1985; Shult *et al.*, 1988). The factors that determine fractionation into different densities are not known, but such observations emphasize the importance of keeping experimental conditions (especially pH and osmolality of the gradient medium) constant. Since it is almost impossible to produce identical conditions from experiment to experiment, it is preferable to compare eosinophils from different sources within, rather than between, experiments.

B Patients with eosinophilia

Increased numbers of hypodense eosinophils are found in the blood of patients with eosinophilia-associated diseases, such as the hypereosinophilic syndrome (HES) (Winqvist *et al.*, 1982; Prin *et al.*, 1983; Peters *et al.*, 1988), parasitism (Prin *et al.*, 1984; DeSimone *et al*, 1982, 1983), allergy (Prin *et al.*, 1983; Fukuda *et al.*, 1985; Shult *et al.*, 1988; Frick *et al.*, 1988a) and neoplasia (Winqvist *et al.*, 1982; Prin *et al.*, 1983; Prin *et al.*, 1984). The density distribution profiles of eosinophils from patients with eosinophilia owing to causes other than HES are heterogeneous with both normal and low density eosinophils; the numbers of hypodense eosinophils are positively correlated with the degree of blood eosinophila (Fukuda *et al.*, 1985; Shult *et al.*, 1988). The density distribution of eosinophils from patients with HES is distinctive in that more than 90% of the peripheral blood eosinophils are hypodense (Peters *et al.*, 1988) and eosinophils have a strikingly low density (1.076 g ml^{-1}). A similar distribution has been observed for eosinophils from a patient with eosinophilic leukaemia (Winqvist *et al.*, 1982). The density distribution of eosinophils may vary and can be related to development of disease symptoms or amelioration of symptoms after drug therapy. In HES, the proportion of normodense eosinophils decreased after glucocorticosteroid therapy, while that of hypodense cells was effectively unchanged (Prin *et al.*, 1983). This interesting result may explain occasional ineffectiveness of glucocorticosteroids in HES. The mean percentage of hypodense eosinophils in allergic rhinitis has been reported to be 30% (Frick *et al.*, 1988a) and an increased percentage of hypodense eosinophils was found more often in patients with moderate to severe symptoms than in subjects without symptoms or with mild disease (Frick *et al.*, 1988a). The relationship between hypodense eosinophils and environmental ragweed-pollen concentration was recently studied in allergic rhinitis (Frick *et al.*, 1988a). Before the onset of ragweed pollination, all patients were asymptomatic and had a normal proportion of hypodense eosinophils in peripheral blood. However, when their blood was re-evaluated during the ragweed-pollen season, the incidence of hypodense eosinophils was increased. This group also reported that the number of hypodense eosinophils increased when late asthmatic responses occurred after antigen inhalation challenge (Frick *et al.*, 1989). Studies of eosinophilia in asthma have reported 35% (Fukuda *et al.*, 1985), 41% (Shult *et al.*, 1988) and 65% (Kloprogge *et al.*, 1989) hypodense eosinophils. Hypodense eosinophils were predominant in affected tissues. In pleural fluids from patients with various lung diseases 80–100% of the eosinophils were hypodense (Winqvist *et al.*, 1982; Prin *et al.*, 1984), whereas in bronchoalveolar lavage (BAL) fluids from asthmatic subjects only 60% were hypodense (Fukuda and Makino, 1989). When contemporary samples of blood and BAL fluids were compared, eosinophils from the BAL fluids consistently showed lower densities.

This conclusion is supported by a study of three subjects experimentally infected with hookworm, demonstrating that the absolute number of eosinophils increased following infection to a peak of about 3000 eosinophils mm^{-3} and the percentage of light-density eosinophils increased from a mean of 34% to 80% (White *et al.*, 1986).

III BIOLOGICAL AND FUNCTIONAL CHARACTERISTICS OF HYPODENSE EOSINOPHILS

Hypodense eosinophils possess a number of properties consistent with classification as activated cells (summarized in Table 1). Biochemically, hypodense eosinophils show increased membrane hexose transport upon contact with zymosan-activated serum (Prin *et al.*, 1983), higher oxygen metabolism both at rest and upon adherence to serum-treated Sephadex (Winqvist *et al.*, 1982) and increased superoxide generation in response to phorbolmyrisitate acetate (PMA) (White *et al.*, 1986); a contradictory result was obtained in one study that showed hypodense eosinophils have a reduced respiratory burst activity (Prin *et al.*, 1984).

When compared with normodense cells from the same subjects, hypodense eosinophils have been reported to produce greater amounts of leukotriene C_4 (LTC_4) if stimulated with IgG-coated particles (Shaw *et al.*, 1985), serum-treated zymosan (Kauffman *et al.*, 1987) or calcium

Table 1 The functional characteristics of hypodense eosinophils.

Surface receptors	Increased expression of CR3, FcγR and FcεR2
Biochemistry	Increased membrane hexose transport, oxygen consumption and superoxide production
	Increased synthesis and secretion of leukotriene C_4, and platelet-activating factor
Mobilization	Increased ability to adhere to vascular endothelial cells
	Increased chemotactic responsiveness
Degranulation	Release of granule protein by stimulation with specific antigen or anti IgE
Cytotoxicity	Enhanced capacity to kill larval helminths and enhanced antibody-dependent cell-mediated cytotoxicity

ionophore A23187 (Kajita *et al.*, 1985). However, one study of eosinophils from patients with asthma, reported a contradictory result, with decreased generation of LTC_4 in hypodense eosinophils compared with normodense eosinophils (Kauffman *et al.*, 1987). After stimulation, numerous cells including the eosinophil produce platelet-activating factor (PAF) (Lee *et al.*, 1984) and hypodense eosinophils from a patient with HES generated at least three times as much PAF in response to A23187 (our unpublished data).

The eosinophil plasma membrane possesses receptors for immunoglobulins, complement and membrane-derived agents (Kay, 1985). Hypodense eosinophils have greater numbers of Fc receptors for IgG and complement receptors than do normodense cells (Winqvist *et al*, 1982) and, more interestingly, show potent cytotoxic activity for antibody-coated target cells (Prin *et al.*, 1983). Human eosinophils also possess Fc receptors for IgE (FcR) and have been shown to participate directly in killing of IgE-coated parasite targets (Capron *et al.*, 1984). This IgE-dependent cytotoxicity seems restricted to hypodense eosinophils and may be linked to an increase in the number of FcR and/or the binding affinity for IgE. It has been reported that hypodense eosinophils show increased FcE receptor expression and tissue eosinophils, particularly hypodense alveolar eosinophils, show an increased proportion of cells bearing cytophilic IgE (Capron *et al.*, 1985a, b).

Eosinophil activation can be determined by measurement of the release of a granule protein, eosinophil peroxidase (EPO). Hypodense eosinophils from filariasis-infected patients in the presence of specific antigen or anti-human IgE were able to release EPO, whilst normodense eosinophils showed no significant release of EPO after IgE-dependent activation (Khalife *et al.*, 1986). Most reports have concluded that hypodense eosinophils are "activated". The two contrary reports of decreased LTC_4 generation (Kauffman *et al.*, 1987) and reduced respiratory burst activity

(Prin *et al.*, 1984) may be explained by postulating that populations of hypodense eosinophils from different sources can be heterogeneous with regard to their responsiveness to activating stimuli. The basic mechanisms underlying responses to different stimuli remain to be determined. Nevertheless, hypodense eosinophils are metabolically and functionally distinct from the normodense eosinophils and may have a greater potential for tissue injury.

The mechanisms by which eosinophils accumulate at inflammatory sites in eosinophil-related pathologic state are not understood. It is generally assumed that eosinophils initially adhere to vascular endothelium, cross the vascular barrier by diapedesis and then migrate towards the site where chemotactic factors originate. When the capacity of eosinophils to adhere to cultured human umbilical vein endothelial cells was measured, hypodense eosinophils showed a significantly higher spontaneous adherence to the endothelial cells than normodense cells. Stimulation with PAF caused higher levels of adherence, although the magnitude of stimulation was similar for both populations (Kimani *et al.*, 1988). Further, in a recent study of eosinophil chemotaxis using a modified Boyden chamber technique, it has been demonstrated that hypodense eosinophils show a significantly greater chemotactic response to PAF than do normodense cells (Fukuda and Makino, 1989). These observations suggest that hypodense cells more readily emigrate from blood vessels into sites of inflammation.

IV MONOCLONAL ANTIBODY AGAINST THE HYPODENSE EOSINOPHIL

Monoclonal antibodies have been prepared in order to assist detection of differences in membrane antigen expression on eosinophils of different density. Mice were immunized with hypodense eosinophils from highly hypereosinophilic patients. One study produced six clones of monoclonal antibodies, which were specific for the plasma membrane of blood eosinophils and neutrophils, eosinophil myelocytes and haemopoietic cell lines (Tai *et al.*, 1985). When those eosinophils, which expressed antigens detected by these antibodies, were examined in relation to the cell density, five of the antigens were preferentially expressed on the intermediate density eosinophils, whilst one was preferentially expressed on hypodense eosinophils. Another group (Capron *et al.*, 1986) prepared a monoclonal antibody (BB10) which bound specifically to hypodense eosinophils and normal platelets, but not to normodense eosinophils. Interestingly, this antibody strongly inhibited IgE-dependent, but not IgG-dependent, eosinophil cytotoxicity against schistosomula targets and IgE rosette formation.

From these lines of evidence, the antibody target is believed to be an eosinophil Fc receptor. Both studies demonstrate that antigen expression distinguishes eosinophils of different density and the monoclonal antibodies have potential as phenotypic markers to identify hypodense cells in human disease.

V MORPHOLOGY OF HYPODENSE EOSINOPHILS

Morphological abnormalities of eosinophils have been reported in patients with eosinophilia, when there is evidence of cytoplasmic vacuolization and partial degranulation (Connell, 1968; Spry and Tai, 1976). These abnormalities have been associated specifically with hypodense eosinophils, isolated by density gradient centrifugation technique. Electron microscopy has revealed that the morphology of hypodense eosinophils varies according to the origin of the cells.

In a recent study, the ultrastructural characteristics of circulating hypodense eosinophils from patients with HES have been compared with those of circulating normodense eosinophils from normal persons (Peters *et al.*, 1988). The number of granules and the number of lucent granule cores per cell did not differ between eosinophils from the two study groups. However, analyses of granule areas in electron micrographs revealed that hypodense eosinophils have significantly smaller individual granules. A decreased ratio of total granule area to cytoplasmic area may explain the low density of the eosinophils from patients with HES. When the major basic protein (MBP) content of eosinophil was measured by radioimmunoassay, hypodense cells were shown to contain significantly less MBP than normodense cells. Furthermore, the MBP content in these cell fractions increased in parallel with increasing density of the eosinophils. This finding, together with the previous observation of decreased eosinophil cationic protein (ECP) in hypodense eosinophils (Winqvist *et al.*, 1982), suggest that decrease in protein content of the cells is an important factor in accounting for the reduced density.

Ultrastructural studies of resident eosinophils suggested a different morphological basis for hypodense eosinophils. The eosinophils in BAL fluid from patients with asthma consistently showed partial or complete lucency of the granule matrix or of the crystalloid core (Metzger *et al.*, 1986; Fukuda and Makino, 1989), indicating that degranulation is an alternative explanation to account for reduced density in eosinophils. However, contemporary samples of eosinophils from peripheral blood

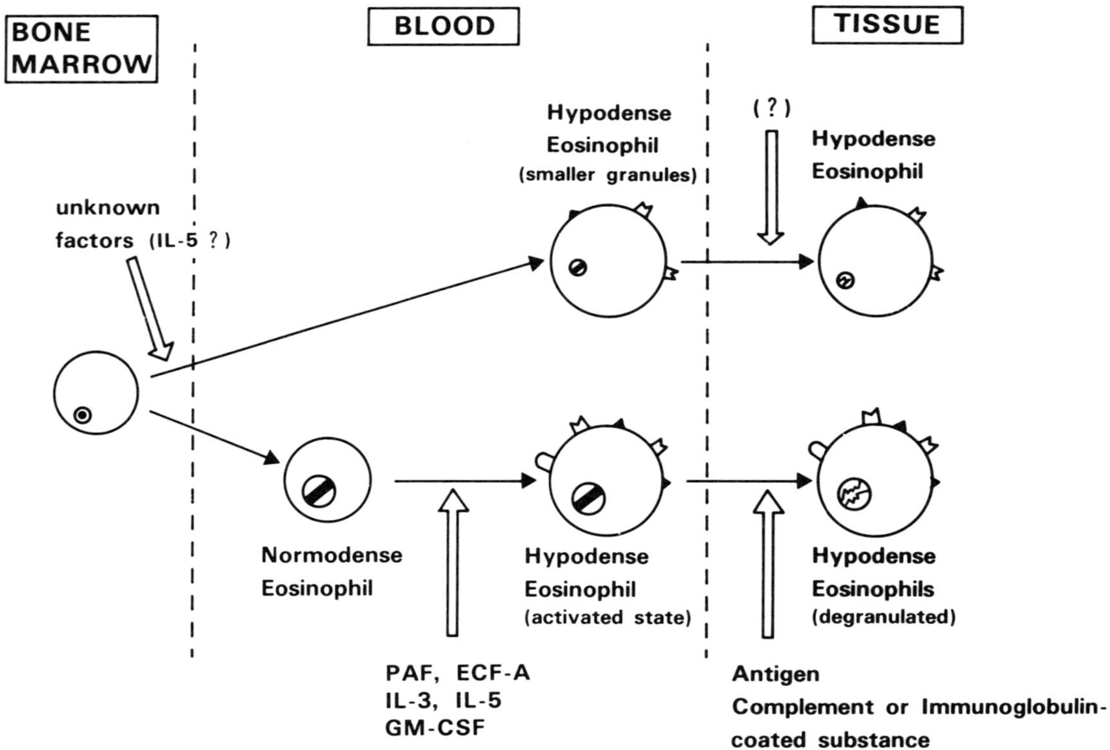

Fig. 1 The hypodense eosinophil hypotheses. See text for explanation.

eosinophils from the same patients had cytoplasmic granules with an ultrastructure characteristic of normal eosinophils, despite the occurrence of a substantial proportion of hypodense eosinophils in the circulation (Fukuda and Makino, 1989). These findings agree with previous observations of near normal ultrastructure of hypodense eosinophils in the blood of patients with asthma (Kauffman *et al.*, 1987; Shult *et al.*, 1988).

VI MECHANISMS OF HYPODENSE EOSINOPHIL GENERATION

The morphological diversity of hypodense eosinophils has led to several hypotheses regarding their generation (Fig. 1). Firstly, hypodense eosinophils may appear in the peripheral blood as a consequence of the release of immature eosinophils from bone marrow. Density distribution analysis of human bone marrow cells using Percoll gradients has revealed a progressive increase in density with maturation of cells within the granulocytic series (Olofsson *et al.*, 1980); myeloblasts peak at 1.062 g ml^{-1}, promyelocytes at 1.073 g ml^{-1}, myelocytes at 1.078 g ml^{-1}, metamyelocytes at 1.080 g ml^{-1} and mature eosinophils at 1.090 g ml^{-1}. If eosinophils were released prior to complete maturation, i.e., during augmented eosinophilopoiesis, eosinophils with lower than normal density and containing immature granules would increase in the circulation. The ultrastructural characteristics of hypodense eosinophils of HES patients, described above, may reflect their cellular immaturity. The mechanisms responsible for the abnormally augmented eosinophilopoiesis in HES is unclear, but it may be due to an increased production of interleukin 5, since this cytokine selectively and potently stimulates the production of eosinophils in cultures of human bone marrow (Campbell *et al.*, 1987).

Secondly, hypodense eosinophils may develop as a consequence of activation. Indeed, when normodense eosinophils were cultured with human recombinant granulocyte/macrophage colony stimulating factor (GM-CSF), interleukin 3 or interleukin 5 in the presence of fibroblasts, the cells became hypodense (Owen *et al.*, 1987; Rothenberg *et al.*, 1988). These hypodense eosinophils had an augmented capacity to generate LTC_4 and to kill *Schistosoma mansoni* larvae, thus demonstrating similar properties to the hypodense eosinophils found in the peripheral blood of eosinophilic patients. These cytokines may, therefore, be responsible for persisting circulating hypodense eosinophils in certain diseases that are characterized by eosinophilia.

Thirdly, hypodense eosinophils may be a consequence of exposure to PAF. The appearance of hypodense eosinophils after antigen inhalation challenge in atopic asthma and the observation of increased numbers of hypodense eosinophils during ragweed-pollen season in ragweed-sensitive allergic rhinitis patients (Frick *et al.*, 1988a) would suggest an involvement of mediators of immediate type hypersensitivity. PAF is known to be released following interaction between allergen and IgE receptors on macrophages (Arnoux *et al.*, 1987) and there is increasing evidence for the involvement of PAF in allergic diseases (Guinot *et al.*, 1987; Barnes *et al.*, 1988; Lellouch-Tubiana *et al.*, 1988). Incubation of normodense eosinophils with chemotactic agents such as PAF and ECF-A tetrapeptide converts them to the hypodense phenotype (Fukuda and Makino, 1989) and also results in many of the features of activated cells, such as enhanced cytotoxicity (Anwar *et al.*, 1980) and receptor expression (Kay and Walsh, 1984). However, stimulation of eosinophils with these agents did not cause release of granule protein, eosinophil-derived neurotoxin (EDN) and a membrane-associated protein, Charcot–Leiden crystal (CLC) protein (Fukuda and Makino, 1989). Thus, stimulated cells mimic the hypodense eosinophils found in the peripheral blood of patients with asthma in that they are not a result of degranulation, but are activated cells. In addition, when volume distribution of eosinophils was determined using a Coulter Counter equipped with a mean cell volume computer and volume channel analyser, an increase in cell volume was observed in the eosinophils exposed to PAF or ECF-A tetrapeptide. Although it is not yet known whether hypodense eosinophils present in the blood of patients with asthma show similar increase in cell volume, the effects of eosinophil chemotactic agents may explain the occurrence of low density eosinophils in hypersensitivity diseases.

In asthma, eosinophil density further decreases following retention within the bronchial tissues. Ultrastructural findings suggest that in such tissue, eosinophils become further activated so as to initiate degranulation. The agents that cause eosinophils to degranulate *in situ* have yet to be identified, but recent studies *in vitro* have suggested the importance of local factors such as antigen (Khalife *et al.*, 1986) and IgA molecules (Ghazaleh and Gleich, 1988). This process may be directly linked to the tissue injury by eosinophils and requires further investigation.

VII CONCLUSION

In eosinophil-associated diseases, including asthma, peripheral blood eosinophils not only increase in number but also become hypodense. Compared to normodense cells, hypodense eosinophils have increased expression of membrane receptors, are metabolically more active, produce more LTC_4 and PAF, show higher ability to migrate towards inflammatory sites, have exclusive capacity to release granule proteins upon immunological stimulation and are more cytotoxic for helminthic larvae. These properties of hypodense eosinophils and the clinical observations of a correlation between the appearance of hypodense eosinophils and disease symptoms suggest that these cells preferentially participate in disease processes and, therefore, have a greater potential than normodense eosinophils to contribute to host defence and to effect tissue injury. The morphology of hypodense eosinophils varies according to their origin. For example, hypodense eosinophils in the peripheral blood of patients with HES are characterized by small granules and obviously differ from those of patients with eosinophilia due to other causes. The question as to whether hypodense eosinophils from different sources comprise a unitary group remains unanswered. Whilst circulating hypodense eosinophils can be described as activated without being degranulated, hypodense eosinophils in tissues show a morphological appearance consistent with degranulation that possibly represents the final consequence of stimulation by various activating agents produced during the disease process. Further investigations of the hypodense eosinophil should provide a better understanding of the role of the eosinophils and eosinophilia in disease.

ACKNOWLEDGEMENT

We are grateful to Miss H. Machida for typing this manuscript.

REFERENCES

Anwar, A.R.E., McKean, J.R., Smithers, S.R. and Kay, A.B. (1980). Human eosinophil- and neutrophil-mediated killing of schistosomula of Schistosoma mansoni *in vitro*. I. Enhancement of complement-dependent damage by mast cell-derived mediators and formyl methionyl peptides. *J. Immunol.* **124**, 1122–1129.

Arnoux, B., Joseph, M. and Simoes, M.H. (1987). Antigenic release of PAF-acether and b-glucuronidase from alveolar macrophages of asthmatics. *Bull. Eur. Physiopathol. Respir.* **23**, 119–124.

Barnes, P.J., Chung, K.F. and Page, C.P. (1988). Platelet-activating factor as a mediator of allergic disease. *J. Allergy Clin. Immunol.* **81**, 919–934.

Bass, D.A., Grover, W.H., Lewis, J.C., Szejda, P., DeChatelet, L.R. and McCall, C.E. (1980). Comparison of human eosinophils from normal and patients with eosinophilia. *J. Clin. Invest.* **66**, 1265–1273.

Campbell, H.D., Tucker, W.Q.J., Hort, Y., Martinson, M.E., Mayo, J., Clutterbuck, E.J., Sanderson, C.J. and Young, I.G. (1987). Molecular cloning and expression of the gene encoding human eosinophil differentiation factor (interleukin-5). *Proc. Natl. Acad. Sci. USA* **84**, 6629–6633.

Capron, M., Spiegelberg, H.L., Prin, L., Bennich, H., Butterworth, A.E., Pierce, R.J., Aliouaissi, M. and Capron, A. (1984). Role of IgE receptors in effector function of human eosinophils. *J. Immunol.* **132**, 462–468.

Capron, M., Kusnierz, J.P., Prin, L., Spiegelberg, H.I., Ovlaque, G., Gosset, P., Tonnel, A.B. and Capron, A. (1985a). Cytophilic IgE on human blood and tissue eosinophils: detection by flow microfluorometry. *J. Immunol.*, **134**, 3013–3018.

Capron, M., Kusnierz, J.P., Prin, L., Spiegelberg, H.L., Khalife, J., Tonnel, A.B. and Capron, A. (1985b). Cytophilic IgE on human blood and tissue eosinophils. *Int. Arch. Allergy Appl. Immunol.* **77**, 246–248.

Capron, M., Jouault, T., Prin, L., Joseph, M., Ameisen, J.C., Butterworth, A.E., Papin, J.P., Kusnierz, J.P. and Capron, A. (1986). Functional study of a monoclonal antibody to IgE Fcε receptor (FcεR2) of eosinophils, platelets, and macrophages. *J. Exp. Med.* **164**, 72–89.

Connell, J.T. (1968). Morphological changes in eosinophils in allergic disease. *J. Allergy* **41**, 1–9.

DeSimone, C., Donelli, G., Meli, D., Rosati, E. and Sorice, F. (1982). Human eosinophils and parasitic diseases. II. Characterization of two cell fractions isolated at different densities. *Clin. Exp. Immunol.* **48**, 249–255.

DeSimone, C., Ferrari, M. and Sorice, F. (1983). LDH isoenzyme distribution in human eosinophils. *Int. Arch. Allergy Appl. Immunol.* **71**, 193–199.

Frick, W.E., Sedgwick, J.B. and Busse, W.W. (1988a). Hypodense eosinophils in allergic rhinitis. *J. Allergy Clin. Immunol.* **82**, 119–125.

Frick, W.E., Sedgwick, J.B. and Busse, W.W. (1989). The appearance of hypodense eosinophils in antigen-dependent late phase asthma. *Am. Rev. Respir. Dis.* **139**, 1401–1406.

Fukuda, T., Dunnette, S.L., Reed, C.E., Ackerman, S.J., Peters, M.S. and Gleich, G.J. (1985). Increased numbers of hypodense eosinophils in the blood of patients with asthma. *Am. Rev. Respir. Dis.* **132**, 981–985.

Fukuda, T. and Makino, S. (1989). Eosinophil heterogeneity. In *Eosinophils in Asthma* (ed. J. Morley). pp. 125–140. Academic Press, London.

Gartner, I. (1980). Separation of human eosinophils in density gradients of polyvinylpyrrolidone-coated silica gel (Percoll). *Immunology* **40**, 133–136.

Ghazaleh, R.A. and Gleich, G.J. (1988). Eosinophil degranulation and IgG subclasses. *J. Allergy Clin. Immunol.* **81**, 209 (Abstract).

Gleich, G.J. and Adolphson, C.R. (1986). The eosinophilic leukocyte: structure and function. *Adv. Immunol.* **39**, 177–253.

Guinot, P., Brambilla, C., Duchier, J., Braquet, P., Bonvoisin, B. and Cournot, A. (1987). Effect of BN 52063, a specific PAF-acether antagonist, on bronchial provocation test to allergen in asthmatic patients, a preliminary study. *Prostaglandins*. **34**, 723–731.

Kajita, T., Yui, Y., Mita, H., Taniguchi, N., Saito, H., Mishima, T. and Shida, T. (1985). Release of leukotriene C4 from human eosinophils and its relation to the cell density. *Int. Arch. Allergy Appl. Immunol.* **78**, 406–410.

Kauffman, H.F., van der Belt, B., de Monchy, J.G.R., Boelens, H., Koeter, G.H. and de Vries, K. (1987). Leukotriene C_4 production by normal-density and low-density eosinophils of atopic individuals and other patients with eosinophilia. *J. Allergy Clin. Immunol.* **79**, 611–619.

Kay, A.B. and Walsh G.M. (1984). Chemotactic factor-induced enhancement of the binding of human immunoglobulin classes and subclasses to neutrophils and eosinophils. *Clin. Exp. Immunol.* **57**, 729–734.

Kay, A.B. (1985). Eosinophils as effector cells in immunity and hypersensitivity disorders. *Clin. Exp. Immunol.* **62**, 1–12.

Khalife, J., Capron, M., Cesbron, J.Y., Tai, P.C., Taelman, H., Prin, L. and Capron, A. (1986). Role of specific IgE antibodies in peroxidase (EPO) release from human eosinophils. *J. Immunol.* **137**, 1659–1664.

Kimani, G., Tonnesen, M.G. and Henson, P.M. (1988). Stimulation of eosinophil adherence to human vascular endothelial cells *in vitro* by platelet-activating factor. *J. Immunol.* **140**, 3161–3166.

Kloprogge, E., de Leeuw, A.J., de Mouchy, J.G.R. and Kauffman, H.F. (1989). Hypodense eosinophilic granulocytes in normal individuals and patients with asthma: generation of hypodense populations *in vitro*. *J. Allergy Clin. Immunol.* **83**, 393–400.

Lee, T.C., Lenihan, D.J., Malone, B., Roddy, L.L. and Wasserman, S.I. (1984). Increased biosynthesis of platelet-activating factor in activated human eosinophils. *J. Biol. Chem.* **259**, 5526–5530.

Lellouch-Tubiana, A., Lefort, J., Simon, M.T., Pfister, A. and Vargaftig, B.B. (1988). Eosinophil recruitment into guinea-pig lungs after PAF-acether and allergen administration: modulation by prostacyclin, platelet depletion, and selective antagonists. *Am. Rev. Respir. Dis.* **137**, 948–954.

Leonard, E.J., Roberts, R.L. and Skeel, A. (1984). Purification of human blood basophils by single step isopycnic banding on Percoll. *J. Leukocyte Biol.* **35**, 169–177.

Metzger, W.J., Richerson, H.B., Worden, K., Monick, M. and Hunninghake, G.W. (1986). Bronchoalveolar lavage of allergic asthmatic patients following allergen bronchoprovocation. *Chest*, **89**, 477–483.

Olofsson, T., Gartner, I. and Olsson, I. (1980). Separation of human bone marrow cells in density gradients of polyvinylpyrrolidone coated silica gel (Percoll). *Scand. J. Haematol.* **24**, 254–262.

Owen, W.F., Jr, Rothenberg, M.E., Silberstein, D.S., Gasson, J.G., Stevens, R.L., Austen, K.F. and Soberman, R.J. (1987). Regulation of human eosinophil viability, density, and function by granulocyte/macrophage colony-stimulating factor in the presence of 3T3 fibroblasts. *J. Exp. Med.* **166**, 129–141.

Peters, M.S., Gleich, G.J., Dunnette, S.L. and Fukuda, T. (1988). Ultrastructural study of eosinophils from patients with the hypereosinophilic syndrome: a morphological basis of hypodense eosinophilis. *Blood*, **71**, 780–785.

Pincus, S.H., Schooley, W.R., Dinapoli, A.M. and Broder, S. (1981). Metabolic heterogeneity of eosinophils from normal and hypereosinophilic patients. *Blood* **58**, 1175–1181.

Prin, L., Capron, M., Tonnel, A.B., Bletry, O. and Capron, A. (1983). Heterogeneity of human peripheral blood eosinophils: variability in cell density and cytotoxic ability in relation to the level and the origin of hypereosinophilia. *Int. Arch. Allergy Appl. Immunol.* **72**, 336–346.

Prin, L., Charon, J., Capron, M., Gosset, P., Taelman, H., Tonnel, A.B. and Capron, A. (1984). Heterogeneity of human eosinophils II. Variability of respiratory burst activity related to cell density. *Clin. Exp. Immunol.* **57**, 735–742.

Prin, L., Capron, M., Gosset, P., Wallaert, B., Kusnierz, J.P., Bletry, O., Tonnel, A.B. and Capron, A. (1986). Eosinophilic lung disease: immunological studies of blood and alveolar eosinophils. *Clin. Exp. Immunol.* **63**, 249–257.

Rothenberg, M.E., Owen, W.F., Jr, Silbestein, D.S., Soberman, R.J., Sheffer, A.L., Austen, K.F. and Stevens, R.L. (1988). Cytokine regulation of human eosinophil viability, density, and function. *J. Allergy Clin. Immunol.* **81**, 209 (Abstract).

Shaw, R.J., Walsh, G.M., Cromwell, O., Moqbel, R., Spry, C.J.F. and Kay, A.B. (1985). Activated human eosinophils generate SRS-A leukotrienes following IgG-dependent stimulation. *Nature* **316**, 150–152.

Shult, P.A., Lega, M., Jadidi, S., Vrtis, R., Warner, T., Graziano, F.M. and Busse, W.W.

(1988). The presence of hypodense eosinophils and diminished chemiluminescence response in asthma. *J. Allergy Clin. Immunol.* **81**, 429–437.

Spry, C.J.F. and Tai, P.C. (1976). Studies on blood eosinophils. II. Patients with Löffler's cardiomyopathy. *Clin. Exp. Immunol.* **24**, 423–434.

Tai, P.C., Bakes, D.M., Barkans, J.R. and Spry, C.J.F. (1985). Plasma membrane antigens on light density and activated human blood eosinophils. *Clin. Exp. Immunol.* **60**, 427–436.

Vadas, M.A., David, J., Butterworth, A.E., Pisani, N.T. and Siongok, T.A. (1979). A new method for the purification of human eosinophils and neutrophils, and a comparison of the ability of these cells to damage schistosomula of *Schistosoma mansoni*. *J. Immunol.* **122**, 1228–1236.

Weller, P.F. (1984). Eosinophilia. *J. Allergy Clin. Immunol.* **73**, 1–11.

White, C.J., Maxwell, C.J. and Gallin J.I. (1986). Changes in the structural and functional properties of human eosinophils during experimental hookworm infection. *J. Infect. Dis.* **154**, 778–783.

Winqvist, I., Olofsson, T., Olsson, I., Persson, A. and Hallberg, T. (1982). Altered density, metabolism and surface receptors of eosinophils in eosinophilia. *Immunology*, **47**, 531–539.

Index